ETHICS & ISSUES
IN CONTEMPORARY NURSING

Second Edition

Margaret A. Burkhardt

PhD, RN, CS, FNP

Alvita K. Nathaniel

MSN, RN, CS, FNP

Dedication
To Joe and Tim

DELMAR

THOMSON LEARNING™

Australia   Canada   Mexico   Singapore   Spain   United Kingdom   United States

DELMAR

THOMSON LEARNING ™

ETHICS & ISSUES
IN CONTEMPORARY NURSING

Second Edition

Margaret A. Burkhardt
PhD, RN, CS, FNP

Alvita K. Nathaniel
MSN, RN, CS, FNP

Health Care Publishing Director:
William Brottmiller

Executive Editor:
Cathy Esperti

Acquisitions Editor:
Matthew Kane

Development Editor:
Deb Flis

Channel Manager:
Tara Carter

Production Editor:
James Zayicek

Executive Marketing Manager:
Dawn F. Gerrain

Editorial Assistant:
Shelley Esposito

For permission to use material from this text or product, contact us by
Tel   (800) 730-2214
Fax   (800) 730-2215

Library of Congress Cataloging-in-Publication Data

Burkhardt, Margaret A.
  Ethics & issues in contemporary nursing / Margaret A. Burkhardt, Alvita K. Nathaniel.— 2nd ed.
    p.   cm.
  Includes bibliographical references and index.
  ISBN 0–7668-3629-0
  1. Nursing ethics. I. Title: Ethics & issues in contemporary nursing. II. Nathaniel, Alvita K. II. Title.

RT85 .B766 2001
174'.2—dc21   2001032503

Notice to the Reader

Publisher does not warrant or guarantee any of the products described herein or perform any independent analysis in connection with any of the product information contained herein. Publisher does not assume, and expressly disclaims, any obligation to obtain and include information other than that provided by the manufacturer.

The reader is expressly warned to consider and adopt all safety precautions that might be indicated by the activities herein and to avoid all potential hazards. By following the instructions contained herein, the reader willingly assumes all risks in connection with such instructions.

The publisher makes no representation or warranties of any kind, including but not limited to, the warranties of fitness for particular purpose of merchantability, nor are any such representations implied with respect to the material set forth herein, and the publisher takes no responsibility with respect to such material. The publisher shall not be liable for any special, consequential, or exemplary damages resulting, in whole or part, from the readers' use of, or reliance upon, this material.

Contents

Preface

*We who lived in the concentration camps can remember the men
who walked through the huts comforting others, giving away their last
piece of bread. They may have been few in number, but they offer
sufficient proof that everything can be taken from a man but one
thing: The last of his freedoms—to choose one's attitude in any given
set of circumstances, to choose one's own way.*
— V. E. Frankl, *Man's Search for Meaning*

As contemporary nurses, we face complex and challenging personal, interpersonal,
professional, institutional, and social issues. Appropriate responses to these issues
are seldom clear. Ethical dilemmas, in particular, involve choices with no clearly correct solutions. We believe that declaring that there is one correct approach to solving
ethical problems risks imposing personal values on others. We must be sensitive to
that possibility and recognize that our responses to dilemmas depend on such variables as contextual factors, patient and family values, relationships, moral development, religious beliefs, spiritual perspective, cultural orientation, and legal constraints.

It is our intention in this book to (1) acknowledge that each person is a moral
agent, (2) raise awareness of the myriad factors that need to be considered when
dealing with ethical decisions, (3) present a decision-making model to help
individuals learn to process information and move toward action, and (4) affirm
nursing as an ethically responsible profession. We present ethical issues from the
perspective of nursing, recognizing that relationships and the authority to make
decisions are affected by contextual factors such as professional status; gender; the
development of the profession; personal ethical stance; social, economic,
institutional, and political climate; and personal and professional empowerment.

Dealing with ethical issues requires skill in the processes of values clarification,
ethical decision making, self-awareness, empowerment, transcultural sensitivity, and
challenging injustice. The text poses questions about contemporary issues and
provides processes for the development of sensitivity and skill in resolving ethical
problems. Highlighting nurses in a variety of settings and roles, exercises and
activities are intended to facilitate self-reflection and awareness of personal
approaches to issues and decision making. Our goal is that you will become
engaged in active learning throughout the text through the use of *Case Presentations*
based on real-life situations, *Ask Yourself* and *Think About It* exercises derived from
thought-provoking material and case presentations, and *Discussion Questions and
Activities*.

Although acknowledging the rich and divergent history of nursing in other
cultures, we have chosen to write primarily from the Western perspective. The
background that we give explains the many factors that lead to social systems which
either encourage or prohibit certain people from critically examining issues and

making authoritative decisions. The book begins with a chapter that explores the impact of historical factors, particularly religion and gender, on the profession of nursing in Western culture. We hope that this will help you to understand more fully the context of nursing and question arbitrary and artificial barriers to ethical decision making.

With a strong groundwork of ethical theories and principles in Part I, subsequent chapters deal with various issues as they pertain to ethics and ethical decision making. As you explore political, professional, legal, social, and gender issues, we encourage you to look at the related ethical questions and to continually move back and forth from the concrete to the abstract, from the general to the specific, from the global to the personal, and from issue to principle—recognizing the interrelatedness of many factors.

While continuing to discuss ethical issues from the perspective of nursing, in this second edition we have attempted to strengthen the thematic layer of holistic caring. Because we feel it is essential to the study of ethics, we have continued to incorporate classical and older philosophical thought, as well as the perspectives of contemporary philosophers and ethicists as we expand our exploration of complex contemporary issues. Overall improvements from the first edition include a change in language and voice to make the content more personal and accessible to students of all levels, and the addition of a second color to highlight various features and make the text more visually appealing. We updated and expanded the text to include a more thorough discussion of modern and contemporary influences on the profession, virtue ethics, the ethics of care, ethics and the law, nurse practice acts and the responsibilities of boards of nursing, palliative care, self-determination, managed care, and complementary therapies. We also added some recent noteworthy cases to our discussions of palliative care, legal issues, and protection of human subjects.

Principled behavior in personal and professional situations is the organizing theme of this text. Beginning with a brief descriptive history of nursing as it relates to ethics, Part I, *Guides for Principled Behavior,* presents ethical theories, models, and principles that serve as guides for principled behavior. Part II, *Developing Principled Behavior,* discusses personal issues, including values clarification, moral development, and eithical decision making. Part III, *Principled Behavior in the Professional Domain,* presents professional and legal overviews and chapters related to specific issues important to contemporary nursing. This section includes discussion about autonomy, authority, accountability, codes of practice, scholarship issues, practice issues related to health care providers, systems within which nurses work, technology, and patient self-determination. Part IV, *Global Issues That Impinge on Nursing Practice,* addresses health care changes and challenges as a background for understanding issues that nurses encounter in the contemporary health care system. Considerations related to political, economic, social, gender, transcultural, and spirituality issues are discussed in light of nursing role, potential dilemmas, and professional practice. Part V, *The Power to Make a Difference,* focuses on developing skills to empower both nurses and patients to make principled choices and act with courage.

Throughout this book, we have chosen to refer to the recipient of nursing care as *patient* rather than *client*. Since nurses function as members of interdisciplinary health care teams and the term *patient* is commonly used by other health providers, using a common language fosters better communication, understanding, and collegiality. In addition, the American Nurses Association (1996) *Nursing's Social Policy Statement* notes that although the term *client* is preferred by some nurses, it implies that the recipient of care is able to choose one nurse from among many, a choice that typically does not occur. We recognize that the term *client, person,* or *individual* may be the better choice in some circumstances and encourage the reader to make that distinction if needed.

Although we have written from the Western perspective, we recognize that our culture is a melding of traditions and people from many other cultures. We have attempted to be sensitive in reflecting transcultural situations and issues. In that vein, you will notice that when referring to the dates of historical events, we have used the designation B.C.E. (Before the Common Era) rather than the more familiar B.C.

This book is meant to be very personal. You should become engaged, examining and questioning your options and values as they relate to real-life situations. As learning is demonstrated by changed behavior, we hope that you will become a more sensitive, capable, courageous, and responsible decision maker and citizen. We believe with Phyllis Kritek (1994) that "the measure of [one's] character and worth is not whether [one has] avoided making poor choices, but how willing [one is] to learn from these errors in an effort to not repeat them, and how [one elects] to attend to their consequences. . . . Finding meaning, discovering that which is of worth, becomes a searching process where everyone's help is welcome" (pp. 21, 33). This book is offered as a guide to help in the process of learning to make sound choices and act in principled ways in both personal and professional realms. As you use this book, we echo the same sentiment voiced by Florence Nightingale in the preface to her *Notes on Nursing:* "I do not pretend to teach her how, I ask her to teach herself, and for this purpose I venture to give her some hints" (1859, preface).

REFERENCES

American Nurses Association. (1996). *Nursing's social policy statement.* Washington, DC: Author.

Frankl, V. E. (1984). *Man's search for meaning* (Rev. ed.). New York: Washington Square Press.

Kritek, P. B. (1994). *Negotiating at an uneven table: A practical approach to working with difference and diversity.* San Francisco: Jossey-Bass.

Nightingale, F. (1859). *Notes on nursing: What it is, and what it is not.* London: Harrison & Sons.

Acknowledgments

The journey of writing a book requires solitude and the companionship and support of many people. We express gratitude to the many friends and colleagues who have encouraged us along the way. Special thanks are due to Mary Jo Butler and Cynthia Persily, who have encouraged scholarship and principled behavior. We are grateful to Barbara C. Banonis, Mary Jo Butler, Sandra L. Cotton, Sr., Barbara Kupchak, Robin Shirley, and Mary Gail Nagai-Jacobson for their chapter contributions, and to Anna Nicoloudakis for secretarial assistance and general support in innumerable ways. Thanks go to all those who gave the time and care to review the manuscript at various stages in the writing process, providing us with helpful comments and guidance.

Finally, we are eternally grateful to our families, Joe Golden and Tim, Josh, and Maggie Nathaniel, for their loving patience, humor, caretaking, and encouragement throughout this challenging and growthful journey.

Contributors

Barbara C. Banonis, MSN, RN
Well-Being Consultant
LifeQuest International
Charleston, WV

Mary Jo Butler, EdD, RN
Former Associate Professor and Director
West Virginia University
School of Nursing, Charleston Division
Charleston, WV

Sandra L. Cotton, MS, RN, C-ANP
Instructor
West Virginia University
School of Nursing
Morgantown, WV

Sr. Barbara Kupchak, PhD, RN-C
Associate Professor
West Virginia University
School of Nursing
Morgantown, WV

Mary Gail Nagai-Jacobson, MSN, RN
Director, Healing Matters
San Marcos, TX

GUIDES FOR PRINCIPLED BEHAVIOR

Part I lays a foundation for nurses to begin critically examining issues and systematically participating in ethical decision making. Examining the history and context of nursing in Western cultures, Chapter 1 gives nurses insight into the profession of nursing as part of an overall social system—focusing specifically on the influence of the practice of religion and the status of women in society on the profession. Recognizing that knowledge of ethical theories and principles can help the nurse to develop a cohesive and logical system for making individual decisions, Chapters 2 and 3 describe philosophical stance, various classic ethical theories, and ethical principles.

CHAPTER 1

Social, Philosophical, and Other Historical Forces Influencing the Development of Nursing

You know that the beginning is the most important part of any work, especially in the case of a young and tender thing; for that is the time at which the character is being formed and the desired impression is more readily taken.

(Plato, *Republic*)

OBJECTIVES

After completing this chapter, the reader should be able to:

1. Discuss the relationship between social need and the origin of the profession of nursing.

2. Briefly discuss the relationship between moral reasoning and the origin of nursing.

3. Describe the mutually beneficial relationship between the broader society and its professions.

4. Explain the effect of a culture's prevailing belief system on the practice of nursing.

5. Identify how historic spiritual beliefs and religious practices influenced evolutionary changes in nursing.

6. Discuss how the historical background of the status of women in various cultures is related to the practice of nursing.

7. Make plausible inferences relating the evolution of the practice of nursing to the current state of the profession.

INTRODUCTION

Nursing has been called the "morally central health care profession" (Jameton, 1984, p. xvi). Although the development of the profession is difficult to trace, moral action is the historical basis for the creation, evolution, and practice of nursing. The spirit and substance of nursing are based on social and individual moral codes. In this chapter, we look at three historical influences on nursing as a moral discipline—social need, spirituality/religion, and the role of women.

Morals and ethics affect nursing on different levels. As nurses, our motivation to care for others is generated by moral reasoning. Collectively, moral beliefs of groups of people produce rules of action, or ethics. These culturally accepted rules are an integral part of both the experience and the profession of nursing. Expressions of ideals, discussions of moral issues, statements of moral principles, and codes of ethics are found throughout the history of nursing. In addition, Jameton (1984) says nursing is morally worthy work since "caring for and treating the sick, and comforting and protecting the suffering, are basic benefits of human culture" (p. 1). As our modern health care technology extends the boundaries of what is possible, all of society is challenged to examine emerging ethical issues. We are faced with ethical tension in a health care system that requires moral decision making, yet sometimes restricts us from legitimate decision-making roles. We examine the history of nursing to help understand our position within the contemporary health care system.

One of our purposes in writing this text is to present nursing ethics in a manner that will encourage empowered decision making. In an examination of nursing empowerment, Fulton (1997) proposes that nurses' perspectives are distorted and constrained by historical forces that impart negative messages. According to Stevens, these distortions and constraints "impede free, equal and uncoerced participation in society" (1989, p. 58). Struggling to cope with impossible situations, nurses continue to believe negative messages about themselves and behave in ways that are neither constructive nor empowered (Roberts, 1983; Hedin, 1986). In other words, we can only understand our present situation in relation to our social and professional history (Harden, 1996). These ideas are related to critical social theory as proposed by Habermas (1971) and Freire (1972). The basic principle of critical social theory is that we can only understand each aspect of a social phenomenon in relation to the history and structure in which it is found. The significance of ideas can be grasped only when we remove ourselves and objectively view them in the context of historical and social practices and entanglements of power and interest (McCarthy, 1990). Habermas (1971) proposes that as individuals we can assess the evidence and fully participate only when we are aware of, and free from, the hidden oppressions that are working on our lives. Insights gained from the study of nursing history enable us to see these conditions for what they are and find ways of interpreting and releasing them in order to move forward. To this end, we present some selected historical and social forces that have shaped the contours of our profession.

It is difficult to establish a clear picture of the development of the profession of nursing through history. Medicine and nursing both emerged from a long history of healers. It is not possible for us to know the exact origin of either profession, since the earliest stages of each are so closely interwoven (Donahue, 1996). Even so, we know that the history of nursing is one in which people—usually women—have attempted to relieve suffering. Selanders writes, "Nursing's history is one of people, both ancient and modern. It has not evolved solely because of one individual or one event or with directed purpose. Rather, nursing's current status represents a collective picture of societal evolution in a health care framework" (Selanders, 1998a, p. 227). From the beginning, the motivation of nurses to care for others came from practical, moral, or spiritual influences. Our history is also the story of a profession inescapably linked to the status of women. The history of healers, and subsequently that of nurses, has gone through many phases and has been an important part of social movements. Ours is a narrative of a professional group whose status has always been affected by the prevalent standards of society (Donahue, 1996).

THE INFLUENCE OF SOCIAL NEED

Helping professions find their origin, purpose, and meaning within the context of culturally accepted moral norms, individual values, and perceived social need. By serving others, and responding to their need, we express moral belief. The term **moral thought** relates to the thoughtful examination of right and wrong, good and bad. Moral reasoning includes any level of this type of thinking. It may be complex and well developed, or it may be rudimentary. Why do we care about moral issues? Some moral philosophers propose that empathy is a motive for moral reasoning and action. For example, if we visualize the suffering of another person, we begin to imagine ourselves suffering. Some describe the desire to help others as a natural outcome of social consciousness and motivation similar to the golden rule, "Do unto others as you would have them do unto you." A universally popular precept, the golden rule is found in some form in most major moral traditions, including those of Jesus, Confucius, and Hillel (Honderich, 1995). Some say that we follow the golden rule both to help someone in need and, to some degree, in the hope that someone will show us consideration if we are unfortunate enough to find ourselves in similar circumstances. On the other hand, if we base our moral reasoning on pure religious belief, we may be motivated by a desire to obey a commandment, fulfill what we believe to be a duty to God, or gain spiritual rewards. Whether our original motivation of ethical action is based on a desire to help others or a religious duty, the outcome of the action is the same: meeting the health needs of others. As the morally central health care profession, nursing has historically responded to human suffering.

It is likely that at least some members of the hypothetical community described in the *Ask Yourself* exercise on the following page will recognize the importance of helping those in need. These people will begin to exercise moral thinking as they examine their beliefs. Ethics will emerge in the form of rules of action that are specifically related to solving the moral problem. Those committed to helping the ill will devise methods to utilize individual abilities to the best advantage, and fairly distribute the burden of providing services and resources. As this example implies, nursing can be described as a profession that exists to meet certain needs of individuals and groups, and thus is a product of the moral reasoning of people in society.

Ask Yourself

What Is the Motivation for Helping?

Imagine a utopian world in which all people are happy and healthy, and have satisfying relationships. There is neither illness nor death. Each person's needs are entirely met without the help of other people. Within this model society, because everyone is satisfied, healthy, and happy, there is no social disorder and no need for any helping profession: no police, doctors, nurses, lawyers, or social workers. Neither is there need for moral discernment. Now, imagine the social disorder that would follow the introduction of serious disease. Individuals who become ill are unable to care for themselves and to meet their own basic needs.

- How does society deal with this problem?
- Are the ill entirely responsible for themselves?
- Do unaffected members of society continue to live the utopian existence, ignoring the suffering of others, or is the whole of society responsible for helping those in need?
- Does society allow the diseased members to suffer, or do healthy members act to help those afflicted, thus altering their own "perfect" lives—and in turn the prevailing social order?

As we will see in later chapters, the needs of society at a given time combined with the technological capabilities and knowledge base determine the existence and parameters of a profession. Societies establish dynamic boundaries of a profession which move and change as needs change. Our profession is a part of society and, to continue to exist, our professional interest must continue to be (and must be perceived as) serving the interests of the "larger whole of which it is a part" (American Nurses Association [ANA], 1980, p. 3). The landmark document *Nursing: A Social Policy Statement* (ANA, 1980) was the profession's first description of its social responsibility. We

Think About It

What Makes People Service Oriented?

- Why do you think people are motivated to help those who are in need?
- The actions of those who choose to help others in specific situations might be described as based on self-interest, altruism, or a combination of other motives. How would you describe the motivation to care for others within the healing professions today?

can use both this document and a subsequent revision, *Nursing's Social Policy Statement* (ANA, 1996), as a framework for understanding the profession's relationship with society and our obligation to those who receive nursing care. These documents express the mutually beneficial relationship between the broader society and its professions as follows:

> A profession acquires recognition, relevance, and even meaning in terms of its relationship to that society, its culture and institutions, and its other members. Professions acquire recognition and relevance primarily in terms of needs, conditions, and traditions of particular societies and their members. It is societies (and often vested interests within them) that determine, in accord with their different technological and economic levels of development and their socioeconomic, political and cultural conditions, and values, what professional skills and knowledge they most need and desire. By various financial means, institutions will then emerge to train interested individuals to supply those needs. Logically, then, the professions open to individuals in any particular society are the property not of the individual but of society. (ANA, 1980, p. 3)

The nursing profession was created by society for the purpose of meeting specific health needs. In response, the profession has made an implicit promise to ensure, by various means, that members are competent to provide the service, and further, that these are the *only* members of society that can qualify to provide the service. The relationship of social need and our motivation to care for others is complementary. It is fortunate that human nature is such that some of us, for whatever reason, are interested in serving others.

SPIRITUAL, RELIGIOUS, AND GENDER INFLUENCES

Spiritual/Religious Influences. The spiritual and religious foundation of past and present cultures determines many aspects of health care. Spiritual belief and religious practice have made major contributions to the moral foundation of nursing and other healing professions; they have also influenced both the gender and, to some degree, much of the activity of healers. Spirituality and religious doctrine have also influenced beliefs about the value of individuals, life, death, and health. Historically, many of the dominant religious institutions made judgments about the origin and essence of healing and described (and sometimes certified) those who would hold positions as legitimate healers. The path that nursing has taken since ancient times has not been smooth. There have been advances and setbacks; libraries have been destroyed; widely diverse groups have held the title of nurse; and those who were the nurses in some early cultures left few records. Nevertheless, nursing in some form has existed in every culture, and has been influenced by spiritual beliefs, religious practices, and related cultural values.

Gender Influences. One of the most critical factors that influences nursing practice is the role of women in society. In every culture women have been healers. Because nursing has generally been a profession of women (from the beginning, 95 percent to 98 percent of nurses have been women), women's status in society is central to determining the extent of freedom and respect granted to nurses. Contours of the profession have been shaped, in large part, by social forces that determine gender roles in society. Gender stereotyping has always been a problem for nurses. As a result of the perception that women are more humane and more caring by nature, they have been viewed as naturally endowed with nursing talents. Even Florence Nightingale wrote, "Every woman . . . has, at one time or another of her life, charge of the personal health of somebody, whether child or invalid—in other words, every woman is a nurse" (Nightingale, 1859, preface). This kind of stereotyping has been both a blessing and a curse to nursing.

Society either allows or fails to allow women to assume roles of authority, roles that allow independent decision making or limited participation in the decision-making process. There were periods in history in which women were the honored sole practitioners of the healing arts, and there were periods in which women were forced into submissive and subservient healing roles.

Ancient Times

According to Jeanne Achterberg (1990), the **cosmology** of a culture indirectly determines specific beliefs about the origin of disease and healing. As the overarching belief system of a culture, cosmology describes the structure, origin, and processes of the universe as viewed by the people of the culture. Cosmology includes beliefs about the gods. The nature of the gods worshiped in any culture directly affect prevailing healing beliefs. Regarding ancient cultures Achterberg says,

> When gods lived in the earth, the whole planet was worshiped as the manifestation of the divine. The rivers, the rocks, and especially humans were the inhabitants of a sacred place. All—what we call living and nonliving alike—was alive and related. All humans breathed the breath of the spirit and drank the waters of the spirit. (p. 188)

Thus, in ancient cultures, the healer was involved with the sacred elements of the earth and the spirit in healing practices.

Early culture viewed the vocation of healer in terms associated with the sacred. In ancient times the position of healer was practiced by those thought to have special spiritual gifts. Through the study of relics, we learn that healing arts in the ancient cultures of Sumer, Denmark, Greece, and others were performed in sacred ceremonies by priests, priestesses, or shamans. These ancient healers represented the embodiment of the cultures' gods on earth (Achterberg, 1990). In ancient Persia there are indications that there were three types of healers: those who healed with the knife, those who healed with herbs, and those who healed with sacred words. Practitioners who used sacred words were considered to have the greatest prestige (Dolan, 1973). Archeological evidence suggests that in all early cultures the position of the healer was associated with the sacred.

Having a great influence on Western thought, early Hebrew teaching codified health practices as an integral part of the religion. The Mosaic health code applied to every aspect of individual, family, and community life. It included principles related to rest, sleep, cleanliness, hygiene, and childbearing (Dolan, Fitzpatrick, & Herrmann, 1983). The code required inspection of food, detection and reporting of disease, methods of disposal of excreta, feminine hygiene, and isolation of those with communicable illness. It specified particular methods of hand washing and care of food. The Hebrew high priest served in the capacity of priest-physician, and the people were admonished to honor him. Thus, for the early Hebrews, that which was "right" to do in regard to health was mandated by religious doctrine.

In ancient times when the reigning deity had a feminine, bisexual, or androgynous nature, women were leaders in the healing arts. Achterberg (1990) reports that many diverse and widely placed cultures left evidence that there was a very early time when women served in the esteemed roles of healer and priestess. As the world became a harsher place, and the gods assumed a masculine nature, women's role as independent, primary healer was taken away.

The Early Christian Era

Arguably the most profound religious influence on healing beliefs and practices in Western civilization occurred with the advent of the Christian era. The effect of Christian belief and organized Christian religion on the history of health and healing is multifaceted. It is interesting to closely examine textbooks on nursing history and recognize divergent opinions among authors. The pendulum swings from authors' bias that presents only the positive aspects of the Christian influence on the history of nursing, to those that condemn Christianity as a destructive, misogynistic force that hindered nursing progress.

In a text on nursing history popular since its original edition in 1916, Dolan writes, "Man and the universe were made to exist in the profound execution of the plan of Creation" (1973, p. 3). Dolan uses the New Testament of the Bible to describe Jesus' message about caring for others in the following way: (1) caring for others represents caring for Jesus; (2) there is spiritual reward to be gained by caring for others; (3) even in a world of selfishness and hatred one should love God and one's neighbor; (4) every person, even the "poorest and most miserable," is an important member of the Kingdom of God; and (5) every person has worth and dignity. As this example shows, nursing texts, in Western culture, often reflect the prevailing influence of early Christian teaching on healing practices and the nursing profession.

Early Christian nurses were frequently women of high social status and often became independent practitioners. Many set aside special places in their homes for hospitality and care of the sick. These places were called Christrooms (Dolan, 1973; Dolan, Fitzpatrick, & Herrmann, 1983). Early Christians exhibited caring and respect for the intrinsic value of each human.

As centuries passed, the path of healing practices assumed a winding course. Jeanne Achterberg describes the first five hundred years after the birth of Christ as the "calm before the storm." She says, "These were fluid times, when religion was a satisfying and exotic blend of ingredients taken from pre-Christian, pagan, and folk traditions" (1990, p. 39). As time passed, war, disease, and the influence of religious dogma effectively altered the course of the healing traditions.

When religious belief moved toward a single male god, women's healing role changed from that of sacred healer to subservient caregiver. By the time Jesus lived, women's place in the healing arts was minimal. Jesus called this into question with an assault on patriarchy. According to Achterberg, Jesus challenged tradition by associating freely with women. He selected the most "compassionate, maternal images from the Jewish tradition, creating a Christian god as androgynous . . . as any male god in history. In some of the early sects, God was even seen as a dyadic being (mother-father), rather than the trinity (father-son-holy spirit)" (1990, p. 38). As a result, women enjoyed renewed acceptance as healers. Their intellect and contribution to the religious movement were respected by the early Christians. This resurgence of power and respectability, however, only lasted for a few centuries after the birth of Christ.

The Middle Ages

As the early Middle Ages began, many people believed that the world was falling into ruin. During this time, disease, large-scale food shortages, and war interacted to produce a predictable sequence: war drove farmers from their fields and destroyed their crops; destruction of the crops led to famine; and the starved and weakened people were easy victims to the onslaught of disease (Cartwright, 1972). The established social structure was deteriorating, and disorganized communities turned to feudalism, monasticism, and, in certain regions, Islam as solutions to the chaos they were experiencing. During this time, monasticism and other religious groups offered the only opportunities for men and women to pursue careers in nursing. Much of hospital nursing was carried out by repentant women and widows called sisters and by male nurses called brothers. Deaconesses, matrons, and secular nursing orders were among the organized groups that had religious foundations and offered nursing services.

According to Dolan, these early nurses believed they were following the command of God to imitate Jesus, who spent his life ministering to those in need. For many, this service was viewed as a means of securing salvation. Dolan quotes the Sisters of Charity founder Saint Louise De Marillac, who wrote in a letter dated 1633, "We do not want those who have no desire to work at their spiritual perfection in the service of God. They should have no motive in coming except the one of serving God and their neighbor" (1973, p. 100). Women who entered nursing orders donated their property and wealth to the Church and devoted their lives to service. Believing that "charity" was synonymous with "love," many early Christians sold their possessions and gave everything to the Church or the poor. Although in many cases "nursing" care was given by slaves or servants, religious orders offered the only route through which respectable women and men could serve as nurses.

The overall belief system of a culture influences the extent to which members accept various healing methods and health care practices. An example of this can be seen in historical accounts of the healing arts in the Middle Ages. The term **empirical** relates to knowledge gained through the processes of observation and experience. Many people, especially those involved with the Church, had deeply anti-empirical beliefs. Consequently, people were more likely to seek healing through religious intervention, touching of religious relics, visiting of sacred places, chanting, and other methods approved by the Church. Because of religious fervor at the time, empirical treatment (particularly if provided by anyone not explicitly sanctioned by the Church), even if it was successful, was thought to be produced by the devil, since the position of the Church was that only God and the devil had the power to either cause illness or promote healing.

Because of increasingly influential Christian doctrine, there was a constant war waged against the flesh. Achterberg (1990) relates that people during the Middle Ages believed that they should "mortify the flesh" in the name of honoring the spirit. There was little attention to physical needs. People were dirty and covered with rashes and "foul eruptions." These problems were made worse by rough, dirty, woolen clothing and the constant presence of ticks and fleas. Thus, as a direct result of religious teaching, health care practices during the Middle Ages actually caused the spread of disease, intensified health problems, and limited effective empirical healing practices.

The Crusades, which began in 1096 and lasted nearly two hundred years, brought many changes in the health of the population. These holy wars led to deplorable sanitary conditions, fatigue, poor nutrition, diarrhea, and the spread of communicable diseases. These health problems led to a need for more hospitals and greater numbers of health care providers. In response to the compelling need, military nursing orders were formed. These orders drew large numbers of men into the field of nursing (Dolan, 1973).

Another direct result of the Crusades was the collection of relics by the Church. Believed to offer the potential of healing miracles, the spoils of war included body parts of Crusade martyrs. Through their sale the Church obtained significant wealth and power. Achterberg (1990) compares this time to an earlier Roman mythology in which large numbers of deities or sainted mortals, their relics, and pilgrimages to their sacred sites were believed to hold the key to health.

For most of the Middle Ages, the Roman Catholic Church held tremendous influence over the people and governments of all European countries. Powerful leaders within the Church determined the appropriateness of various healing practices. Official credentialing of physicians, nurses, and midwives was left in the hands of the Church. Even after civic legislation became common, the Church continued to enforce the law and monitor practitioners (Achterberg, 1990). As we will see in the following section, this power was also used to enforce religious doctrine related to the status of women in society.

Accounts of the actual treatment of patients in early times vary. In some hospitals operated by religious orders, patients were treated as welcome guests. People sometimes pretended to be ill to be admitted. In contrast, there are reports that some groups of patients were treated inhumanely, even by members of nursing orders. If these nurses believed their duty was to God and to the spiritual rather than physical needs of the patients, they may have been less attentive to physical, emotional, and comfort needs.

For centuries the treatment of the mentally ill was based on the idea that they were possessed by devils or that they were being punished for their sins (Dolan, 1973). They were often put in chains, starved, and kept under filthy conditions. There was even a time when it was thought that torture was useful in driving out madness. Because the public perception of mental illness was based on religious beliefs related to demon possession and punishment for sin, the mentally ill were treated inhumanely.

During the Middle Ages, the status of women also declined. In many ways this was directly related to Church doctrine. St. Thomas Aquinas, ironically known within the Church as the "angelic doctor" (Donahue, 1996), wrote that one should "only make use of a necessary object, woman, who is needed to preserve the species or to provide food and drink. . . . Woman was created to be man's [helper], but her unique role is in conception . . . since for all other purposes men would be better assisted by other men" (Thomas Aquinas as cited by Achterberg, 1990, p. 68). Centuries earlier, another Church leader, St. Jerome, frequently recognized for his support of matrons in their calling as nurses, remarked that "woman is the gate of the devil, the path of wickedness, the sting of the serpent, in a word a perilous object" (Heer, 1961, p. 322). These religious leaders were setting the stage for the persecution of women, which would last for hundreds of years and leave a persistent legacy of misogyny.

During the Middle Ages, religious and Church-sanctioned secular nursing orders afforded the only legitimate avenue for women wishing to be nurses. The Church popularized the ideals of virginity, poverty, and a life of service. By the end of the thirteenth century, an estimated 200,000 women served as nurses within these orders (Achterberg, 1990). Caring for pilgrims in improvised infirmaries and clinics, women's nursing orders were particularly welcome during the Crusades. As was often the case, these orders were subordinate to the men's communities (Donahue, 1996). Nevertheless, some speculate that within the structure of the Church, these women exercised a degree of independence and autonomy. There is no doubt that they made a great contribution to the health care of the time.

During the Middle Ages, the Church and the newly formed medical profession were actively engaged in the elimination of lay female healers. Women were excluded from universities. Except for those devoting their lives to serving in religious nursing orders, women were not allowed by the Church to practice the healing arts. During a revival of learning in the thirteenth century, the Church imposed strict controls on the new profession of medicine and officially prohibited women from its practice (Achterberg, 1990, p. 15). Nevertheless, some women continued to secretly practice the healing arts, both within and outside the home. They used knowledge handed down for generations, intuitive knowledge, and empirical knowledge.

It was a popular religious view that women were essentially evil by nature. The pain of childbirth was believed to be punishment for Eve's transgression, and served the purpose of reminding women of their original sinful nature. Those who dared provide pain relief to others during childbirth were severely punished (Achterberg, 1990). One can only speculate about the role of empathy in caring for laboring women during these difficult times. Later, the Original Sin of Eve would be used to justify torturing and murdering thousands of women during the witch hunts.

Although the medical profession was officially sanctioned by the Church, and male physicians were beginning to be trained in the university setting, there was scant scientific knowledge. The physician relied solely on superstition (Ehrenreich & English,

1973). University-trained physicians used bloodletting, astrology, alchemy, and incantations. Their patients were almost exclusively wealthy. Physicians' treatments were usually ineffective, often dangerous, and inaccessible to the majority of the poor.

Peasant women were often the only healers for people who had no doctors and suffered bitterly from poverty and disease (Ehrenreich & English, 1973). These folk healers had extensive knowledge about cures that had been handed down for generations via oral tradition. They constantly improved their practice through empirical methods of observation, trial, and evaluation. While physicians continued to rely on superstition, these women developed an extensive understanding of bones and muscles, herbs, drugs, and midwifery (Barstow, 1994; Ehrenreich & English, 1973). Some authorities believe these peasant folk healers were actually practicing some form of magic or witchcraft (Barstow, 1994). Others speculate that women were honoring the old pagan religions, and worshiping the old gods who (to Church authorities) assumed the persona of the devil (Achterberg, 1990). It is likely that these women were simply assuming caring and curing roles in a manner that was consistent with prevailing folk belief. After all, almost everyone in medieval Europe believed in the reality of magic (Barstow, 1994). This atmosphere set the stage for Church-sanctioned crimes against women in the form of the witch hunts.

In its sweep across Europe, the witch hunts lasted from the fourteenth to the seventeenth century. The atmosphere that led to the witch hunts was a critical mixture of war, disease, and poverty, combined with religious fervor, superstition, and political unrest. The witch trials were accomplished through an organized partnership among Church, state, and the emerging medical profession. Women, particularly women healers, represented a political, religious, and sexual threat to both Church and state. An atmosphere of superstition and widespread belief in magic set the stage that would allow terrible crimes to be perpetrated against women (Achterberg, 1990; Barstow, 1994; Ehrenreich & English, 1973).

Armed with papal authorization to purge Germany of witches, Dominican inquisitors, Kramer and Sprenger, wrote *Malleus Maleficarum* (Barstow, 1994). In this witch hunters' manual, Kramer and Sprenger expressed virulent anti-feminine and anti-sexual opinions. They claimed that women are "liars, more superstitious than men, more impressionable, wicked minded, and in need of constant male supervision" (Barstow, 1994, p. 172). They wrote, "If a woman dare to cure without having studied she is a witch and must die" (Kramer & Springer as cited by Ehrenreich & English, 1973, p. 19); "No one does more harm to the Catholic Church than midwives" (p. 13). They also wrote, "When a woman thinks alone, she thinks evil. . . . Women are intellectually like children" (Barstow, 1994, p. 172). Kramer and Sprenger defined witchcraft as treason against God, and described it as female rebellion. According to Barstow, "the document reeks with fear and hatred of women, concluding with thanks to God 'who has so far preserved the male sex from so great a crime'" (1994, p. 62). The most authoritative document used by witch hunters, the *Malleus Maleficarum* was printed in four languages and at least twenty-nine editions between the years of 1486 and 1669 C.E.

What were the crimes of which the women were accused? Any woman who treated an illness, even if she applied a soothing salve to the diseased skin of her child, was likely to be accused of witchcraft. If the treatment failed, she was thought to have cursed the patient. If the treatment succeeded, she was believed to be in consort with the devil. Although women were permitted to practice midwifery (no one else wanted to do it), these women were in danger of being accused of witchcraft if anything went wrong with either mother or baby.

Ask Yourself

Healing or Witchcraft?

Imagine yourself the parent of a small child in the sixteenth century. You believe the Church doctrine about the origin of the knowledge of healing. Your family and neighbors are aware of the growing problem of witchcraft in the region. Your child becomes ill and you recall a remedy that your mother used successfully with the same ailment.

- Will you openly attempt to alleviate your child's suffering and risk being accused of witchcraft?
- How would you feel having to make this decision?

No one knows how many women were killed during the witch trials. When records were kept, they were abysmal. Often names were not used, and occasionally the verdict and sentence were not recorded. The most authoritative estimate of the number of executions is 200,000, although some estimates are as high as 10 million. Women comprised 85 percent to 95 percent of those killed (Barstow, 1994). During the twelfth century in Russia, when looking for witches, authorities simply rounded up all the women in an area. Some small European towns were left with one woman or no women at all (Achterberg, 1990; Barstow, 1994; Ehrenreich & English, 1973).

It is difficult to comprehend the effect of the witch hunts on European society. Women had silently watched the public humiliation, torture, disfigurement, and death of other women. Barstow believes that this public acknowledgment of the evil nature of the female sex left all women humiliated and frightened. Because both the accused and those viewing the proceedings were powerless to prevent the torture and executions, the witchcraze served to undermine women's belief in the ability and power of women. Indeed, this was likely the inference made by all of society. Achterberg writes, "women were never again given full citizenship in any country, nor was their role in the healing professions reinstated" (1990, p. 98). Even after the end of this terrible time, women were prohibited from independent healing professions by law in every country in Europe. This created a climate by which, under the protection and patronage of the ruling classes, males became the authoritative medical professionals (Ehrenreich & English, 1973). Although accounts of the witch hunts are absent in most popular nursing history texts, these events probably influenced the future of the profession more than any other single factor. As Ehrenreich and English write, "It was to become a theme of our history" (1973, p. 6).

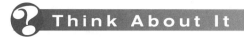

Who Has the Right to Make Ethical Decisions?

Ethical decision making is not the sole domain of the physician. Nurses may be better prepared and have more opportunity to discuss ethical dilemmas with patients and families.

- Can you describe an instance in which the physician assumed the authority to make an ethical decision, denying nurses (and perhaps the patient and family) participation in the decision-making process?

- If you feel you have an important contribution to make in a particular circumstance, and your opinion is not considered, how do you react?

- How do you think nurses can overcome the strong heritage of subjugation?

The Renaissance and the Reformation

The sixteenth century heralded the beginning of two great movements: the Renaissance and the Reformation. Resulting from a revolutionary spirit and quest for knowledge, the Renaissance produced an intellectual rebirth that began the scientific era. The Reformation was a religious movement precipitated by the widespread abuses that had become a part of Church life and doctrinal disagreement among religious leaders (Donahue, 1996).

The Renaissance gave birth to the scientific revolution and a new era in the healing arts. Beginning its gradual escape from the control of the Church, the scientific community made advances in mathematics and the sciences. René Descartes is credited with proposing a theory that quickly altered philosophic beliefs about the separation of mind and body. He proposed that the universe is a physical thing, and that everything in the universe is like a machine, which can be analyzed and understood. Descartes further theorized that the mind and body are separate entities (Durant, 1926), and that people are set against a world of objects that they must seek to master (McCarthy, 1990). Based on Descartes' work, **Cartesian philosophy** began to replace religious beliefs related to the physical and spiritual realms of humankind. As a direct result, a separation was created between the acts of caring and curing in the healing arts. The arrival of this philosophy, while elevating the sciences and making scientific inquiry possible, did not improve the status of nursing. Achterberg identifies this time as an important turning point. Regarding Cartesian philosophy, she says, "When spirit no longer is seen to abide in matter, the reverence for what is physical departs. Hence medicine no longer regarded itself as working in the sacred spaces where fellow humans find themselves in pain and peril, and where transcendence is most highly desired" (1990, p. 103). As Cartesian philosophy became popular, nurses' place in the health care system became limited to the "caring" realm. Caring was given lower priority than curing within the hierarchy of the healing arts. Some would argue that this legacy remains with nursing yet today.

The Reformation produced a split in the Church. Brought about by widespread abuses and differences in belief among Church leaders, a struggle between Catholic and Protestant groups spread across Europe. As a result, Catholicism lost its power in many countries. According to Donahue (1996), laws and customs in Protestant countries discouraged the humane care of the "downtrodden and the weak" (p. 193). Religious nursing orders were driven out of hospitals. Many were ultimately closed. It was during this era that hospitals became places of horror. There was no qualified group to take the place of the religious nursing orders. Unqualified and undesirable women were assigned nursing duties. Conditions were at their very worst between 1550 and 1850, known as the "Dark Period of Nursing," when convalescent patients, prostitutes, prisoners, and drunkards provided hospital nursing care (Donahue, 1996).

Although the world was changing, the witch hunts lasted well into the Reformation. Following the end of the witch trials, the day-to-day life of women changed little. Although released from the grip of fear produced by the witch hunts, women continued to live in subordination to men. For the most part, they were not allowed to be legitimate members of any profession. In the nineteenth century, nursing leaders began to emerge who would contribute to improving the status of nurses.

THE MODERN ERA

Nursing as we known it today began to emerge in the modern era. Known as the founder of modern nursing, Florence Nightingale (1820–1910) in her life and writing reflects the influence of the Renaissance and Reformation. Even though she was devoutly religious, Nightingale worked to free nursing from the bonds of the church, which she called "an over busy mother" (Roberts & Group, 1995). As a person, Nightingale remains an enigma. She saw nursing as a profession separate from the Church, yet she began her career as the result of a mystic experience (Simkin, 2001). According to Nightingale, God spoke to her four times, calling her into his service when she was sixteen-years old (Selanders, 1998b). Her experience in the Crimean War was the direct result of her second revelation, which she termed a call from God (Showalter, 1981; Dossey, 2000). Although she was opposed to using church affiliation as a criterion for admission to nursing programs, her religious beliefs were evident in her dealings with students, whom she admonished to work, work, work, because "if there is no cross, there is no crown" (Achterberg, 1990; Selanders, 1998b). In addition, Nightingale's description of nursing as "caring for the mind and the body" implies a rejection of Descartes' philosophy on the separation of these two human spheres.

Florence Nightingale became a model for all nurses. She was a nurse, statistician, sanitarian, social reformer, and scholar. She was politically astute, intelligent, and single-minded. Contrary to accepted Victorian social order, Nightingale addressed moral issues with courage and conviction. Having strong opinions on women's rights, she was not hesitant to challenge the established male hierarchy. Nightingale argued for the removal of restrictions that prevented women from having careers (Simkin, 2001). Her writings instructed nurses to "do the thing that is good, whether it is 'suitable for a woman' or not" (Nightingale, 1859, p. 76). Although some argue that Nightingale was not a feminist, her writings indicate that she felt women should have a more important place in the social structure. She wrote, "Passion, intellect, moral activity—these three have never been satisfied in woman. In this cold and oppressive conventional atmosphere, they cannot be satisfied" (Nightingale, 1852/1979, p. 29). It is certain that she did not ascribe to the popular Cartesian notion that women do not have minds and souls, and are put on the earth solely for man's purpose and pleasure (Roberts & Group, 1995).

Another of nursing's great modern leaders is Lavinia Lloyd Dock (1858–1956). Considered a radical feminist, Dock actively engaged in social protest, picketing, and parading for women's rights (Roberts & Group, 1995). She was concerned with the many problems plaguing nursing, warning that male dominance in the health field was the major problem confronting the nursing profession. Lavinia Dock's contemporaries ignored her concerns and twentieth- and twenty-first-century nurses have found themselves fighting the same battles.

The mid-1900s heralded great advances for nurses. During these decades nurses moved into spheres of professional, social, and political responsibility. Although recurrent themes of paternalism and subjugation continued to affect the nursing profession, twentieth-century women became more politically active. The woman's movement encouraged political, social, and economic action to correct the wrongs suffered by women. Roberts and Group (1995) write that "Nurses' consciousness of their subordinated and oppressed group status became heightened, propelling some nurses to advocate radical role-breaking, risk-taking behaviors" (p. 187). The profession gained acceptance as a legitimate health care force. In 1958 the first liaison committee was established between the ANA and the AMA. An historic joint conference was held between the groups in 1964. Participating in federal policy making, the nursing profession was represented as Medicare was signed into law in 1965 and later enjoyed federal legislation that authorized Medicare reimbursement for nurse practitioners and clinical specialists in 1997 (Zolot & Nelson-Hogan, 2000).

No longer forced into roles of subjugation in the last half of the twentieth century, many nurses claimed legitimate authority to provide independent health care services and assume institutional and political leadership positions. Perceiving a health care crisis of growing proportions, and recognizing a need for comprehensive, accessible, and affordable health care, society challenged established institutions to foster greater use of nurses in expanded roles. Encouraged by a society in which health care had become a scarce resource, nurse practitioners, nurse midwives, and other advanced nurses began to assert themselves as independent professionals.

Thus entering the twenty-first century, nursing in Western culture is shaped by religious/spiritual and cultural influences of the past. As a tapestry woven of one piece over time, nursing owns the heritage of those early times. Although many nurses have overcome social and institutional barriers to practice as full members of the healing professions, others continue to struggle within patriarchal, institutional hierarchy. Recognizing the legitimate need for both the caring and curing aspects of healing, nurses are charged with working together to improve their status and to ensure that the problems of the past are not repeated. Today's health care system is one that is experiencing rapid change. Managed care and other health care reform programs offer nurses opportunities and challenges. The position of the professional nurse within these systems is far from assured. Recalling lessons from the past, nurses remain acutely aware of threats to newly won professional recognition.

SUMMARY

Nursing is a profession that was created by society for the purpose of meeting specific perceived health needs. The profession belongs to society and therefore is bound by the duty to competently meet the needs for which it was created. Individual nurses, therefore, have a duty to fulfill the promise the profession has made to society.

In all cultures, the profession has been profoundly influenced by various aspects of spirituality and the practice of religion. Both the nature of the healer and the healing act have been influenced by the prevailing cosmology. Until the past two centuries, healing was strongly associated with the sacred. Religious institutions have influenced the parameters and membership of the profession—by either including or excluding particular groups.

In every culture women have been healers. Because nursing is primarily a profession of women, the status of women in society has been an important factor in determining the role of nurses in the health care system. Women's status in society directly determines the freedom they are given to become educated, to think and act independently, and to participate fully in the healing arts. There were periods in history in which women were allowed freedom and responsibility, and there were dark periods in which women lived in subjugation. Nursing today is at a crossroads, free of many of the restrictions of the past, yet not fully franchised as a profession with power and authority.

CHAPTER HIGHLIGHTS

- Throughout history, spiritual beliefs, religious practice, cultural norms, and political factors have influenced evolutionary changes in nursing. These factors continue to influence the practice of nursing today.
- Social need is the criterion for the existence of all professions.
- Moral thinking originates as individuals or groups desire to meet the needs of others.
- The practice of nursing is focused on meeting the health care needs of others; therefore, the practice of nursing originates in moral thinking.
- Professions exist to meet the needs of society.
- Society grants professionals the exclusive right to practice within defined parameters.
- Professionals have a reciprocal duty to society to practice competently.
- Because nursing is primarily a profession of women, the social status of women affects the status of the profession.
- The status of the nursing profession determines members' ability to practice with freedom and responsibility.

DISCUSSION QUESTIONS AND ACTIVITIES

1. Talk with nurses, physicians, and ministers. Ask their opinions about why some people choose to help others in need. In class, analyze and compare the responses.

2. Discuss the historical developments that caused the separation of the professions of medicine and nursing. How were the distinctions drawn as to the boundaries of the professions? How would you change the boundaries today?

3. Search the World Wide Web for information on Florence Nightingale. A letter pertaining to her own health, in her handwriting, can be viewed at http://www. uab.edu/reynolds/flo.html. Pictures and a short history can be found at http://www.sparticus.schoolnet.co.uk/REnightingale.htm.

4. What is the relationship between the role of women in history and the status of nurses?

5. What is the relationship between the role of women today and the status of nurses?

6. Search out a few retired nurses. Ask them to describe the relationship between nurses and physicians in the mid-1900s. How was this related to the roles of women in society during the same time period?

7. Discuss the relationship between the role of nurses in the health care system today and their role in ethical decision making in the clinical setting.

8. Discuss the challenges that the profession of nursing faces related to attaining or maintaining an authoritative role in the health care system of the future.

REFERENCES

Achterberg, J. (1990). *Woman as healer*. Boston: Shambhala Publications.

American Nurses Association. (1980). *Nursing: A social policy statement*. Kansas City, MO: Author.

American Nurses Association. (1996). *Nursing's social policy statement*. Washington, DC: Author.

Barstow, A. L. (1994). *Witchcraze: A new history of the European witch hunts*. San Francisco: HarperCollins Publishers.

Cartwright, F. F. (1972). *Disease and history*. New York: Dorset Press.

Dolan, J. A. (1973). *Nursing in society: A historical perspective* (13th ed.). Philadelphia: Saunders.

Dolan, J. A., Fitzpatrick, M. L., & Herrmann, E. K. (1983). *Nursing in society: A historical perspective* (15th ed.). Philadelphia: Saunders.

Donahue, M. P. (1996). *Nursing: The finest art*. St. Louis, MO: Mosby.

Dossey, B. M. (2000). *Florence Nightingale: Mystic, visionary, healer*. Springhouse, PA: Springhouse.

Durant, W. (1926). *The story of philosophy*. New York: Washington Square Press.

Ehrenreich, B., & English, D. (1973). *Witches, midwives, and nurses: A history of women healers*. New York: The Feminist Press.

Freire, P. (1993). *Pedogogy of the oppressed* (New rev. 20th Anniversary ed.). New York: Continuum.

Fulton, Y. (1997). Nurses' views on empowerment: A critical social theory perspective. *Journal of Advanced Nursing, 26,* 529–536.

Habermas, J. (1971). *Communication and the evolution of society.* Boston: Beacon Press.

Harden, J. (1996). Enlightenment, empowerment and emancipation: The case for critical pedagogy in nurse education. *Nurse Education Today, 16*(1), 32–37.

Heer, F. (1961). *The medieval world.* New York: New American Library.

Hedin, B. A. (1986). A case study of oppressed group behavior in nurses. *Image: Journal of Nursing Scholarship, 18*(2), 53–57.

Honderich, T., ed. (1995).*The Oxford companion to philosophy.* Oxford, England: Oxford University Press.

Jameton, A. (1984). *Nursing practice: The ethical issues.* Englewood Cliffs: Prentice-Hall.

McCarthy, T. (1990). The critique of impure reason. *Political Theory, 18*(3), 437–469.

Nightingale, F. (1979). *Cassandra.* Old Westbury, NY: Feminist Press. (Original work published in 1852).

Nightingale, F. (1859). *Notes on nursing: What it is, and what it is not.* London: Harrison & Sons.

Plato. *Republic.*

Roberts, J. I., & Group, T. M. (1995). *Feminism and nursing: An historical perspective on power, status, and political activism in the nursing profession.* Westport, CT: Praeger.

Roberts, S. J. (1983). Oppressed group behavior: Implications for nursing. *Advances in Nursing Science, 5*(4), 21–30.

Selanders, L. C. (1998a). Florence Nightingale: The evolution and social impact of feminist values in nursing. *Journal of Holistic Nursing, 16*(2), 227–243.

Selanders, L. C. (1998b). The power of environmental adaptation: Florence Nightingale's orginial theory for nursing practice. *Journal of Holistic Nursing, 16*(2), 247–263.

Showalter, E. (1981). Florence Nightingale's feminist complaint: Women, religion, and suggestions for thought. *Journal of Women in Culture and Society, 6,* 395–412.

Simkin, J. *Florence Nightingale.* Retrieved January 14, 2001, from the World Wide Web at: http://www.sparticus.schoolnet.co.uk/REnightingale.htm.

Stevens, P. E. (1989). A critical social reconceptualization environment in nursing: implications for methodology. *Advances in Nursing Science, 11*(4), 56–68.

Zolot, J. S., & Nelson-Hogan, D. (2000). News. *American Journal of Nursing, 100*(10), 32–37.

CHAPTER 2

Ethical Theory

Within Siddhartha there slowly grew and ripened the knowledge of what wisdom really was and the goal of his long seeking. It was nothing but a preparation of the soul, a capacity, a secret art of thinking, feeling and breathing thoughts of unity at every moment of life. This thought matured in him slowly, and it was reflected in Vasudeva's old childlike face: harmony, knowledge of the eternal perfection of the world, and unity.

(Hesse, 1971, p. 131)

OBJECTIVES

After completing this chapter, the reader should be able to:

1. Discuss the purpose of philosophy.
2. Define the terms moral philosophy and ethics.
3. Discuss the importance of a systematic study of ethics to nursing.
4. Discuss the importance of ethical theory.
5. Describe utilitarianism.
6. Describe deontological ethics, defining the terms categorical imperative and practical imperative.
7. Define the terms virtue and virtue ethics.

INTRODUCTION

At its core, nursing deals with issues and situations that have elements of ethical or moral uncertainty. A spiraling dependence on technology and the resulting longer lifespans and higher health care costs, coupled with increasing professional autonomy, creates an atmosphere in which we are faced with problems of ever-increasing complexity. We need to be able to recognize situations with ethical and moral implications, and make coherent and logical ethical decisions based upon recognized ethical principles and theory. This text will prepare you to examine issues and come to logical, consistent, and thoughtful ethical decisions. The study of ethics will make you more rational, responsible, self-reliant, and effective.

Nurses need to be able to recognize ethical components of practice and engage in a structured ethical decision-making process. This requires four basic elements. First, we must have willingness and courage to participate in work that is emotionally painful. Ethical problems deal with issues of great significance to those involved and, by their very nature, have no easy or obvious solutions. Second, we must have a solid knowledge base that prepares us to identify circumstances that involve ethical components. Knowledge and insight of personal values, cultural norms, moral development, and ethical theory are necessary for the practicing nurse. Third, we must be sensitive, patient, and insightful. Recognition of subtle clues that may indicate when a situation is laden with ethical components demands that we are attentive to all facets of the predicament. This requires time, focused attention, and sensitivity. Fourth, we need to be knowledgeable and adept in making logical, fair, and consistent decisions. Ethical decision making models offer a variety of methods for coming to rational conclusions. Each of these four components must be present for us to participate effectively in ethical decision making.

CASE PRESENTATION

Nursing Students Face an Ethical Dilemma

Tonya and Lydia are two senior nursing students assigned to work in the intensive care unit with a critically ill patient. The patient, Mr. Dunn, is an eighty-seven-year-old retired ironworker. He lives alone in an old two-story frame house. Mr. Dunn is diabetic. He is nearly blind and has moderately advanced prostate cancer and Alzheimer's disease. Mr. Dunn was admitted to the intensive care unit after he was discovered unconscious in his home by a neighbor. At that time he was ketoacidotic and had a very severe necrotic wound on his left leg. The surgeon attending Mr. Dunn is planning amputation of his left leg but has been unable to get consent from either Mr. Dunn or his next of kin, a niece who lives out of town.

Tonya is proud of her efficiency as a nursing student. She makes rapid decisions. Tonya insists that Mr. Dunn must have the amputation. She boldly suggests to the physician that he have a surrogate appointed for Mr. Dunn so that the surgery can proceed. The course is clear to her. Lydia, on the other hand, is not certain of the correct course of action. She talks to Mr. Dunn and his niece about his condition. She wonders if the amputation is the best solution to his problem. She thinks about what his quality of life will be after the surgery. She worries about his ability to care for himself and about his state of mind should he be forced to live in a nursing home. She thinks about what she would want for her father if he were in the same situation. Lydia falls asleep at night pondering these thoughts. She does not know how to go about solving the problem. Tonya is impatient with Lydia. She sees no benefit to the time and energy spent worrying about this problem when the solution is apparent to her. She dislikes wasting her time talking to Lydia about these concerns.

In this example, we see nurses at both extremes. Tonya makes quick decisions. In all likelihood she fails to recognize the ethical nature of the problem, the bearing the outcome may have on the people involved, or the conflicting possible solutions. She has great pride in her ability to make decisions, and has confidence in the correctness of those decisions. Lydia, being more insightful and sensitive, recognizes intuitively that the problem presents no clear solution. She is troubled by the situation, but has no tools with which to deal with the predicament. Each of these nurses will benefit from a study of nursing ethics.

Think About It

Facing Ethical Dilemmas

- What alerts you to the presence of an ethical dilemma?
- How do you feel when confronted with difficult ethical decisions?
- To what degree do you think nurses should become involved in making decisions such as the one described in the situation above?
- With which qualities of each nurse do you identify?

Ethics and Nursing

Nursing is a profession that deals with the most personal and private aspects of people's lives. From the beginning of time, and by definition, nurses, whether called healers, caretakers, nurturers, or nurses, have cared for those in need in a very personal and intimate way. Nurses are attentive to patients' needs over long periods of time. They may have made home visits and may know patients' families. They may care for patients at their bedside for hours and days on end. It is through the intimacy and trust inherent in the nurse-patient relationship that nurses become critical participants in the process of ethical decision making.

As participants in a dynamic profession, we are faced with ethical choices that affect the profession itself. For example, as the needs and demands of society change, boundaries of the domain of nursing contract and expand. This forces us to make decisions about such issues as the delegation of traditional nursing functions to non-nurse caregivers and the expanding boundaries of nursing. Because nursing is self-regulated, we are called on to review and discipline peers. This holds many ethical implications as we attempt to balance desires to advance the profession, protect the public, and maintain professional cohesiveness.

Nurses may also be called to take part in decision making on a broader scale. More than ever before, we are participating as members of policy-making bodies. Community, state, and national task forces, committees, and boards of advisors are among those health care decision-making groups in which nurses have become integral and respected members. It is imperative that nurses participating in decision making at this level be aware of the ethical implications of the decisions, particularly those dealing with distribution of goods and services. These decisions are at the very heart of our society's beliefs about the value of the individual and, as such, compel those involved to cautiously deliberate every decision. A working knowledge of ethical theory will help us make clear and consistent decisions.

PHILOSOPHY

Philosophy is the intense and critical examination of beliefs and assumptions. It is both natural and necessary to humanity. Philosophy gives coherence to the whole realm of thought and experience. It offers principles for deciding what actions and qualities are most worthwhile. Philosophy may also show inconsistency in meaning and context (Kneller, 1971). There are many philosophical schools of thought. Because of the nature of philosophy, it is impossible to verify philosophic beliefs or theories; nevertheless, the study of philosophy helps give order and coherence to beliefs and assumptions. It gives shape to what would otherwise be a random chaos of thoughts, beliefs, assumptions, values, and superstition.

Philosophers examine questions dealing with life's most important aspects. Typical questions include the following: What is the meaning of life? Is there a God? What is reality? What is the essence of knowledge? How can something be known? How can one describe the relationships among persons, or between humans and the Divine? What is happiness? What is the ideal or virtuous human character? How can one understand human beliefs, values, and morals? Questions such as these have been asked by the most widely studied philosophers. Buddha asked, "How can one find the path that leads to the end of suffering?" Confucius asked, "What is the remedy for social disorder?" Socrates asked, "How should one live?" Through the centuries philosophy has concerned itself with topics that define the essence of human life. Martin Buber said, "With soaring power [man] reaches out beyond what is given him, flies beyond the horizon and the familiar stars, and grasps a totality" (1965, p. 61).

Ayn Rand, author and social philosopher, expressed her thoughts eloquently when she wrote the following:

A philosophic system is an integrated view of existence. As a human being, you have no choice about the fact that you need a philosophy. Your only choice is whether you define your philosophy by a conscious, rational, disciplined process of thought and scrupulously logical deliberation—or let your subconscious accumulate a junk heap of unwarranted conclusions, false generalizations, . . . undefined wishes, doubts and fears, thrown together by chance, but integrated by your subconscious into a kind of mongrel philosophy and fused into a single weight: self doubt, like a ball and chain in the place where your mind's wings should have grown. (1982, p. 5)

Raphael (1994) describes philosophy as essentially divided into two branches: the philosophy of knowledge and the philosophy of practice. The philosophy of knowledge is attentive to critical examination of assumptions about matters of fact and argument. Included in this branch are epistemology (the study of knowledge), metaphysics (the study of ultimate reality), the philosophy of science, philosophy of the mind, and philosophical logic. Philosophy of practice, on the other hand, focuses on the critical examination of assumptions about norms or values and includes ethics, social and political philosophy, and the philosophy of the law. It is the philosophy of practice, particularly moral philosophy, that provides a groundwork for discussion of many of the troubling issues facing nurses.

Ethical theory provides a framework for cohesive and consistent ethical reasoning and decision making. This chapter is devoted to an examination of the two ethical theories that have had the greatest influence on contemporary bioethics: utilitarianism and deontology. A description of virtue or character ethics is also included. There are many ethical theories, some more sound than others, and some consisting of combinations of other theories. Theories related specifically to resource allocation, such as libertarianism, are described in Chapter 15. Nurses who are interested in a more detailed examination of specific theories should read works by the original theorists as well as analysis by contemporary writers.

MORALS/ETHICS

Ethics is concerned with the study of social morality and philosophical reflection on its norms and practices. Moral issues are those which are essential, basic, or important, and deal with important social values or norms, such as respect for life, freedom, and love; issues that provoke the conscience or such feelings as guilt, shame, self-esteem, courage, or hope; issues to which we respond with words like *ought, should, right, wrong, good, bad*; and, issues that are uncommonly complicated, frustrating, unresolvable, or difficult in some indefinable way (Jameton, 1984, p. 4). Morality refers to traditions or belief about right and wrong conduct (Beauchamp & Walters, 1999). Morality is a social and cultural institution with a history and code of learnable rules. Morality exists before we are taught its rules—we learn about them as we grow up (Beauchamp, 2001). **Moral philosophy** is the philosophical discussion of what is considered good or bad, right or wrong, in terms of moral issues.

Ethics, addresses the question, "What should I do in this situation?" Ethics offers a formal process for applying moral philosophy. The study of ethics gives us a groundwork for making logical and consistent decisions. These decisions may be based upon morality or formal moral theory. In the end, though, ethics does not tell us what we ought to do. We must decide that for ourselves.

Philosophical Basis for Ethical Theory

Unlike mathematics or other empirical sciences, there are no apparent absolute rules governing ethics. Mathematicians can say for certain that two plus two always equals four, regardless of the time factors, circumstances, feelings, or beliefs of those involved in the calculations. Ethical rules are less clear and difficult or impossible to prove. For example, while some people believe that killing for any reason is always wrong, others might argue that euthanasia can be beneficial either for the individual or the society, that abortion to save the life of the mother is permissible, or that killing during war is justified. There are reasonable arguments, based upon opposing viewpoints, that support any of these beliefs. How can rational people reach such different conclusions? The answer to this question may lie in the particular perspectives of the persons involved.

Ethical theories are derived from either of two basic schools of thought: naturalism or rationalism. An examination of these perspectives will help clarify the various theories.

Ask Yourself

What Is Your Code of Ethics?

- Do you believe that there are some actions that are absolutely wrong in all circumstances? Give examples.
- Do you believe that you have an innate knowledge of right and wrong?
- How did you learn right and wrong? What was the influence of your parents? Society? Other forces?
- What are your thoughts about how beliefs concerning right and wrong originate? To what degree do you believe that rules about right and wrong originate from a universal source? From within oneself?

Naturalism. **Naturalism** is a view of moral judgment that regards ethics as dependent upon human nature and psychology. Naturalism attributes differences in moral codes to social conditions, while suggesting that there is a basic congruence related to the possession, by nearly all people, of similar underlying psychological tendencies (Raphael, 1994). These similarities suggest that there is universality (or near-universality) in moral judgment. This viewpoint allows each group or person to make judgments based upon feelings about particular actions in particular situations. It further suggests that most people's judgments in similar circumstances will be much alike. Naturalism does not explain aberrant, selfish, or cruel choices that are made by apparently rational people.

Naturalism holds that, collectively, all people have a tendency to make similar ethical decisions. Though there are many value differences among cultures, the variations are not as great as they may seem. Most people desire to be happy, to experience pleasure, and to avoid pain. There seems to be a natural tendency to sympathize with the wishes and feelings of others and, as a consequence, to approve of helping people in need. Raphael outlines similarities among cultures:

> All societies think that it is wrong to hurt members of their own group at least (or to kill them unless there are morally compelling reasons); that it is right to keep faith; that the needy should be helped; that people who deliberately flout the accepted rules should be punished. (1994, p. 16)

Raphael points to **sympathy** as a motivating factor in moral decision making. Sympathy is sharing, in imagination, of others' feelings. This entails imagining ourselves in the shoes of the other and consequently sharing their feelings. Sympathy involves such feelings as pleasure, the tendency to warm toward one who has pleased another, pain, and the tendency to feel hostile toward one who has caused pain to another. Sympathy, according to some, is a natural tendency and is the basis for moral reasoning.

Rationalism.   The opposing school of thought is **rationalism.** Rationalists argue that feelings or perceptions, though they may seem similar in many people, may not actually be similar. Rationalists believe there are absolute truths that are not dependent upon human nature. They argue that ethical values have an independent origin in the nature of the universe or in the nature of God, and can be known to humans through the process of reasoning. Rationalists believe there are truths about the world that are necessary and universal, and that these truths are superior to the information that we receive from our senses (Raphael, 1994).

To rationalists, moral rules are necessarily true. Rationalists see the knowledge gained through the senses as only contingently true (Raphael, 1994). For example, the grass is perceived as green, but the color may be different—or may be seen as different by some. One who feels bad when hearing of the misfortune of another may not feel the same way about all others. On the other hand, moral or ethical rules, originating from a higher source and being free of the variances in human nature, are always true. For example, rationalists argue that it is good to help those in need, and the truth of this maxim will not change based upon different circumstances or perceptions.

The differences in the two schools of thought revolve around the question of the origin of ethics. Is ethics a matter of feeling, or of reason? Are individuals free to make ethical choices based upon predictable human nature, or is the foundation of ethics based upon universal or theologic truth? The comparison between naturalism and rationalism is seen clearly in the study of ethical theories. We are challenged to consider these two viewpoints when reading ethical theory.

THEORIES OF ETHICS

Moral philosophy is the branch of philosophy that examines beliefs and assumptions about the nature of certain human values. Ethics is the practical application of moral philosophy; that is, given the moral context of good or bad, right or wrong, "What ought one to do in a given situation?" The philosopher reveals an integrated global vision in which elements, like pieces of a puzzle, have a logical fit. By developing theories of ethics, the philosopher hopes to explain values and behavior related to cultural and moral norms. Each theory is based upon the particular viewpoint of the individual philosopher, and maintains, within itself, philosophical consistency. The discussion related to naturalism and rationalism explains, in part, one basic difference among moral philosophers. We chose utilitarianism and deontology for inclusion in this chapter because they are complete and integrated and are the major theories central to medical, nursing, and bioethics.

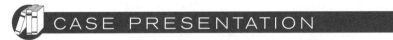

CASE PRESENTATION

Conflicting Duties

Ms. Washington is director of a local hospice service. Unrelated to her work with hospice, she serves on a statewide advisory board that makes recommendations about allocation of Medicaid services. In response to a dramatic decrease in federal appropriations, the board is mandated to recommend funding cuts to specific programs. Ms. Washington and other board members are asked to choose between eliminating funding for adolescent well-child screening programs that serve tens of thousands of youth, or eliminating a single costly program that provides catastrophic assistance to only a few individuals. Because of her experience with hospice care, Ms. Washington recognizes the importance of programs to help with catastrophic illness; however, she is hesitant to advise eliminating a program that is proven to help large numbers of children.

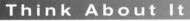

Think About It

Resolving Conflicting Duties

- To what degree does Ms. Washington have a primary duty to see that catastrophic programs benefiting her hospice patients continue to be funded?
- As an advisory board member, what is Ms. Washington's responsibility to the large number of adolescents who would be denied health care if the well-child program for adolescents were no longer funded?
- What basis should Ms. Washington use for making her decision?
- How would you decide what to do in this situation?

The preceding case implies the differences among various ethical theories. Remember, there are no clear answers in ethical dilemmas. The reader's basic viewpoint is reflected in responses to the questions. In many instances answers are inconsistent, perhaps illustrating a need to identify and strengthen a cohesive ethical basis for practice.

Utilitarianism

Utilitarianism, sometimes called **consequentialism,** is a form of teleological theory. Telos comes from the Greek and literally means end. Utilitarianism is the moral theory that holds that an action is judged as good or bad in relation to the consequence, outcome, or end result that is derived from it. Utilitarianism is an important ethical philosophy that has its basis in naturalism. According to the utilitarian school of thought, right action is that which has greatest **utility** or usefulness. No action is, in itself, either good or bad. Utilitarians hold that the only factors that make actions good or bad are the outcomes, or end results, that are derived from them.

Utilitarianism is a broad term that relates to a number of important theories. One of the first utilitarians was the Roman philosopher Epicurus, whose teachings date to about 200–300 B.C.E. Epicurus believed that both good and evil lie in sensation, pleasure being good and pain being evil. He taught that pleasure can be gained by living a life of moderation, courage, and justice, and by cultivating friendship. Epicurus also believed that deities dwell apart from humans, and are not concerned with the state of human existence; therefore, humans control their own destinies (Honderich, 1995).

There was a rebirth of interest in utilitarian philosophy in the late eighteenth and early nineteenth centuries. Jeremy Bentham (1748–1832), a leading political philosopher, is considered to be the father of modern utilitarianism. According to Bentham's theory, actions can be considered to be right when they increase happiness and diminish misery, and can be considered to be wrong when they have the opposite effect. Following is Bentham's definition of the "principle of utility":

> By utility is meant that property in any object, whereby it tends to produce benefit, advantage, pleasure, good, or happiness . . . or . . . to prevent the happening of mischief, pain, evil, or unhappiness to the party whose interest is considered: if that party be the community in general, then the happiness of the community: if a particular individual, then the happiness of that individual. (Bentham, 1948, p. 2)

Bentham attempted to create a science derived from the principle of utility. He proposed that we should measure the product of an act in terms of the value of a proposed pleasure. Six criteria used to measure the pleasure included intensity, duration, certainty, propinquity (nearness in place or time), fecundity (the chance of it being followed by sensations of the same kind), and purity (the chance of it not being followed by sensations of the opposite kind). Bentham proposed that each criterion be given a value, and that the sum of the values related to the pleasure be weighed against a similar sum of values related to the pain that might result from any given act. The person should act in accordance with a mathematical formula, resolving ethical decisions based upon the sum total of the value of a given act.

Though many critics describe Bentham as having a hedonistic tendency (his theory is often referred to as hedonistic utilitarianism), it is clear from his writings that his interest extended far beyond physical pleasure. He wrote that *pleasure* is synonymous with many other terms such as *good, profit, advantage, benefit*, and so forth. In fact, his interest in the common good of the community refutes those who charge that his theory is hedonistic. He describes a type of justice in which action should have a tendency to augment the happiness of the community as a whole, rather than diminish it.

John Stuart Mill (1806–1873) was a leading nineteenth-century British moral philosopher. Like Bentham, Mill was a utilitarian. He described utilitarianism in terms of judging acts according to the end result. He wrote, "All action is for the sake of some end; and rules of action, it seems natural to suppose, must take their whole character and color from the end to which they are subservient" (Mill, 1910, p. 2). The phrase *the end justifies the means* relates to Mill's theory. According to Mill, the only right actions are those that produce the greatest happiness. His "greatest happiness principle" holds that the right action in conduct is not the agent's own happiness, but the happiness of all concerned. He further believed that sacrifice is good only when it increases the total sum of happiness. For Mill, the object of virtue is the multiplication of happiness. He cautioned, however, that we must carefully attempt to avoid violating the rights of some people in the process of maximizing the happiness of others.

Mill defined his concepts in ways that make the meaning of this theory clearer. He described happiness as a state of pleasure that is not restricted to physical pleasure alone. In fact, Mill made a strong argument in favor of prioritizing pleasure, with intellectual pleasure having greater priority than physical or hedonistic pleasure. Further, Mill condemned those who chose sensual indulgences to the injury of health. He described the greatest sources of physical and mental suffering as "indigence, disease, and the unkindness, worthlessness, or premature loss, of objects of affection" (Mill, 1910, p. 14).

Although Mill disagreed with the notion that rules of ethics are edicts from God, he related utilitarianism to Judeo-Christian doctrine. He believed utilitarianism to be in the spirit of the golden rule, "do unto others as you would have them do unto you" (Random House et al., 1987). Thus, the Golden Rule depicts the ideal perfection of the utilitarian morality. Mill further wrote that the happiness of humankind is certainly within the interest of a benevolent God, and that people are given the opportunity to make ethical choices according to these precepts. Interestingly, similar versions of the golden rule are common to most major religions and moral traditions (Honderich, 1995).

CASE PRESENTATION

Making Decisions Based Upon the Situation

Many years ago, as a junior nursing student, Mary was assigned to observe the labor and delivery department of a small rural hospital. As frequently occurs in small towns, the nurses and physicians were acquainted with many of the women—they knew their backgrounds, home situations, and so forth. During her second day on the unit, Mary attended the delivery of a set of premature twins. Unhappy that she was pregnant again, the thirty-five-year-old mother had nine living children and two previous miscarriages. After delivering the tiny babies, the physician walked to a nearby room and placed them on a metal utility table. He turned and said to those in attendance, "Nobody is to touch them. She doesn't need any more babies."

Because these babies were very premature, it is unlikely they would have survived in the best of situations; nevertheless, the nurses struggled with the moral implications. This example raises many ethical questions, and illustrates a case of paternalism and utilitarianism taken to the extreme.

Think About It

Does the End Justify the Means?

- Utilitarianism holds that an action is judged as good or bad in relation to the consequences or outcomes that are derived from it. If the physician were thinking in terms of utilitarianism, what could have been the arguments to support his actions?

- Assume that the twins were rescued. Name as many possible outcomes as you can imagine.

- Name four arguments in support of, and four arguments in opposition to, the physician's decision?

- Considering her position as student in the hospital, what were Mary's options?

- What thoughts would have gone through your mind if you were in the situation?

Although the works of Bentham and Mill are the most frequently quoted, there are many other utilitarian theories. There are two basic types of utilitarianism. **Act-utilitarianism** suggests that people choose actions that will, in any given circumstance, increase the overall good. **Rule-utilitarianism,** on the other hand, suggests that people choose rules that, when followed consistently, will maximize the overall good.

Act-utilitarianism.   Act-utilitarianism allows for different, sometimes opposing, action in different situations. For example, while act-utilitarians probably believe that it is best to tell the truth (or keep promises, or avoid killing, and so on), they recognize that there are times when the overall consequences will be better for everyone concerned if this guideline is not followed, even if the rights of some individuals are violated (Beauchamp & Childress, 1994; Smart, 1997). Act-utilitarians recognize that tenets should be used as rough guidelines rather than strict rules.

Rule-utilitarianism.   Rule-utilitarianism, on the other hand, suggests that people should act according to rules that tend to maximize happiness and diminish unhappiness. Rule-utilitarianism requires that people tell the truth (keep promises, avoid killing, and so on) in all circumstances, because the overall good is maximized by consistently following such rules. An example of rule-utilitarian thinking regarding truth telling comes from the writing of Dr. Worthington Hooker, a prominent nineteenth century figure in medical ethics:

> The good, which may be done by deception in a few cases, is almost as nothing, compared with the evil which it does in many, when the prospect of its doing good was just as promising as it was in those in which it succeeded. And when we add to this the evil which would result from a general adoption of a system of deception, the importance of a strict adherence to the truth in our intercourse with the sick, even on the ground of expediency, becomes incalculably great. (Beauchamp & Childress, 1994, p. 51)

The argument of this rule-utilitarian was that even though the patient's health is sometimes maximized through the use of deception, a widespread use of deception will eventually cause more harm than good. Thus, though rule-utilitarians recognize that in some instances good might result from a particular act, in the end, the overall good is maximized by the following of strict rules in all situations.

Though utilitarianism is a widely accepted ethical theory, there are a few problems inherent in its use. Utilitarianism does not give sufficient thought to respect of persons. In fact, it is possible that harm can be done to minority groups or individuals in the name of overall good. It gives little recognition to the principle of autonomy, particularly when we consider utilitarian decision making relative to distributive justice. Critics argue that utilitarianism sacrifices rights of individuals in favor of the overall good.

Even though there are problems inherent in utilitarianism, this ethical theory captures the imagination as an attractive moral philosophy. Its appeal lies in the simple precept of promoting happiness for as many people as possible. It is particularly useful as a method of deciding issues of distributive justice.

Ask Yourself

Is Utilitarianism Useful?

- What useful guidelines does utilitarianism provide in terms of distributing resources?
- To what degree is it permissible to sacrifice the rights of one to provide for the welfare of many?
- To what degree is it permissible to sacrifice the rights of many to provide for the welfare of one?

Deontology

Deontological theories of ethics are based upon the rationalist view that the rightness or wrongness of an act depends upon the nature of the act, rather than its consequences. The term **deontology** is taken from the Greek word for duty. Occasionally, deontology is called **formalism;** some writers refer to this type of ethical theory as **Kantianism.** Kantianism is based upon the writings of the German philosopher

Immanuel Kant, who shaped many deontological formulations. For the purpose of this chapter, the terms *deontology* and *Kantian ethics* are used interchangeably.

Kant was born at Königsberg, Prussia, in 1724. After an uninspiring academic career, he surprised the world with his groundbreaking ethical theory. Late in his life, Kant published volumes of philosophical writings that shook the religious and political systems of his day, and continue to have strong influence on contemporary ethical philosophy. Kant contended that ethical rules are universal, and that humans can derive certain consistent principles to guide action. The awareness of these moral rules is the product of pure reason, rather than experience, as the naturalists would maintain. Kant asserted that moral rules are absolute and apply to all people, for all times, in all situations. He believed that ethical rules could be known by rational humans. Knowledge of the right course of action in any given situation could be obtained by following a maxim that he called the **categorical imperative.** *Categorical* refers to moral rules that do not admit exceptions; imperative denotes a command that is derived from principle. Kant said there is only one categorical imperative:

> Act only according to that maxim by which you can at the same time
> will that it should become a universal law. (1959, p. 39)

In other words, no action can be judged as right which cannot reasonably become a strict law. As an example, Kant related a moral problem in which a man needs money to feed his family. He knows that he will not be able to repay it, but sees that nothing will be lent to him if he does not promise to repay it at a certain time. In order to satisfy himself that the act of breaking the promise to repay the money is morally correct, the man asks himself the question, "Should every person always make promises which they know will not be fulfilled?" Through reasoning the man can see that this could not become a universal law, because no one would ever believe what has been promised. As a consequence, promise making would hold no meaning. Kant gave similar examples of situations related to suicide, squandering of talent, and helping others. Rather than compile a list of specific ethical rules, Kant proposed that each rational person should use the test of the categorical imperative to guide actions.

Following the categorical imperative, Kant also described the **practical imperative:**

> Act so that you treat humanity, whether in your own person or that
> of another, always as an end and never as a means only. (1959, p. 47)

To treat another person as an end, according to Kant, is to make his or her ends your own, and to act toward his or her purposes as you naturally do toward your own. Raphael (1994) makes the point that Kant's practical imperative automatically shows that domination of one person over another is morally wrong. Domination makes no allowance for the dominated person's power of decision making. He also notes that acting toward another as you would toward yourself mandates that, whenever possible, you must help people who need help. The practical imperative requires that we must fulfill certain duties owed to others.

When the categorical imperative and the practical imperative are merged, there is a strong implication that each person is a member of a *realm of ends*—a politically organized society. Kant calls this "a systematic union of rational beings through common objective laws" (1959, p. 51). This requires that we should act as members of a community of equal and autonomous individuals, and that each member treat all others as moral beings. Each person should have regard for the desires of others, and allow them freedom of decision. In Kantian theory, there is an inherent recognition that all people are equal and equally competent to make universally legislative decisions. According to Raphael (1994), "Kantian ethics is in fact an ethics of democracy. It requires liberty, equality, and fraternity" within a politically organized society (p. 57).

Deontology also implies that ethics are derived from fulfilling duties. One must act for the sake of duty or obligation. Kant believed that all *imperatives of duty* can be deduced from his categorical imperative (one should act as if one's actions could become universal law for all people) and must also comply with his practical imperative (treat all people as ends, none as means to an end). He also believed that an action done from duty has its moral worth based upon reverence for the law and doing one's duty, rather than the results or outcomes of the act (Paton, 1961). Most professional codes of ethics are based upon Kantian principles. Nurses' codes of ethics stress the importance of fulfilling duties that are inherently owed to patients, and the importance of preserving the dignity and autonomy of each individual patient.

There are some acknowledged problems with the practical application of Kantian or deontological ethics. Kantianism is exceptionless and rigid. It does not assist us in choosing among conflicting alternatives or principles and, in fact, may actually present a conflict between two equally compelling duties. In addition, it seems reasonable to speculate that the automatic disregard of the consequences of any given action can occasionally lead to disastrous results.

Like utilitarianism, deontology is an attractive ethical theory. It is, in fact, a most popular foundation for many contemporary beliefs. It provides clear guidelines for judging the rightness or wrongness of action. It recognizes the dignity and autonomy of individuals, and allows all people equal consideration. It serves as a basis for much of the contemporary ethical thinking that guides health care delivery.

CASE PRESENTATION

Weighing Rights and Duties in Questions of Justice

Sumiko is the home health nurse for Mrs. B. Her patient is an eighty-nine-year-old widow who lives in the home that she and her husband shared until his death five years earlier. She suffers from severe rheumatoid arthritis and has a new colostomy. The colostomy was performed as a last resort for severe ulcerative colitis. Mrs. B. is unable to care for herself because of the advanced state of her arthritis. Her daughter, son-in-law, and two teenage grandchildren moved into her home to take care of her daily needs. After many months, the family feels that caring for the elderly woman has become an unbearable burden. They ask Sumiko to help arrange long-term care in a local nursing home. Mrs. B. wants to continue to live in her home.

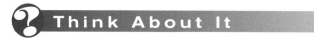

Think About It

Whose Rights Are More Important?

- Does Mrs. B. have the right to stay in her home, even if the entire family is made unhappy by her presence?
- According to Kantian ethics, what factors must the family consider in deciding?
- Kantian ethics is duty-oriented. Assuming that a Kantian basis for ethical decision making is used, to whom does Sumiko owe a duty?
- To what degree should the rights of the other family members bear on the decision that Sumiko makes?
- How does the ANA *Code for Nurses with Interpretive Statements* offer Sumiko guidance as she responds to this situation?
- Apply the categorical imperative to Sumiko's decision.
- Whose decision is this to make? Why?
- What would you do if you were Sumiko? On what basis would you make your decision?
- How might cultural factors influence decisions in this situation?

Virtue Ethics

Virtue ethics, sometimes called **character ethics,** represents the idea that individuals' actions are based upon a certain degree of innate moral virtue. First noted in the writings of Homer, and subsequently in the works of Plato, Aristotle, and early Christian thinkers, Western moralism emerged with the idea of cardinal virtues: wisdom, courage, temperance, justice, generosity, faith, hope, and charity (Kitwood, 1990). Modern and contemporary writers also include such virtues as honesty, compassion, caring, responsibility, integrity, discernment, trustworthiness, and prudence. Though nearly absent in nursing ethics texts in the past twenty years, virtue ethics is reemerging as an important framework for examining moral behavior.

The concept of virtue ethics presents a challenge to deontological and utilitarian theories. These theories conceive of the demands of morality similarly; ethics provides guidelines to action which begins with the question, "What morally ought we to do?" (Beauchamp, 2001). In contrast, virtue ethics does not ask this question; instead, it posits that the basic function of morality is the moral character of persons. Beauchamp (2001) suggests that virtue should not be thought of as a moral requirement, because this confuses it with a principle or rule. Rather, we could say that virtue is a character trait that is socially valued. A *moral* virtue is a character trait that is morally valued such as truthfulness, kindness, or honesty. A person with moral virtue has both consistent moral action and a morally-appropriate desire.

The term "ethics" was derived from Aristotle's word *ethika*, which refers to matters having to do with character. Aristotle (384–332 B.C.E.) considered goodness of character to be produced by the practice of virtuous behavior, rather than virtuous acts being the end result of a good character. According to Aristotle, virtues are tendencies to act, feel, and judge that are developed from a natural capacity by proper training and exercise. He believed that practice creates a habit of acting in a virtuous way, and that virtue can be learned and improved. Virtue, according to Aristotle, depends on "clear judgment, self-control, symmetry of desire, and artistry of means" (Durant, 1926, p. 75). He considered virtue to be the fruit of intelligent pursuit. "It is not the possession of the simple [person], nor the gift of innocent intent, but the achievement of experience in the fully developed [person]" (Durant, p. 75). He considered excellence to be won by training and habituation, and believed that virtuous character is created by repeatedly acting in a virtuous manner. Aristotle's traits of a virtuous character provided three criteria:

1. Virtuous acts must be chosen for their own sake.

2. Choice must proceed from a firm and unchangeable character.

3. Virtue is a disposition to choose the mean.

The *golden mean* of virtuous behavior, for Aristotle, meant practicing moderation: avoiding both excess and deficiency. Aristotle did not list a number of moral principles. For him, the basic moral question is not "what should one do" but rather "what should one be" (Mayo, 1958).

Phillipa Foot adds another perspective to Aristotle's concept of a virtuous person. Foot proposes that virtue lies not only in engaging in virtuous acts, but also in will. She defines will as "that which is wished for as well as what is sought." According to Foot, a positive or moral will is sometimes the necessary ingredient in success. She says,

> sometimes one man succeeds where another fails not because there is some specific difference in their previous conduct but rather because his heart lies in a different place; and the disposition of the heart is part of virtue. What this suggests is that a man's virtue may be judged by his innermost desires as well as by his intentions and this fits with our idea that a virtue such as generosity lies as much in someone's attitudes as in his actions. (1997, p. 330)

According to Foot, virtue is not like a skill or an art. It cannot merely be a practiced and perfected act: it must actually engage the will. In other words, an act, though apparently kind or generous, for example, cannot be considered to be virtuous if the intention is not good. Although Aristotle's idea of virtue is one of hope (everyone has the capacity to learn virtuous action), Foot makes the road to virtuous character less easily traveled.

Focal Virtues. In the discussion of virtue as related to biomedical ethics, Beauchamp and Childress define character as being "comprised of a set of stable traits that affect a person's judgment and action" (1994, p. 463). Like Aristotle, these authors suggest that although people have different character traits, all have the capacity to learn or cultivate those that are important to morality. Beauchamp and Childress propose that there are four focal virtues that are more pivotal than others in characterizing a virtuous person: compassion, discernment, trustworthiness, and integrity.

Compassion. **Compassion** is the ability to imagine oneself in the situation of another. Beauchamp and Childress (1994) define the term in the following manner: "The virtue of compassion is a trait combining an attitude of active regard for another's welfare with an imaginative awareness and emotional response of deep sympathy, tenderness, and discomfort at the other person's misfortune or suffering" (p. 466). This virtue embodies internalizing of the golden rule. Compassion is so important that many times the patient's need for a compassionate and caring presence outweighs the need for technical care. We must be careful, however, that compassion does not impede our ability to make objective decisions.

Discernment. The virtue of **discernment** is related to the classical concept of wisdom. "The virtue of discernment rests on sensitive insight involving acute judgment and understanding, and it eventuates in decisive action" (Beauchamp & Childress, 1994, p. 468). Discernment gives us insight into appropriate actions in given situations. It requires sensitivity and attention attuned to the demands of a particular context. For example, a discerning nurse will recognize when a patient needs comfort and reassurance rather than privacy. Discernment requires that we continually strive to recognize and understand important nuances in human behavior.

Trustworthiness. **Trustworthiness** is another focal virtue for nurses. "Trust is a confident belief in and reliance upon the ability and moral character of another person. Trust entails a confidence that another will act with the right motives in accord with moral norms" (Beauchamp & Childress, 1994, p. 469). Trustworthiness is measured by others' recognition of the nurse's consistency and predictability in following moral norms. In practical terms, trustworthiness is accounted for in the reputation we have among coworkers. This virtue is important for us in relationships with patients, physicians, and other nurses.

Integrity. **Integrity** is perhaps the cardinal virtue. **Moral integrity,** according to Beauchamp and Childress (1994), means soundness, reliability, wholeness, and an integration of moral character. It also refers to our continuing to follow moral norms over time. It is "the character trait of a coherent integration of reasonably stable, justifiable moral values, together with active fidelity to those values in judgment and action" (p. 473). A person with integrity has a consistency of convictions, actions, and emotions and is trustworthy. Integrity is compromised when the nurse acts inconsistently or in a way that is not supported by professed moral beliefs. Deficiencies in moral integrity may include such vices as hypocrisy, insincerity, and bad faith.

Virtue Ethics in Nursing. How does the concept of virtue or character ethics fit with nursing as a principled profession? It is likely that principled behavior, while not the sole domain of a good moral character, is more likely to occur in the presence of one. Certainly Florence Nightingale thought virtue was an important trait of the good nurse. Traditionally recited by graduating nurses, the Nightingale Pledge implies virtue of character as nurses promise purity, faith, loyalty, devotion, trustworthiness, and temperance. It is reasonable to say that good character is the cornerstone of good nursing, and that the nurse with virtue will act according to principle. If Aristotle was correct in his belief that virtue can be practiced and learned, then we can learn, through practice, those acts which, by their doing, create a virtuous person.

SUMMARY

Ethical theory helps us understand the origin and process of ethical and moral thinking and behavior. Two important theories are particularly important to nursing ethics. The ethical theory of utilitarianism was developed in part by Jeremy Bentham, and later refined by John Stuart Mill. Utilitarianism suggests that ethical decisions should be made in regard to the outcome or end result. Accordingly, no action in itself is inherently right or wrong. This theory also provides for the greatest good for the greatest number. Utilitarianism is particularly useful in situations of distributive justice but tends to ignore the rights of the minority or the individual.

Deontology, or Kantian ethics, was initially developed by Immanuel Kant. This theory, through the use of the categorical imperative, assists one in making ethical decisions. The categorical imperative demands that the agent ask the question, can this action be a law for all people in all circumstances? Additionally, the theory presents the practical imperative, which requires that we treat all individuals as if they were ends only, rather than means. Kantian ethics provides clear guidelines for making ethical decisions, but does not provide for making decisions when there are conflicting duties or obligations.

Virtue, or character, ethics, as described by Aristotle, describes each person as capable of practicing and learning virtue through repetition of virtuous acts. Thus, the virtuous person is one in whom virtue is habituated. Virtue ethics complements other ethical theories, and can be used to nurture or predict character in individuals. Ethical theories can help us understand ethical decision-making models, and assist in developing a cohesive and logical system for making individual decisions.

CHAPTER HIGHLIGHTS

- Philosophy is the intense and critical examination of beliefs and assumptions.
- Moral philosophy is the philosophical discussion of what is considered to be good or bad, right or wrong.
- Ethics is a formal process for making logical and consistent decisions, based upon moral philosophy.
- As the morally central health care profession, nursing requires astuteness of moral and ethical issues.
- Ethical theories explain values and behavior related to cultural and moral norms.
- Utilitarianism holds that right action is that which has the greatest utility or usefulness, and no action is in itself either good or bad.
- Deontology is based upon the rationalist view that the rightness or wrongness of

an act depends upon the nature of the act, rather than the consequences that occur as a result of it.

- Kantianism is a particular deontological theory developed by Immanuel Kant.
- The categorical imperative is the Kantian maxim requiring that no action can be judged as right which cannot reasonably become a law by which every person should always abide.
- The practical imperative is the Kantian maxim requiring that one treats others always as ends and never as a means.
- Virtue ethics, usually attributed to Aristotle, represents the idea that individuals' actions are based upon innate moral virtue.

DISCUSSION QUESTIONS AND ACTIVITIES

1. Go to the Kennedy Institute of Ethics web site at: http://www.georgetown.edu/research/kie/. Do a literature search through BIOETHICSLINE for recent articles on ethical theory. Report your findings to the class.

2. Describe the differences in beliefs about the origin of ethical rules.

3. Describe a hypothetical situation in which an ethical dilemma exists, and discuss solutions to the dilemma in terms of act-utilitarianism and rule-utilitarianism.

4. Identify specific health care funding policies, and discuss them in terms of utilitarian theory.

5. Identify different ethical codes, including professional codes, that are based upon Kantian or deontological ethics.

6. Describe a real or hypothetical situation in which there is an ethical dilemma. Relate a solution to the dilemma, using the rule of the categorical imperative.

7. List and describe the virtues that you feel are important for nurses.

8. Consider the following situation: Two nursing students are discovered to have cheated on several assignments. After being questioned by the instructor, both students deny having cheated, even though the evidence is irrefutable. Discuss these students in terms of virtue ethics and Kantian ethics. Do these students have integrity? Do these students have the character to become good nurses? How would you apply the categorical imperative?

REFERENCES

Beauchamp, T. L. (2001). *Philosophical ethics* (3rd ed.). Boston: McGraw Hill.

Beauchamp, T., & Childress, J. (1994). *Principles of biomedical ethics* (4th ed.). New York: Oxford University Press.

Beauchamp, T. L., & Walters, L. (1999). *Contemporary issues in bioethics*. Belmont, CA: Wadsworth.

Bentham, J. (1948). *An introduction to the principles of moral legislation*. New York: Hafner Press.

Buber, M. (1965). *The knowledge of man: A philosophy of the interhuman*. New York: Harper & Row.

Durant, W. (1926). *The story of philosophy*. New York: Washington Square Press.

Foot, P. (1997). Virtues and vices. In C. Sommers & F. Sommers, eds., *Vice and virtue in everyday life: Introductory readings in ethics* (4th ed., pp. 328–343). Fort Worth, TX: Harcourt Brace College. (Reprinted from P. Foot, *Virtues and vices*, Berkeley, CA: University of California Press)

Hesse, H. (1971). *Siddhartha*. New York: Bantam.

Honderich, T., ed. (1995). *The Oxford companion to philosophy*. New York: Oxford University Press.

Jameton, A. (1984). *Nursing practice: The ethical issues*. Englewood Cliffs, NJ: Prentice-Hall.

Kant, I. (1959). *Foundations of the metaphysics of morals* (L. W. Beck, trans.). Indianapolis: Bobbs-Merrill.

Kneller, G. F. (1971). *Introduction to the philosophy of education*. (2nd ed.). New York: John Wiley & Sons.

Mill, J. S. (1910). *Utilitarianism*. London: Dent & Sons.

Paton, H. J., trans. & ed. (1961). *The moral law*. London: Hutchinson & Co.

Rand, A. (1982). *Philosophy: Who needs it?* New York: Bobbs-Merrill.

Random House, et al. (1987). *The Random House Dictionary of the English Language* (2nd ed., unabridged). New York: Random House.

Raphael, D. D. (1994). *Moral philosophy* (2nd ed.). New York: Oxford University Press.

Smart, J. J. C. (1997). Utilitarianism. In C. Sommers & F. Sommers, eds., *Vice and virtue in everyday life: Introductory readings in ethics* (4th ed., pp. 110–123). Fort Worth, TX: Harcourt Brace College. (Reprinted from J. J. C. Smart & B. Williams, eds., *Utilitarianism: For and against,* New York: Oxford University Press)

CHAPTER 3

Ethical Principles

The quality of mercy is not strain'd
It droppeth as the gentle rain from heaven
Upon the place beneath. It is twice blest:
It blesseth him that gives, and him that takes.
(William Shakespeare, *The Merchant of Venice*)

OBJECTIVES

After completing this chapter, the reader should be able to:

1. Discuss the principle of autonomy in terms of patients' rights, informed consent, parentalism, and noncompliance.

2. Discuss the principle of beneficence as it relates to nursing practice.

3. Define the principle of nonmaleficence, and weigh actions in terms of harm and benefit.

4. Relate the principle of veracity to nursing practice.

5. Examine the principle of confidentiality in nursing practice, recognizing legal implications and reasonable limits to confidentiality.

6. Discuss the principle of justice as it relates to the delivery of health care goods and services.

7. Relate the principle of fidelity to nursing's promise to society.

8. Discuss situations in which there is a conflict between two or more ethical principles.

INTRODUCTION

Ethical issues are commonly examined in terms of a number of **ethical principles**. Ethical principles are basic and obvious moral truths that guide deliberation and action. Major ethical theories utilize many of the same principles, though either the emphasis or meaning may be somewhat different in each. For example, autonomy is a dominant principle in deontological theory but is less important in utilitarian theory. It is vital for nurses to understand ethical principles and be adept at applying them in a meaningful and consistent manner. (See Figure 3–1.) It is the authors' contention that consistent adherence to principle is an important basis for ethical practice in nursing. This chapter examines the following ethical principles: autonomy, beneficence, nonmaleficence, veracity, confidentiality, justice, and fidelity.

Figure 3–1 **Principles of Ethics**

Autonomy
Beneficence
Nonmaleficence
Veracity
Confidentiality
Justice
Fidelity

Respect for Persons

All of the principles discussed in this chapter presuppose that nurses have respect for the value and uniqueness of persons. Occasionally viewed as an ethical principle in its own right, **respect for persons** implies that one considers others to be worthy of high regard. Certainly, genuine regard and respect for others serves as the cornerstone of any caring profession. Discussion of the ethical principles in this chapter is based upon the belief that we value the principle of respect for persons.

AUTONOMY

The word **autonomy** literally means self-governing. Autonomy is a word that is frequently used, yet poorly understood. We are told to respect the autonomy of patients, but are given little guidance in understanding the meaning of this abstract concept. The term is more frequently used as a contrast to undesirable states such as dependency, coercion, paternalism, thoughtlessness, and habit (Jameton, 1984). We are expected to understand the concept and be advocates to ensure the maintenance of autonomy for all patients.

Aveyard (2000) suggests that the ambiguous use of the term autonomy should be replaced by a concept with a specific meaning and working definition. The term *autonomy* denotes having the freedom to make choices about issues that affect one's life. Autonomy is closely linked to the notion of respect for persons, and is an important principle in cultures where all individuals are considered to be unique and valuable members of society. In cultures that do not regard all members as being of equal worth or that respect social structure above individual rights, autonomy is less important. Autonomy implies that each person has the freedom to make decisions about personal goals. It is a state in which each of us is free to choose and implement our own decisions, free from lies, restraint, or coercion (Edge & Groves, 1994, p. 31). In societies where slavery exists, where women are expected to be subservient to men, where minority races are not respected, or where children are exploited, the notion of autonomy is meaningless. Autonomy cannot thrive in a climate that does not allow for either the independent planning of personal goals or the privilege of examining and choosing options to meet goals.

Implied in the concept of autonomy are four basic elements. First, the autonomous person is respected. It is logical that those choosing the nursing profession would inherently value and respect the unique humanness of others. This element is essential to assuring autonomy. Second, the autonomous person must be able to determine personal goals. These goals may be explicit and of a global nature, or may be less well defined. For example, the patient with an ankle injury may have a goal to return to athletic play within two weeks of the injury, or may simply wish to be pain free. In each case the patient develops personally chosen goals that are consistent with a particular lifestyle. Third, the autonomous person has the capacity to decide on a plan of action. The person must be able to understand the meaning of the choice to be made and deliberate on the various options, while understanding the implications of possible outcomes. Imagine, for example, ordering from a restaurant menu written in a language you do not understand. You have the freedom and responsibility to make a choice, but cannot make a meaningful choice without an understanding of the various foods offered. When we believe that a patient is not able to comprehend the meaning of choices, goals, or outcomes, we say that the person is incompetent to make decisions, or lacks decision-making capacity. There are certain groups of patients that are generally thought of as unable to make informed choices. Children, fetuses, and the mentally impaired are among these groups. Fourth, the autonomous person has the freedom to act upon the choices. In situations where persons are capable of formulating goals, understanding various options, and making decisions, yet are not free to implement their plans, autonomy is either limited or absent. Autonomy may be limited in situations where the means to accomplish autonomously devised plans do not exist. An example is seen in the case of the indigent person who does not have access to health care insurance. This person may choose to have, for example, a pancreas transplant in lieu of insulin injections, but does not have the financial means to meet this goal. In order to assure autonomy, each of the four elements must be present to a reasonable degree.

A number of intrinsic factors may threaten patient autonomy. The patient's role is a dependent one. The patient seeks health care assistance because of a real or perceived need and, as a result, can be thought of as being dependent upon the health care provider. The role of the health care professional, on the other hand, is one of power. This power is based upon knowledge and authority and is inherent in the role. This complementary relationship, while a necessary one, can lead to violations of patient autonomy.

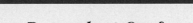

Ask Yourself

Is the Patient Role a Dependent One?

- Describe a time when you or a family member experienced the role of hospitalized patient.
- How did you or your family member feel when interacting with members of the health care team who were dressed, while you or your family member were in pajamas or a hospital gown or, worse yet, naked?
- Describe the degree to which you or your family member were able to maintain dignity and autonomy.

Health care professionals are often insensitive to the way in which the health care industry systematically dehumanizes and erodes the autonomy of consumers. Patients are forced to comply with rules that require them to be and act dependent. Immediately upon admission to a hospital, patients are disrobed, asked questions about personal and private matters, forced to relinquish money and belongings, and expected to remain in a bed, emphasizing the dependency of the patient role. Patients are placed in rooms with doors that are seldom closed and asked to wear pajamas. Workers, who are strangers to patients, freely enter and leave the patients' rooms, making privacy impossible. Regardless of patients' personal habits or knowledge of their own health care, they are forced to bathe at certain times, eat at certain times, take medications at certain times, and are often prohibited from practicing self-care measures that may have been their habits for many years. Patients are expected to follow each plan that is made. Otherwise, they will be labeled difficult or *noncompliant*. For all the lip service given the importance of autonomy, health care professionals are often guilty of creating a climate of dependency for patients—of coercing otherwise autonomous, intelligent, and independent adults essentially into a very dependent role.

Recognizing Violations of Patient Autonomy

Often, nurses and other health care workers fail to recognize subtle violations of patient autonomy. This especially occurs when nurses perceive choices to be self-evident. At least four factors are related to this failure. First, nurses may falsely assume that patients have the same values and goals as themselves. This state of mind compels some nurses to believe that the only reasonable course of action is the one that is consistent with their own values. This leads to faulty conclusions. For example, if an elderly person chooses to stay in her own home, even though to others she seems to be incapable of caring for herself, the choice might be viewed as unreasonable and might become grounds to believe the patient incompetent to make decisions. In other words, "If you don't make the choices that seem correct to me, you must be incompetent to make decisions." In truth, the elderly person may recognize that life is drawing to a close and may want to remain in familiar surroundings, maintain dignity, remain independent, and prevent needless depletion of her life savings. The decision is based upon her thoughtful consideration of the consequences of staying home versus the consequences of living in a long-term care facility. There are some who would insist that she should be allowed to stay at home, even if she places herself at considerable danger, as long as she does not jeopardize the autonomy of others.

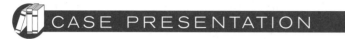

CASE PRESENTATION

Noncompliance Versus Autonomy

Cora is a forty-five-year-old woman who looks years older than her stated age. She has very limited monthly income and no health insurance. Cora smokes two and one-half packs of cigarettes per day. She has severe COPD with constant dyspnea and frequent exacerbations. The nurse who sees her at a local free clinic is interested in at least preventing further problems, and speaks to Cora often about the importance of quitting smoking. The situation becomes very frustrating for all involved when Cora returns repeatedly for increasingly severe problems, having failed to quit smoking. Cora, of course, becomes labeled as noncompliant. During a particularly severe exacerbation, the nurse says to Cora, "You know you are committing suicide by continuing to smoke." Cora's reply is, "You don't understand. I live alone. I have no money, no friends, no family, and will never be able to work. I know the damage I'm doing, but smoking is the only pleasure I have in life." (Nathaniel, 2000)

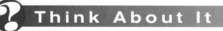

Think About It

Do Nurses Coerce Patients?

- In attempting to persuade Cora to stop smoking, to what degree is the nurse disallowing Cora's right to autonomy?
- Does Cora have the right to choose to continue smoking?
- If rights and responsibilities are correlative, how should the clinic respond to Cora's continuing to smoke? Would you suggest that the clinic continue to serve Cora, even though she is not following the plan of care?
- To what degree is coercion employed in situations such as Cora's? Is coercion an appropriate strategy?
- What would you do?

The second cause of failure to recognize subtle violations of patient autonomy lies in our failure to recognize that individuals' thought processes are different. Discounting a particular decision as incorrect may not take into consideration the fact that people process information in different ways. For example, there are those whose thought processes are very logical and methodical; others think in ways that are creative and free-flowing. It is particularly important to recognize these types of differences when several people are working together to come to a common decision. What is obvious to one will not be obvious to all—not necessarily because of a difference in values, knowledge base, or intellect, but because of different backgrounds and styles of thinking (Harrison & Bramson, 1982). This is an important consideration when collaborating with patients, families, and other professionals.

The third cause of failure to recognize subtle violations of patient autonomy lies in our assumptions about patients' knowledge base. It is easy for us to forget that we have gained a specialized body of knowledge through our programs of basic nursing education and extensive work experience. Knowledge about basic anatomy and physiology, disease process, the mechanism of action of drugs, and so forth is so ingrained in our minds that it is easy to presume everyone has at least some of the same type of knowledge. We often assume patients have more knowledge than is reasonable for them to have. Consequently, we may discount or criticize patients' decisions, even though flaws lie in the patients' level of knowledge, rather than the appropriateness of decisions. Recall that an understanding of the choices, outcomes, and implications are inherently necessary for autonomous decision making. The nurse must accurately assess the patient's level of understanding in order to assure autonomy.

The fourth cause of our failure to recognize subtle violations of patient autonomy lies in the unfortunate fact that in some instances the "work" of nursing becomes the major focus. This produces a climate of industrious habit. As we go about our work—doing procedures, giving medications, writing care plans, and trying to keep up a frantic pace—attentiveness to assuring patient autonomy is sometimes neglected. In today's climate of advanced technology, fiscal uncertainty, staffing reductions, and bottom-line management, we should guard against focusing on work rather than caring.

Autonomy for patients is more frequently discussed in terms of larger issues, such as informed consent, paternalism, compliance, and self-determination. Let us review this principle as related to these and other recurrent themes.

Informed Consent

Informed consent relates to a process by which patients are informed of the possible outcomes, alternatives, and risks of treatments, and are required to give their consent freely. It assures the legal protection of a patient's right to personal autonomy in regard to specific treatments and procedures. The concept of informed consent is one that has come to mean that patients are given the opportunity to autonomously choose a course of action in regard to plans for medical care. This is usually discussed in relation to surgery and complex medical procedures. Informed consent will be discussed in more depth in Chapter 11.

Paternalism/Parentalism

Paternalism is a gender-biased term that literally means acting in a *fatherly* manner. The traditional view of paternal actions includes such role behaviors as leadership, benevolent decision making, protection, and discipline. As commonly used in nursing, the term *paternalism* carries negative connotations, particularly related to implied dominant male versus submissive female roles. The term *parentalism*, a nongender term that parallels the meaning of paternalism while avoiding gender-bias, is used in the subsequent discussion.

In the health care arena, the concept of parentalism translates to professionals who restrict others' autonomy, usually to protect that person from perceived or anticipated harm. Parentalism is appropriate when a patient is judged to be incompetent or to have diminished decision making capacity. As advocates, we choose to do for the patient that which it is reasonable to believe the patient would choose for self, if that were possible. For example, we assume that a person would choose to be protected from injury. Within that context, and believing a patient to be incompetent, we may be justified in restraining an elderly person who is likely to fall or wander off if left unrestrained. We can consider parentalism a form of advocacy when we combine genuine concern for the patient with a well-founded belief that the patient is unable to make autonomous decisions.

The risk of harm is not enough by itself to judge a person incompetent. Virginia Henderson, the well-known nursing leader and author, recounts her experience as a hospitalized patient:

> I was in the room with another patient, and I couldn't stand being in bed any longer, and I would sit in a chair. This nurse came in and saw me sitting in the chair, and she said "Ms. Henderson if you keep doing that, we are going to have to tie you down" . . . I thought, You just try it. . . . (Goldsmith, 1992, p. 4)

Even though Ms. Henderson was ninety-four years old at the time of her hospitalization, she was certainly competent to make decisions for herself. Patients who are competent must be allowed to act autonomously—even if the choices can be predicted to cause them harm or render them incompetent (Quinn & Smith, 1987). The exception can be made that even competent persons cannot be allowed to act in a way that would cause harm to others.

The term *paternalism* generally evokes negative sentiments among nurses. This is due in part to a recognition that in the past patients' autonomy was frequently violated in the name of beneficence. Professionals sometimes make the dangerous assumption that they are uniquely qualified to make health care decisions by virtue of their professional knowledge and, further, that professional knowledge is the only knowledge needed to make decisions for patients. "Health care professionals often [believe they] understand better than patients do the full clinical implications of health risks, for they have seen the clinical results of its total actual results" (Quinn & Smith, 1987, p. 37). This kind of thinking allows us to ignore multiple factors that might be unrelated to physical outcomes, yet affect the whole person. These factors include, among others, economic considerations, lifestyle, values, role, culture, and spiritual beliefs. In making decisions, all possible factors must be taken into consideration. This dictates that the patient must be autonomously engaged in the decision-making process.

It is interesting to compare discussion of the concept of paternalism in the nursing and medical literature. Nursing literature generally describes paternalism in a negative way. Nurses often think of paternalism as behavior that precludes autonomy. Medical literature, on the other hand, discusses paternalism as a benevolent quality. The following passage illustrates this point:

> In its strong version, the principle of paternalism justifies restricting someone's autonomy if by doing so we can benefit her. In such a case, our concern is not only with preventing the person from harming herself, but also with promoting her good in a positive way. The principle might be appealed to even in cases in which our actions go against the other's known wishes. (Munson, 1992, p. 43)

The differences between the nursing and medical community in relation to beliefs about paternalism probably relate to historical, cultural, and gender factors. Interdisciplinary discussion is needed in order to reach a consensus about the appropriateness of paternalism in health care decision making. Use of the term *parentalism* avoids negative gender reference and should be used in discussion.

Ask Yourself

Who Should Make Decisions?

- How do you feel when someone else makes a decision about you without your input?
- Since nurses and doctors know more about the science of health care, when, if ever, is it appropriate for them to make decisions about the health care regimen without participation of the patient?

Noncompliance

The term **noncompliance** is generally thought of as denoting an unwillingness of the patient to participate in health care activities. This commonly entails lack of participation in a regimen that has been planned by the health care professional but must be carried out by the patient. Examples of such activities include taking medication as scheduled, maintaining a therapeutic or weight loss diet, exercising regularly, and quitting smoking. Use of the term *noncompliance* is just as likely to represent failure of the nurse as that of the patient. Discussion about noncompliance and care of the noncompliant patient centers around two basic factors. First, the autonomous participation of the patient in the health care plan is essential to success. When patients are fully aware of the choices in health care therapies and the consequences of nontreatment and are encouraged to make health care decisions, they are more likely to assume ownership of them and, as a result, to participate in care. Often nurses formulate plans of care that are consistent with a scientific base of knowledge but seem unreasonable to the patient. The nurse is amiss if the patient is not an autonomous participant in the formulation of the plan. Second, nurses and other health care professionals must assess patients' abilities to follow plans of care. Patients may be unable to comply with plans of care for a variety of reasons including lack of resources, lack of knowledge, lack of support from family members, psychological factors, and cultural beliefs that are not consistent with the proposed plan of care. An example of patients' inability to comply with a plan of care is seen every day in physicians' offices and emergency departments. Often patients are given prescriptions for medications that are prohibitively expensive. When they return with the same symptoms, not having taken the prescribed medication, they are invariably labeled as noncompliant. The problem is not one of compliance, but rather health care professionals' negligence in assessing patients' ability to follow a plan of care.

What are we to do when patients are well informed and apparently able to follow plans of care, yet do not? One hears stories of physicians who refuse to continue to care for patients who do not comply with instructions-smoking cessation, for example. In a climate of limited resources, this is a question worthy of contemplation. Codes of ethics for nurses universally support respect for individuals and individual choice, and are not restricted by considerations of social or economic status (ANA, 2001; ICN, 2000; Canadian Nurses Association, 1997). Further, the nurse must not be affected by patients' individual differences in background, customs, attitudes, and beliefs. Because health care practices are an integral part of patients' backgrounds, customs, and beliefs, refusal to participate in a plan of care, regardless of the outcome, is the prerogative of the patient, and must not affect the care given by the nurse. Ultimately, choices about health care practices belong to patients. If allowed to choose, patients should not be labeled in a negative way for choices with which nurses do not agree. It is not appropriate for professionals who express the belief that all competent patients have the right to autonomous choice to make value judgments about the choices made, and subsequently label patients as noncompliant (Nathaniel, 2000).

BENEFICENCE

The principle of **beneficence** is one that requires nurses to act in ways that benefit patients. There is no controvesy as to whether nurses are obligated to act beneficently—beneficent acts are morally and legally demanded by our professional role (Beauchamp & Walters, 1999). The objective of beneficence provides nursing's context and justification. It lays the groundwork for the trust that society places in the nursing profession, and the trust that individuals place in particular nurses or health care agencies. Perhaps this principle seems straightforward, but it is actually very complex. As we think about beneficence certain questions arise: How do we define beneficence—what is *good*? Should we determine what is good by subjective, or by objective, means? When people disagree about what is good, whose opinion counts? Is beneficence an absolute obligation and, if so, how far does our obligation extend? Does the trend toward unbridled patient autonomy outweigh obligations of beneficence? As Veatch (2000) asks, "Is the goal really to promote the total well-being of the patient? Or is the goal to promote only the *medical* well-being of the patient?" (p. 41) We must keep these questions in mind as we practice.

The ethical principle of beneficence has three major components. (See Figure 3–2.) It maintains, first, that we ought to do or promote good (Beauchamp & Childress, 1994). Even with the recognition that *good* might be defined in a number of ways, it seems safe to assume that the intention of nurses in general is to do good. Questions arise when, in particular situations, those involved cannot decide what is *good*. For example, consider the case of a patient who is in the process of a lingering, painful, terminal illness. There are those who believe that life is sacred and should be preserved at all costs. Others believe that death is preferable to a life of pain and dependence. The definition of *good* in any particular case will determine, at least in part, the action that is to be taken.

Figure 3–2 **Beneficence**

> Do or Promote Good
> Prevent Harm
> Remove Evil or Harm

The principle of beneficence also maintains that we ought to prevent evil or harm (Beauchamp & Childress, 1994). In fact, some believe that doing no harm, and preventing or removing harm, is more imperative than doing good. All codes of nursing ethics require us to prevent or remove harm. For example, the International Council of Nurses (ICN) *Code of Ethics for Nurses* (2000) says, "The nurse takes appropriate action to safeguard individuals when their care is endangered by a co-worker or any other person." Similarly, the Canadian Nurses Association *Code of Ethics for Registered Nurses* (1997) says,

> Nurses give primary considerations to the welfare of clients and any possibility of harm in future care situations when they suspect unethical conduct or incompetent or unsafe care. When nurses have reasonable grounds for concern about the behavior of colleagues in this regard, or about the safety of conditions in the care setting, they carefully review the situation and take steps, individually or in partnership with others, to resolve the problem.

Likewise, the American Nurses Association (ANA) *Code of Ethics for Nurses* (2001) is very clear about the nurse's responsibility in these situations: "As an advocate for the patient, the nurse must be alert to and take appropriate action regarding any instances of incompetent, unethical, illegal or impaired practice by any member of the health care team or the health care system or any action on the part of others that places the rights or best interests of the patient in jeopardy." In regard to removing harm the ANA *Code of Ethcis for Nurses* (2001) is very specific. Steps include the following: expressing concern to the person carrying out the questionable practice, reporting the practice to the appropriate authority within the institution, and if not corrected, reporting the problem to other appropriate authorities, such as practice committees of the pertinent professional organizations or licensing boards.

NONMALEFICENCE

The principle of **nonmaleficence** is related to beneficence. This principle requires us to act in such a manner as to avoid causing harm to patients. Included in this principle are deliberate harm, risk of harm, and harm that occurs during the performance of beneficial acts. Most ethicists today tend toward the Hippocratic tradition which says, first do no harm (the principle of nonmaleficence), placing this principle above all others. It is obvious that we must not commit acts that cause deliberate harm. This principle prohibits, for example, experimental research that assumes negative outcomes for the participants, and the performance of unnecessary procedures for economic gain or solely as a learning experience. Nonmaleficence also means avoiding harm as a consequence of doing good. In such cases, the harm must be weighed against the expected benefit. For example, sticking a child with a needle for the purpose of causing pain is always bad—there is no benefit. Giving an immunization, on the other hand, while causing similar pain, results in the benefit of protecting the child from serious disease. The harm caused by the pain of the injection is easily outweighed by the benefit of the vaccine. In day-to-day practice, we encounter many situations in which the distinction is less clear, either because the harm caused may appear to be equal to the benefit gained, because the outcome of a particular therapy cannot be assured, or as a result of conflicting beliefs and values. For example, consider analgesia for patients with painful terminal illness. Narcotic analgesia may be the only type of medication that will relieve very severe pain. This medication, however, may result in dependence and can hasten death when given in amounts required to relieve pain. Cammon and Hackshaw (2000) offer another common example. Orders for patients to have nothing by mouth before procedures and tests are common practice, unquestioned by most nurses. The authors cite examples in which elderly patients were denied food for up to six days as tests and procedures were completed. The consequences of starvation in the elderly are unquestionable, yet the practice of following NPO orders for long periods of time is seldom questioned. As nurses, we must be alert to situations such as these in which harm may outweigh benefit, taking into account our own values and those of patients.

CASE PRESENTATION

Beneficence Versus Nonmaleficence

A middle-aged nurse recounts an incident that she believes relates to the principle of nonmaleficence. As a senior nursing student she was responsible for the care of a man who had a shotgun wound to his abdomen. Surgery had been performed, and the surgeon was unable to adequately repair the damage. The man was not expected to survive the day. He was, however, awake and strong, though somewhat confused. He had a fever of 107° Fahrenheit. He was receiving intravenous fluids and had continuous nasogastric suction. The man begged for cold water to drink. The physician ordered nothing by mouth in the belief that electrolytes would be lost through the nasogastric suction if water were introduced into the stomach. The student had been taught to follow the physician's orders. She repeatedly denied the man water to drink. She worked diligently—giving iced alcohol baths, taking vital signs, monitoring the intravenous fluids, and being industrious. He begged for water. She followed orders perfectly. After six terrible hours she turned to find the man quickly drinking the water from one of his ice bags. She left the room, stood in the hallway, and cried. She felt she had failed to do her job. As a result of the gunshot wound, the man died the next morning. Today her view of the situation is different.

Think About It

Weighing Harm Against Benefit

- Was this patient harmed? Discuss your answer.
- What was the benefit of the nothing by mouth order?
- Discuss whether the harm of thirst or the benefit of maintaining nothing by mouth should take precedence.
- What other ethical principles are relevant?
- Why did the student experience such extreme distress?

This case illustrates the difficulty encountered when attempting to honor the principles of beneficence and nonmaleficence.

VERACITY

The term **veracity** relates to the practice of telling the truth. Truthfulness is widely accepted as a universal virtue. Most of us were taught as children to always tell the truth. Philosophers, in general, favor openness and honesty. The philosophers most frequently cited in nursing literature, Immanuel Kant and John Stuart Mill, agree in favor of truth telling. Nursing literature promotes honesty as a virtue and truth telling as an important function of nurses. However, there are some differences in perspective among health care professionals. Bioethicists disagree on the absolute necessity of truth telling in all instances.

Ask Yourself

Is Truth Telling Always Beneficent?
- What situational variables influence how you feel about giving placebos?
- If your goal is to be beneficent and if the patient would benefit from a placebo, is deception justifiable if it will help the patient?
- What principles are in conflict when giving placebos?

We can support nurses' practice of telling the truth in many ways. Truth telling engenders respect, open communication, trust, and shared responsibility. It is promoted in all professional codes of nursing ethics.

A very general interpretation of the ideas of the contemporary philosopher Martin Buber (1965) suggests that true communication between people can take place only when there are no barriers between them. Lying or deception creates a barrier between people and prohibits both meaningful communication and the building of relationships. Recognizing that communication is the cornerstone of the nurse-patient relationship, an argument can be made that nurses must be truthful in order to communicate effectively with patients.

Violating the principle of veracity shows lack of respect. Telling lies, or avoiding disclosure, implies that the specific function of the nurse or other person involved assumes prominence over the patient or, at the very least, the autonomy of the patient. Jameton (1984) suggests that manipulating information for the purpose of controlling others is like using coercion to control them. In essence this keeps them from participating in decisions on an equal basis. Used to benefit the patient, it is parentalism; used against the patient, it is fraud (Myers, 2000).

Jameton (1984) also suggests that deceiving others may constitute an unnecessary assumption of responsibility. When unfortunate consequences occur, the one responsible for the deception can also be assumed to be responsible for consequences. On the other hand, when bad consequences occur after we have reported the truth, we can attribute responsibility to unfortunate circumstances.

Truth telling engenders trust. We can make the argument that truth telling is imperative in assuring that patients continue to trust nurses and other health care professionals. It is by virtue of the trust in these relationships that patients are willing to suspend some measure of autonomy and seek help in meeting health care needs. Without this trust the nurse-patient relationship would be destroyed.

Veracity has been described as desirable by the American Hospital Association in the *Statement on a Patient's Bill of Rights* (1975). According to the second statement of this document, patients have the right to obtain complete, current information concerning diagnosis, treatment, and prognosis in terms they can be reasonably expected to understand. Though this position relates specifically to physicians' responsibility of disclosure, there are implications for nursing as well. As patient advocates, nurses are responsible for assuring that patients' rights are honored.

As with other principles, there is a dramatic discrepancy between nursing and medical literature in regard to veracity. Recognizing that nearly all health care is an interdisciplinary effort, and that disclosure of information to patients involves both nurses and physicians, it is important for us to understand the medical perspective.

Physicians often make the claim that patients do not want bad news, and that truthful information has the potential to harm them. In the name of beneficence, some physicians proceed with either nondisclosure or outright lies. Lipkin (1991) argues that physicians should sometimes deceive their patients or withhold information from them. It is his view that patients do not have sufficient information about how their bodies function to interpret medical information accurately, and sometimes do not want to know the truth about their illness. Joseph Ellin (1991) discusses special considerations that have been posed by the medical profession in relation to truth telling. He suggests that it does not seem beneficent to adopt an ethic of absolute veracity in which it is an obligation to cause avoidable anguish to someone who is already ill, especially when hope and positive outlook may promote healing and help prolong life. He writes, "One could hope to avoid this dilemma by holding that the duty of veracity, though not absolute, is to be given very great weight, and may be overridden only in the gravest cases . . ." (p. 82). Ellin draws a distinction between lying and deception: lying is the purposeful telling of untruths, whereas deception is usually accomplished through nondisclosure. He argues that there is an absolute duty to avoid lying to patients; however, there is no duty not to deceive. Examples he gives include withholding information about a poor prognosis or giving placebo medication. Consider the following situation: A mother of four is admitted to the emergency department after an automobile accident in which two of her children are killed. Recognizing that she is in very serious condition, according to Ellin, it would be appropriate to avoid telling her of the death of her children. If, however, she asks about their condition, she must be told the truth.

Ask Yourself

Is the Truth Sometimes Harmful?

- Do you think it is acceptable to deceive a patient in order to prevent unnecessary suffering?
- How would you feel if you were a patient and the health care team and your family conspired to deceive you—if, for example, you were ill and you had a bleak prognosis?

Bok (1991) examines the practice of physicians deceiving patients in the name of beneficence. She writes that lying to patients has historically been seen as an excusable act. "Some would argue that doctors, and only doctors, should be granted the right to manipulate the truth in ways so undesirable for politicians, lawyers, and others" (p. 75). In fact, truth telling has never been a principle that was given consideration in the medical literature. Veracity is absent from virtually all oaths, codes, and prayers. Even the Hippocratic Oath makes no mention of truthfulness. The 1847 version of the American Medical Association Code of Ethics endorses some forms of deception by stating that the physician has a sacred duty to avoid "all things which have a tendency to discourage the patient and to depress his spirits" (Bok, 1994, p. 1683).

Nursing and medicine view veracity from two different perspectives. It is clear that physicians have traditionally seen disclosure or nondisclosure to be a facet of care within their control that can have implications for patient welfare. To withhold bad news is often considered a beneficent act if disclosure of the information is predicted to harm the patient. Nursing, on the other hand, upholds veracity as supporting individual rights, respect for persons, and the principle of autonomy. Recognition of the viewpoint of others is imperative for professionals who must collaborate. Chapter 4 discusses methods of making decisions about ethical problems when there are differences of perspective among those involved.

CONFIDENTIALITY

Confidentiality is the ethical principle that requires nondisclosure of private or secret information with which one is entrusted. Support for this principle is found in codes and oaths of nursing and medicine dating back many centuries. Nursing codes of ethics require that we maintain confidentiality of patient information. According to the ICN *Code of Ethics for Nurses* (2000), "The nurse holds in confidence personal information and uses judgement in sharing this information." Similarly, the ANA *Code of Ethics for Nurses* (2001) and the Canadian Nurses Association *Code of Ethics for Registered Nurses* (1997) direct nurses to maintain confidentiality. Confidentiality is the only facet of patient care mentioned in the Nightingale Pledge. This oath has been recited for decades by graduating nurses: "I will do all in my power to elevate the standard of my profession and will hold in confidence all personal matters committed to my keeping and all family affairs coming to my knowledge in the practice of my profession." Physicians do not escape the promise of confidentiality. The Hippocratic Oath is very clear: "Whatever, in connection with my professional practice, or not in connection with it, I see or hear, in the life of men, which ought not to be spoken of abroad, I will not divulge, as reckoning that all such should be kept secret." Though there are compelling arguments in favor of maintaining confidentiality, there is disagreement about the absolute requirement of confidentiality in all situations.

The ability to maintain privacy in one's life is an expression of autonomy. The capacity to choose what others know about us, particularly intimate personal details, is important, because it enables us to maintain dignity and preserve a measure of control over our own lives. Markus and Lockwood discuss the importance of privacy:

> Privacy is thus a value closely related to, and perhaps ultimately grounded on, the value of personal autonomy. To take this value of privacy seriously is to subscribe to a number of familiar precepts. It means that we should be reluctant to pry, that we should respect personal confidences, and that when we enter into relationships with others that render us privy to sensitive or intimate personal information, we should be [careful] about passing this information on, even in the absence of any specific request not to do so. (1991, p. 349)

Thus, maintaining confidentiality of patients is an expression of respect of persons and, in many ways, is essential to the nurse-patient relationship. Consider the following case presentation.

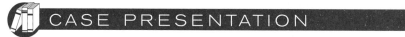 CASE PRESENTATION

Making the Best Choice

Lora is a seventeen-year-old cheerleader. She comes to the local family planning clinic requesting birth control pills. Lora is a very attractive, neat, and pleasant patient. In the process of completing the initial physical examination, the nurse practitioner finds evidence of physical abuse, including a recent traumatic perforated ear drum. Lora hesitantly and tearfully admits that her biological father slapped her across her left ear prior to her coming to the clinic. She reports that she recently moved into his home after living most of her life with her mother and stepfather. She tearfully reports that her stepfather was sexually abusive to her and that she wishes to remain with her biological father. She says that she can tolerate being slapped around occasionally, and she does not want to get her biological father in trouble or be forced to move back to her stepfather's home. State law requires that the nurse report any suspicion of child abuse. Both codes of ethics and federal law require that the nurse maintain confidentiality.

Think About It

To Tell or Not to Tell

- What are the principles involved?
- Does the nurse's obligation to report the incident of child abuse supersede the obligation to maintain confidentiality-particularly considering that the patient requested confidentiality? What if Lora was fourteen years old?
- What are the options for the nurse?
- What are the possible outcomes of the different options?
- Does Lora's autonomy outweigh the nurse's responsibility to report the abusive situation?

There are at least two basic ethical arguments in favor of maintaining confidentiality. The first of these is the individual's right to control personal information and protect privacy. The second argument is one of utility.

This right to privacy flows from autonomy and respect for persons. On one level, patients have the right to expect that personal and private information will not be shared unnecessarily among health care providers. Patient information is not an appropriate topic for elevator or dinner conversation. It is most likely that violations of this nature were what authors had in mind when writing early creeds and oaths that promise confidentiality. Nurses and other professionals often casually discuss private patient matters. On another level, nurses must keep in mind the number of people who have legitimate access to patient records. In a hospital situation, patient charts are accessible to many personnel. Nurses, physicians, dieticians, respiratory therapists, utilization review staff, financial officers, students, secretaries, physical therapists, and others have legitimate reason to view patient records. Information of a sensitive and private nature that the patient intends for the nurse alone can become widely known in a large health care facility. Care must be taken in choosing information to be recorded in patients' charts. Special care must be taken to avoid inadvertent breaches of confidentiality (Erlen, 1998) including those involved with electronic records (Muldoon, 1996). It is important for nurses to be aware of the many threats to patient confidentiality.

Confidentiality is particularly important when revelation of intimate and sensitive information has the potential to harm the patient. Harm can take various forms such as embarrassment, ridicule, discrimination, deprivation of rights, physical or emotional harm, and loss of roles or relationships. Consider the plight of many AIDS victims whose diagnoses have become public knowledge. Confidentiality is particularly important when dealing with vulnerable populations (Winston, 1988).

The second argument is one of utility. If patients suspect that health care providers reveal sensitive and personal information indiscriminately, they may be reluctant to seek care. Government policy makers recognize this problem. Because of the intimate and private nature of reproductive health issues, confidentiality of those seeking family planning services, for example, is mandated. Those caring for AIDS patients also recognize the need to maintain confidentiality. According to Winston (1988), many who work with AIDS patients find such arguments particularly compelling, believing that disclosure of patients' antibody status or a diagnosis of AIDS would have a "chilling effect," discouraging those in high-risk groups from seeking care. There are other diagnoses, such as mental illness, alcoholism, and drug addiction that, if revealed, could lead to public scorn, and subsequently discourage others from seeking care.

Limits of Confidentiality

Should the principle of confidentiality be honored in all instances? There are arguments that favor questioning the absolute obligation of confidentiality in certain situations. These arguments include theories related to the principles of harm and vulnerability (Winston, 1988). The harm principle can be applied when the nurse or other professional recognizes that maintaining confidentiality will result in preventable wrongful harm to innocent others. Mandatory premarital testing for syphilis, for example, is intended to prevent the spread of a serious communicable disease to innocent babies and spouses. In this instance, society chooses to override the privacy of the individual to protect the health of the innocent. Though directing nurses to maintain confidentiality, the ANA *Code of Ethics for Nurses* (2001) recognizes that duties of confidentiality are not absolute and may need to be modified to protect the patient, other innocent people, and in cases of mandatory disclosure for public safety.

In rare instances, case law supports the harm principle. In July of 1976, the California Supreme Court ruled that a psychologist, Dr. Lawrence Moore, and his superior, Dr. Harvey Powelson, and the agency for which they worked were liable in the wrongful death of Tatiana Tarsoff. Prosenjit Poddar killed Tatiana Tarsoff in October of 1969. According to Tatiana's parents, two months earlier Poddar confided his intention to kill Tatiana to his psychologist, Dr. Moore. Though Dr. Moore initially tried to have his patient involuntarily committed, Dr. Powelson intervened and allowed Poddar to return home. Neither Tatiana nor her parents were informed of the patient's threats. The court found that the defendants were responsible for the wrongful death of Tatiana because they knew in advance of the patient's intentions. The obligation to protect the innocent third party superseded the obligation to maintain confidentiality. According to the majority opinion in this case, the duty to warn arises from a special relation between the patient and the psychologist that imposes a duty to control the patient's conduct (Tobriner, 1991).

Foreseeability is an important consideration in situations in which confidentiality conflicts with the duty to warn. The nurse or other health care professional should be able to reasonably foresee harm or injury to an innocent other in order to violate the principle of confidentiality in favor of a duty to warn. This consideration precludes blanket disclosure of private information that might predict harm to others. The Tarasoff case exemplifies reasonable application of the harm principle. Subsequent court cases support the decision in the Tarasoff case. Courts have found that privacy is not absolute and is subordinate to the state's fundamental right to enact laws that promote public health.

The harm principle is strengthened when one considers the vulnerability of the innocent (Haggarty, 2000). The duty to protect others from harm is stronger when the third party is dependent on others or is in some way especially vulnerable. This duty is called the vulnerability principle. Vulnerability implies risk or susceptibility to harm when vulnerable individuals have a relative inability to protect themselves (Winston, 1988). For example, nurses have an absolute duty to report child abuse. Because children are dependent and vulnerable, they are at greater risk of harm. Coupling of the harm principle with the vulnerability principle produces a rather strong argument for abandoning the principle of confidentiality in certain instances.

Think About It

Can Nurses Violate Confidentiality?

- How do you think confidentiality and the harm and vulnerability principles can be reconciled?
- How would you feel if a relative contracted HIV from a source who public health officials knew was infected, and had reason to believe would infect your relative, but neglected to warn?
- How would you feel if you were HIV infected and your health care provider violated your right to confidentiality?

Actions that are considered ethical are not always found to be legal. Though there is an ethical basis for subsuming the principle of confidentiality in special circumstances, and there is some legal precedent for doing so, there is legal risk to disclosing sensitive information. There is dynamic tension between the patient's right to confidentiality and the duty to warn innocent others. Nurses need to recognize that careful consideration of the ethical implications of actions will not always be supported in bureaucratic and legal systems.

JUSTICE

Justice is the ethical principle that relates to fair, equitable, and appropriate treatment in light of what is due or owed to persons, recognizing that giving to some will deny receipt to others who might otherwise have received these things. Within the context of health care ethics, the relevant application of the principle focuses on distribution of goods and services. This application is called **distributive justice.** Unfortunately, there is a finite supply of goods and services, and it is impossible for all people to have everything they might want or need. One of the primary purposes of governing systems is to formulate and enforce policies that deal with fair and equitable distribution of scarce resources.

Decisions about distributive justice are made on a variety of levels. The government is responsible for deciding policy about broad public health access issues, such as children's immunization and Medicare for the elderly. Hospitals and other organizations formulate policy on an institutional level and deal with issues such as how decisions will be made concerning who will occupy intensive care beds and which types of patients will be accepted in emergency rooms. Nurses and other health care providers frequently make decisions of distributive justice on an individual basis. For example, having assessed the needs of patients, nurses decide how best to allocate their time (a scarce resource).

There are three basic areas of health care that are relevant to questions of distributive justice. First, what percentage of our resources is it reasonable to spend on health care? Second, recognizing that health care resources are limited, which aspects of health care should receive the most resources? Third, which patients should have access to the limited health care staff, equipment, and so forth? (Jameton, 1984).

In making decisions of distributive justice, one must ask the question, "Who is entitled to these goods or services?" Philosophers have suggested a number of different ways to choose among people. Figure 3–3 lists some of the ways that people have historically made these types of decisions.

Figure 3–3 **Distributive Justice**

To each equally
To each according to need
To each according to merit
To each according to social contribution
To each according to the person's rights
To each according to individual effort
To each as you would be done by
To each according to the greatest good to the greatest number

There are those who believe that all should receive equally regardless of need. On the surface, nationalized health care systems would seem to meet this criterion, since all citizens are eligible for the same services. However, because some citizens would necessarily require more health care services than others, nationalized systems also meet the criterion of need. German philosopher, Friedrich Nietzsche, had a different perspective. He believed that there are superior individuals, and that society's goal should be to enhance these "supermen." For Nietzsche, the choice of distribution was a clear one—to each according to his present or future social contribution (Durant, 1926). To each according to that person's rights indicates a libertarian viewpoint, and to each as you would be done by is a reflection of the golden rule. The idea that each should receive according to effort is a common belief in our culture and indicates the traditional "work ethic." Entitlement programs in the United States generally award benefits based upon a combination of need and the greatest good that can be accomplished for the greatest number of people. Chapter 15 discusses the application of the principle of distributive justice in greater detail.

FIDELITY

The ethical principle of **fidelity** is often related to the concept of faithfulness and the practice of keeping promises. Society has granted nurses the right to practice nursing through the processes of licensure and certification. "The authority for the practice of nursing is based on a social contract that acknowledges professional rights and responsibilities as well as mechanisms for public accountability" (ANA, 1995, p. 3). The process of licensure is one that ensures no other group can practice within the domain of nursing as defined by society and the profession. Thus, to accept licensure and become legitimate members of the profession mandates that nurses uphold the responsibilities inherent in the contract with society. Members are called to be faithful to the society that grants the right to practice—to keep the promise of upholding the profession's code of ethics, to practice within the established scope of practice and definition of nursing, to remain competent in practice, to abide by the policies of employing institutions, and to keep promises to individual patients. To *be* a nurse is to *make these promises*. In fulfilling this contract with society, nurses are responsible to faithfully and consistently adhere to these basic principles.

On another level, the principle of fidelity relates to loyalty within the nurse-patient relationship. It gives rise to an independent duty to keep promises or contracts (Veatch, 2000) and is a basic premise of the nurse-patient relationship. Problems sometimes arise when there is a conflict between promises that have been made and the potential consequences of those promises in cases in which carrying them out will cause harm in other ways. Though fidelity is the cornerstone of a trusting nurse-patient relationship, most ethicists think there are no absolute, exceptionless duties to keep promises—that, in every case, harmful consequences of the promised action should be weighed against the benefits of keeping the promise.

SUMMARY

As we participate in meeting the health care needs of society, we must be constantly aware of ethical implications inherent in many situations. Each nurse must develop a philosophically consistent framework from which to base contemplation, decision, and action. It is this framework that gives shape to our concept of various ethical principles. The principles discussed in this chapter presuppose nurses' innate respect of persons. Ethical principles include autonomy, beneficence, nonmaleficence, veracity, confidentiality, justice, and fidelity.

CHAPTER HIGHLIGHTS

- Ethical principles are basic and obvious moral truths that guide deliberation and action.
- All ethical principles presuppose a basic respect for persons.
- Autonomy denotes having the freedom to make choices about issues that affect one's life.
- Various intrinsic and extrinsic factors threaten patient autonomy.
- The principle of beneficence maintains that one ought to do or promote good, prevent evil or harm, and remove evil or harm.
- The principle of nonmaleficence requires one to avoid causing harm, including deliberate harm, risk of harm, and harm that occurs during the performance of beneficial acts.
- The principle of veracity relates to the universal virtue of truth telling.
- Confidentiality is the ethical principle that requires nondisclosure of private or secret information with which one is entrusted.
- Justice is the ethical principle that relates to fair, equitable, and appropriate treatment in light of what is due or owed to persons, recognizing that giving to some will deny receipt to others who might otherwise have received these things.
- Fidelity is the ethical principle that relates to faithfulness and promise keeping.

DISCUSSION QUESTIONS AND ACTIVITIES

1. Find the ANA *Code of Ethics for Nurses* on the ANA website at: http://nursing world.org.htm. Read the code and discuss how the various statements relate to the principles discussed in this chapter.

2. Read the following hypothetical situation and answer the questions that follow:
   An elderly gentleman presents himself to the emergency department of a small community hospital. The patient has contractures and paralysis of his left hand; he apparently has complete expressive and at least partial receptive aphasia. Upon questioning, the man takes off his right shoe and points to his right great toe and grimaces, apparently indicating a problem in that area. The nurse is unable to gather any further information from him because of his difficulty in communicating. In attempting to help him, she asks if he has a neighbor or friend accompanying him. He shakes his head, indicating that he is alone. Curious, the nurse asks him how he came to the hospital. The patient smiles and proudly produces a driver's license from his shirt pocket. Subsequently, the nurse leaves the room and returns a few minutes later to find that the patient left the hospital, having received no care. The nurse suspects that because of his current physical condition the man is unsafe to drive a motor vehicle.

   - What are the ethical implications in this situation?
   - What ethical principles are involved?

- Should the nurse pursue avenues to locate the patient and ensure that he is not endangering himself or others by driving? Would this be a breach of confidentiality? Autonomy?
- How does the nurse express fidelity in this situation?
- What is the beneficent action?

3. Describe situations you have witnessed in which decisions were made for patients in a paternalistic manner. Discuss your perception of the appropriateness of parentalism in given situations.

4. Read the following hypothetical case and answer the questions that follow:

Martha is a seventy-five-year-old woman who has terminal cancer of the bladder. During the course of her therapy, she sustains third-degree radiation burns to her lower abdomen and pelvic area. Her wounds are extensive and deep, involving her abdominal wall, bladder, and vagina. The physician orders frequent medicinal douches and wound irrigations. These treatments are very painful, and the patient wants the treatments discontinued but is too timid to actually refuse them. The physician will not change the order.

- Discuss the situation in terms of beneficence and nonmaleficence.
- How does this patient express her autonomy?
- What is the nurse's responsibility in assisting the patient to maintain autonomy?
- How does the nurse deal with conflicting loyalties and principles?

5. Do you think health care professionals should disclose information to patients related, for example, to a poor prognosis, even though the information may cause distress? Discuss your views in depth.

6. Jameton (1984) says that for nurses to be less than competent is unethical. Discuss this statement in terms of fidelity.

7. Read the following hypothetical case and answer the questions that follow:

Nels Gruder is a forty-year-old disabled truck driver. He was injured several years ago in a trucking accident. He subsequently has had back surgery but continues to have severe pain. He has been seen by every local neurosurgeon and, for one reason or another, is not pleased with the care he has gotten. Because of the seriousness of his initial injuries, there is little doubt that Mr. Gruder has chronic back pain. Even though the local emergency room policy of not prescribing narcotic analgesics for chronic pain is clearly stated on signs in the waiting area, Mr. Gruder comes there frequently complaining of severe back pain. He reports a history of gastric ulcers and allergy to nonsteroidal anti-inflammatory drugs (NSAIDs). The nurse practitioner who sees Mr. Gruder is faced with a man who is in obvious pain. She wishes to help him relieve the pain he is experiencing. At the same time she realizes that narcotic analgesia is not appropriate for this type of problem, and is unable to prescribe NSAIDs because of his reports of gastric ulcers and allergy. He says he has tried exercises and a local pain clinic, neither of which was effective. He is aware of the emergency room policy regarding narcotic analgesics for chronic pain, but he comes there in desperation. He insists that his pain is relieved only by narcotic analgesia.

- What ethical principles are involved?
- Does the benefit of pain relief outweigh the harm potentially caused by long-term narcotic analgesic use for this patient?
- Should Mr. Gruder's perceived need for narcotic pain medications be honored even though the nurse practitioner feels he has a problem with drug dependence?
- How does the nurse do what she thinks is right and yet respect Mr. Gruder's autonomy?
- Is it important whether or not the nurse's actions please the patient?

REFERENCES

American Hospital Association. (1975). *Statement on a patient's bill of rights.* Chicago: Author.

American Nurses Association. (1995). *Nursing's social policy statement.* Washington: Author.

American Nurses Association (2001). *Code of ethics for nurses.* Washington, DC: Author.

Aveyard, H. (2000). Is there a concept of autonomy that can usefully inform nursing practice? *Journal of Advanced Nursing, 32*(2), 352–358.

Beauchamp, T., & Childress, J. (1994). *Principles of biomedical ethics* (4th ed.). New York: Oxford University Press.

Beauchamp, T. L., & Walters, L. (1999). *Contemporary issues in bioethics.* Belmont, CA: Wadsworth.

Bok, S. (1991). Lies to the sick and dying. In T. A. Mappes & J. S. Zembaty, eds. *Biomedical ethics* (pp. 74–81). New York: McGraw Hill.

Bok, S. (1994). Truth telling. In W. Reich, ed., *Encyclopedia of bioethics* (pp. 1682–1686). New York: Macmillan.

Buber, M. (1965). *The knowledge of man: A philosophy of the interhuman.* New York: Harper & Row.

Cammon, S. A., & Hackshaw, H. S. (2000). Are we starving our patients? *Ameican Journal of Nursing, 100*(5), 43–46.

Canadian Nurses Association (1997). *Code of ethics for registered nurses.* Author.

Durant, W. (1926). *The story of philosophy.* New York: Washington Square Press.

Edge, R. S., & Groves, J. R. (1994). *The ethics of health care: A guide for practice.* Albany, NY: Delmar.

Ellin, J. S. (1991). Lying and deception: The solution to a dilemma in medical ethics. In T. A. Mappes & J. S. Zembaty, eds., *Biomedical ethics* (pp. 81–87). New York: McGraw-Hill.

Erlen, J. A. (1998). The inadvertent breach of confidentiality. *Orthopedic Nursing, 17*(2), 47–50.

Goldsmith, J., ed. (1992). Virginia Henderson, RN: Humanitarian and scholar. *Reflections, 18*(1), 4–5.

Haggarty, L. A. (2000). Informed consent and the limit of confidentiality. *Western Journal of Nursing Research, 22*(4), 508–514.

Harrison, A. F., & Bramson, R. M. (1982). *Styles of thinking.* New York: Doubleday.

International Council of Nurses (2000). *The ICN code of ethics for nurses.* International Council of Nurses, Geneva Switzerland. Retrieved January 23, 2001 from the World Wide Web: http://icn.ch/indes.html/

Jameton, A. (1984). *Nursing practice: The ethical issues.* Englewood Cliffs, NJ: Prentice-Hall.

Lipkin, M. (1991). On lying to patients. In T. A. Mappes & J. S. Zembaty, eds., *Biomedical ethics* (pp. 72–73). New York: McGraw-Hill.

Markus, A., & Lockwood, M. (1991). Is it permissible to edit medical records? *British Medical Journal, 303,* 349–351.

Muldoon, J. D. (1996). Confidentiality, privacy and restriction for compute-based patient records. *Hospital Topics, 74*(3), 32–37.

Munson, R. (1992). Major moral principles. In *Intervention and reflection: Basic issues in medical ethics* (4th ed., pp. 31–45). Belmont, CA: Wadsworth.

Myers, M. T., Jr. (2000). Lysing for patients may be a violation of federal law. *Archives of Internal Medicine, 160*(4), 2223–2224.

Nathaniel, A. (2000). An examination of ethical principles as they relate to noncompliance. Continuing education case study. Sigma Theta Tau International Honor Society of Nursing. Retrieved January 13, 2001 from the World Wide Web: http://www.nursingsociety.org/

Quinn, C. A., & Smith, M. D. (1987). *The professional commitment: Issues and ethics in nursing.* Philadelphia: Saunders.

Shakespeare, W. The merchant of Venice.

Tobriner, M. O. (1991). Majority opinion in Tarsoff v. Regents of the University of California. In T. A. Mappes & J. S. Zembaty, eds., *Biomedical ethics* (pp. 165–169). New York: McGraw-Hill.

Veach, R. (2000). *The basics of bioethics.* Upper Saddle River, NJ: Prentice Hall.

Winston, M. E. (1988). AIDS, confidentiality, and the right to know. *Public Affairs Quarterly, 2,* 91–104.

DEVELOPING PRINCIPLED BEHAVIOR

Recognizing that values and beliefs are culturally relative, Part II describes theories related to moral development and values clarification. This section examines the process of ethical decision making and its application to clinical situations. Because personal values and moral developoment influence perceptions and decisions, readers are encouraged to become aware of their own values and to examine personal levels of moral development in light of the different theories presened in Part I. Benefiting from this knowledge, readers can begin to be more sensitive to the perspectives, decision making abilities, and tendencies of other people and to acnkowledge the influence of their own values and moral development on various decision making processes.

CHAPTER 4

Values Clarification

As your actions are informed by your awareness of values, your thinking and your ideas are shaped and changed by your experiences with those actions.

(Chinn, 1995, p. 3)

OBJECTIVES

After completing this chapter, the reader should be able to:

1. Define and differentiate personal values, societal values, professional values, organizational values, and moral values.

2. Discuss how values are acquired.

3. Discuss self-awareness as a tool for living an ethical life.

4. Explain the place of values clarification in nursing.

5. Explain the valuing process.

6. Describe values conflict and its implications for nursing care.

7. Describe the interaction between personal and institutional values.

8. Discuss the importance of attending to both personal values and patient values.

INTRODUCTION

Principled behavior flows from personal values that guide and inform our responses, behaviors, and decisions in all areas of our life. Ethical decision making requires self-awareness and knowledge of ethical theories and principles. Such awareness of self includes knowing what we value or consider important. The branch of philosophy that studies the nature and types of values is called **axiology**, a word that comes from the Greek for worth or worthy. Axiology includes the study of values in art, known as aesthetics, in human relations and conduct, known as ethics, and in relation to beliefs regarding relationship with the Divine, known as religion. This chapter discusses the importance of being aware of personal values and how these values influence the way we relate to self and others within personal and professional arenas.

WHAT ARE VALUES?

Values are ideals, beliefs, customs, modes of conduct, qualities, or goals that are highly prized or preferred by individuals, groups, or society. Omery (1989) notes that the fundamental nature of values includes a pattern of a "subjective, strongly motivational preference or disposition toward a person, object, or idea that is more likely to be manifest in an affective situation . . . and [is] more likely to be mobilized by the individual in a hierarchical order" (p. 500). Values, which are learned in both conscious and unconscious ways, become part of a person's makeup. When we are faced with choices, our preferences and their hierarchy becomes evident. For example, if both comfort and appearance are valued in how we dress, the hierarchy becomes evident when we choose to wear the more restrictive suit rather than the more relaxed dress for a professional interview. Our values influence choices and behavior whether or not we are conscious that the values are guiding the choices. Values provide direction and meaning to life and a frame of reference for integrating, explaining, and evaluating new experiences, thoughts, and relationships. Values may be expressed overtly, as espoused behaviors or verbalized standards, or they may manifest in an indirect way through verbal and nonverbal behavior.

Moral Values

As discussed in Chapter 2, individual cognitive evaluation of right and wrong, good, and bad, is reflective of **moral thought.** Flowing from this, preferences or dispositions reflective of right or wrong, should or should not, in human behavior are considered **moral values** (Omery, 1989). Moral values constitute a special case of values because the particular circumstances that call them forth deal with ethical issues or dilemmas. These values may be acquired within contexts such as the family, through our religious or philosophical orientation, or through our profession.

ACQUIRING VALUES

Personal ethical behavior flows from values held by an individual that develop over time. Cultural, ethnic, familial, environmental, educational, and other experiences of living help to shape our values. We begin to learn and incorporate values into our beings at an early age and continue the process throughout our lives. As noted previously, values are acquired in both conscious and unconscious ways. Values may be learned in a conscious way through instruction by parents, teachers, religious ministers and educators, and professional and social group leaders. Many values are formally adopted by groups and are written in professional codes of ethics, religious doctrines, societal laws, and statements of an organization's philosophy. Socialization and role modeling, other ways values are acquired, lead to more subconscious learning. Some values stay with us for much of our lives, and others may change or be altered in response to our own development and experiences. "The most important step in values formation is one's freedom to choose those values that are most cherished and to relinquish those that have little meaning" (Seroka, 1994, p. 11).

Because values become a part of who we are, they often enter into decision making in less than conscious ways. We constantly make judgments that reflect our values, though not always realizing that we have a given set of values or that these values are affecting our decisions (Davis, Aroskar, Liaschenko, & Drought, 1997; Engebretson & Headley, 2000; Simon, Howe, & Kirschenbaum, 1995). Becoming more aware of one's values is an important step in being able to make clear and thoughtful decisions. Knowing one's own values in a conscious way, and being able to help others to name their values clearly, are particularly important in the area of ethical decision making.

Ask Yourself

How Have Your Values Developed?

Think of three ideals or beliefs that you prize in your personal life. Try to trace each belief or ideal back to the earliest time in your life when you were aware of its importance or presence.

- When and how did you learn to view each belief or ideal as important?
- How have they changed or evolved over time?
- Where do you find your support for them?
- How prevalent do you think these beliefs or ideals are among other people?
- What do you think of people who hold different beliefs or ideals?
- Think of a time in your life when one of these beliefs or ideals has been challenged. How did you feel? How did you react?

SELF-AWARENESS

Ethical relationships with others begin with self-knowledge and the willingness to express that awareness to others honestly and appropriately. Self-knowledge is an ongoing, evolving process that requires us to make a commitment to know the truth about ourselves. This is not an easy commitment to make. Although the truth can be painful at times, paradoxically, it can also set us free. We must remember that what we believe to be the truth is always colored by our perceptions, and can change over time (Covey, 1990). Keep in mind that most situations are not black or white. All sides are present in each situation. Like the aperture of a camera, what we see in any situation depends upon how close or far we are standing and the angle from which we are looking. From this perspective, there can be many views of a situation, depending upon how many people are picturing it. Understanding the truth of a situation is usually more accurate if people appreciate that there can be different views and openly share these perspectives (Banonis, 1997).

The term **values clarification** refers to the process of becoming more conscious of and naming what we value or consider worthy. It is an ongoing process that is grounded in our capacity for reflective, intelligent, self-directed behavior (Gaydos, 2000; Keegan, 2000). By focusing time, energy, and attention to reflecting on our values, we shed light on our personal perspective and discover our own answers to many concerns and questions. Developing insight into our values improves our ability to make value decisions. No one set of values is appropriate for everyone; we must appreciate that values clarification may lead to different insights for different people (Engebretson & Headley, 2000; Gaydos, 2000). Engaging in values clarification promotes a closer fit between our words and actions, enabling us to more clearly "walk our talk," thus enhancing personal integrity. As noted in Chapter 3, **integrity** refers to adherence to moral norms that is sustained over time. Trustworthiness and a consistency of convictions, actions, and emotions is implicit in integrity. It is only to the extent that we appreciate our own values that we can truly understand the values of another.

Since values include dimensions of knowing and of feeling, the process of becoming more clear about what we hold dear needs to address both the cognitive and the affective domains. Through analyzing our behavior and becoming more in touch with our feelings, we learn to discern which choices are rational and which are the result of preconditioning (Seroka, 1994). Assessment of personal values requires a readiness and willingness to take an honest look at our ideals and behaviors, at our words, actions, and motivation, and at the congruencies and incongruencies among them. Moving toward the point of choosing our own values, rather than merely acting out prior programing, is a goal of the process.

Enhancing Self-Awareness

Self-awareness is the ultimate tool for living a personally ethical life. Values clarification and **self-awareness** go hand in hand. The first and most important step in awareness of the self is the conscious intention to be aware. Being conscious of our thoughts, feelings, physical and emotional responses, and insights in various situations can promote appreciation of our values. Conversely, by identifying and analyzing personal values, we become more self-aware (Burkhardt & Nagai-Jacobson, 2002; Rew, 1996; 2000). We can enhance insight by developing the ability to step back and see what is going on in any situation, being aware of ourself and our reactions in the present moment. Self-awareness can begin with as simple an act as tuning in to our breathing, noting its rate, rhythm, depth, and other characteristics without any effort to change it. It is a way of becoming conscious of an act that usually occurs quite unconsciously. Another way to become more aware is to pay attention to how we are feeling physically and emotionally in any given situation-to name the feelings without judging them. We might ask, "What do I think I am reacting to here, and can I identify where that reaction comes from?" For example, when you see a beautiful sunset, you might note a feeling of peace, exhilaration, or relaxation, and realize you are responding to beauty, with an ensuing memory that your mother was always one to be observant of beauty in her world. You thus recognize that you learned this value, at least in part, from your mother. Introspection, observation, reflection, meditation, journaling, art, writing, therapy, reading, discussion groups, and feedback assist us in expanding self-awareness.

Individual reflection and discussion with another person or in small groups help us to become more aware of and to analyze our values. Group discussion enables us to react and to hear the reactions of others. Such processes may lead us to see more clearly those values we have accepted because of programming, and to articulate better those values we have chosen. These processes may also lead us to modify our perspective based on the insights of others. Other tools that open our perspective include: taking the other side of a debate, interviewing people with differing opinions, walking in another's shoes and defending their position, and asking for feedback on your positions. Another way to look at values is to ask general questions like "If I knew I would die in six weeks, what would I be doing today?" or "If I had to leave my house and could only take three things with me, what would they be?" or "Where would I like to be five/ten/twenty years from now?"

Simon and colleagues (1995) suggest that the valuing process includes three areas:

Prizing and cherishing one's beliefs and behaviors, which includes knowing what one does and does not support and communicating this to others;
Choosing one's beliefs and behaviors by evaluating values received from others, which includes examining alternatives and their consequences then deciding what is one's own;
Acting on these beliefs with a consistent pattern that reinforces actions supportive of the values.

The intent of values clarification is to help us become more aware of our own values and the valuing process in our lives; it does not aim to impose or instill particular values in our lives.

Journaling.   Kolkmeier (1995) describes **journals** as "records that are kept on a periodic or regular basis and contain factual material and subjective interpretations of events, thoughts, feelings, and plans" (p. 336). For many people, keeping a diary or journal of experiences and personal reactions to situations is a useful tool in developing awareness. A number of books such as those by Progoff (1992), Adams (1990), Kahn (1996), and Baldwin (1991) are available to guide someone new to journaling. Figure 4–1 offers guidelines that may help students utilize the journaling process to gain insight into personal values. The following are a few general considerations that may enhance the ability to gain insight through journaling. When writing in a journal, let your thoughts flow as freely as possible without censoring or judging what you are writing. Allow yourself time and privacy when you are journaling, and keep the journal in a place where you feel comfortable that you control who has access to it. Commit to journaling on a regular basis. Recognize that journaling is a personal process, so go with your style. If a format such as that suggested in Figure 4–1 helps you, go for it! If not, write as the thoughts flow from you.

Figure 4–1 **Journaling for Values Awareness**

- Describe a situation in your personal or professional experience in which you felt uncomfortable or felt that your beliefs or values were being challenged, or in which you felt your values were different from others involved.
- As you record the situation, include how you felt physically and emotionally at the time you experienced the situation.
- Write down your feelings as you remember the situation. Are your reactions now any different from when you were actually in this situation?
- What personal values do you identify in the situation? Try to remember where and from whom you learned these values. Do you totally agree with the values, or is there anything about them that you question or wonder about their validity?
- What values do you think were being expressed by others involved? Where are they similar or different from your values?
- What do you think you reacted to in the situation?
- Can you remember having similar reactions in other situations? If yes, how were the situations similar or different?
- How do you feel about your response to the situation? Is there anything you would change if you could repeat the scene? Rewrite the scene with the changes. What might be the consequences of these changes?
- How do you feel with the new scenario?
- What do you need to do to reinforce behaviors, ideals, beliefs, or qualities that you have identified as personal values in this situation? When and how can you do this?

VALUES IN PROFESSIONAL SITUATIONS

Values clarification is important to nurses in several ways. To know and appreciate our own value system provides a basis for understanding how and why we react and respond in decision-making situations. Knowing our own values enables us to acknowledge similarities and differences in values when interacting with others, which ultimately promotes more effective communication and care. Commitment to developing more awareness of personal values enables us to be more effective in facilitating the process with others. In the professional realm, these others may be staff, patients, families, or institutions.

Values Conflict.   When personal values are at odds with those of patients, colleagues, or the institution, internal or interpersonal conflict may result. This can subsequently affect patient care. Dealing in an effective way with **values conflict** requires conscious awareness of our own values, as well as awareness of the perceived values of the others involved. Such awareness enables the nurse to be more alert to situations in which the behaviors of others are judged according to their own values, or in which personal values are being imposed upon another. When differences in values are identified, the nurse can choose to respond to the other's viewpoint, in a way that seeks understanding and common ground, rather than reacting in a "knee-jerk" fashion. In this way the integrity of the caring relationship can be maintained.

The following case presentation provides an example of values conflict. As you read the case, think about the values that are evident in the situation. Put yourself in the position of each of the participants and ask yourself what you might do if you were in their shoes.

CASE PRESENTATION

A Conflict of Values

Nine-year-old Benton is a patient on the pediatric unit with a diagnosis of terminal stage Ewing's sarcoma. He has three sisters, aged seven, six, and three, who are presently being cared for by a grandmother. His father is self-employed and works long hours. His mother has never worked outside the home. Both parents have high school educations, and their primary activities outside of family are church-related. They belong to a small nondenominational rural church and state that they hold fast to what is taught in the Bible and put their faith in the word of God.

Prior to his illness, Benton, a healthy child, had been brought to the clinic only for acute health concerns. The family does not have health insurance. Shortly after entering second grade two years ago, he began limping. The family attributed the limp to a playground injury. When he continued to complain of pain and the limp persisted after three months, his mother took him to a local health clinic. Above-the-knee amputation followed diagnosis, but metastasis was evident in nine months. Chemotherapy has only been palliative.

The physician has discussed Benton's poor prognosis with the parents, recommending comfort care. The parents say they want everything possible to be done for him, and the father conducts nightly prayer sessions at Benton's bedside, affirming that God is healing Benton. Although Benton has asked whether he is going to die, his father refuses to allow staff to speak with him regarding fears or concerns about his condition. When asked what Benton has been told, the father responds, "He knows God is trying us and we must have faith." The mother, who appears less confident of a healing, is there twenty-four hours a day. She supervises Benton's care relentlessly, at times irritating staff with questions and demands. She keeps a notebook record of her son's care, including medication, times of care, intake and output, and personal assessments. Although Benton used to talk to staff, he now appears frightened and remains quiet, sleeping off and on.

Think About It

Dealing with Values Conflict

Respond to these questions from the vantage point of the nurse in the situation:

- What is your first personal reaction to this situation? Identify your values relative to the situation.
- What do you perceive to be the values of the others involved?
- Identify value incongruencies that might lead to conflict. Give specific examples of how such a conflict can potentially affect patient care.
- Describe specific nursing interventions aimed at managing the conflict in a professional manner, and give examples of how nursing codes would guide such actions.
- Describe your own strengths and limitations as you consider dealing with this situation.

Impact of Institutional Values

Nurses need to be conscious of both the spoken and unspoken values in their work settings. Values of individual institutions and organized health care systems that are explicitly communicated through philosophy and policy statements are called **overt values.** Values may also be implicit in expectations that are not in writing. Implicit or **covert values** are often identified only through participation in or controversies within the setting (Omery, 1989). When seeking employment, nurses should identify congruencies or incongruencies between personal values and those of the institution, because accepting employment implies committing to the value system of the organization. Consider, for example, a nurse, Anton, who accepts a position at a health center because the center publicizes a commitment to providing quality care to all patients. Within two months he notices that patients with Medicaid cards are kept waiting longer than those with private insurance, and are treated rudely by many of the staff. When he initiates teaching with the Medicaid patients, he is told not to waste his time because "those people won't change their ways." Overtly, the health center is committed to quality care for all patients; however, the covert values reflect different attitudes toward and levels of care for those on public assistance. Anton's values of providing quality care for all may prompt a variety of responses in this situation. He may compromise his values if he wants to get along with other staff and do well in the job, he may expend much energy challenging the covert value system, or he may decide that he cannot continue to work in this system.

Ask Yourself

How Should Values Influence Job Selection?

Maria, a recently divorced mother of three, desperately needs to return to work, but nursing jobs in her area are scarce. There is one opening at a women's health clinic that performs abortions. The job, which has excellent salary and benefits, including on-site child care, looks great to Maria, except that abortions are against her religious and personal beliefs. A friend who works at the clinic said that, unless they are short staffed, Maria would not have to assist with abortions if she had objections.

- What dilemmas are evident in this situation?
- What are the value incongruencies?
- What are your values related to this situation?
- What factors should Maria consider in deciding whether to take the job?

Schoof notes that what one believes and how one thinks about a job is important, and has a direct impact on job performance. Such internal belief systems tend to shape a person's thinking and direct them to do what they think is right, regardless of the employer's philosophy. Schoof suggests that it is better to identify what is valued by the employer, that is, where they stand and what they pay attention to and reward, and then to decide if one can work in that environment. As an example, he indicates that there are three primary ways to approach patient care: focus on meeting patient needs (intrinsic care), focus on doing all the tasks (extrinsic care), and focus on following the rules (systemic care) (personal communication, February 12, 1996). If there is a conflict between our values regarding patient care and the values of the institution, physician, and family we may experience moral distress. **Moral distress** is the reaction to a situation in which there are moral problems that seem to have clear solutions, yet we are unable to follow our moral beliefs because of external restraints. This distress is often evidenced in anger, dissatisfaction, frustration, and poor performance in the work setting.

Gingerich and Ondeck (1993) describe one process for defining and making organizational values more explicit. This process includes determining what is valued by staff, board members, management, and physicians regarding the elements of the organization's philosophy and identifying specific expectations for each group. Exercises focused on self-awareness, clinical priorities, and opinions about value-laden issues are conducted within each of the groups to develop awareness of and consensus around the values. This allows all involved to have an investment in the value system.

The Hartman Value Profile is another approach to looking at values within an organization (Hartman, 1967; Edwards & Davis, 1991; H. Schoof, personal communication, 1996). The process involves having the institution select a number of employees representing two groups within the organization: those considered to be the *shining stars*, and those considered least satisfactory. Those identified complete the profile, which is a forced ranking, from best to worst or most despicable, of eighteen items relating to how persons perceive the world around them and eighteen items related to how they perceive their inner selves. Patterns are identified by analyzing the participants' responses utilizing a computerized mathematical system that identifies how each item compares with the others that are ranked. The resulting information provides a profile of the underlying values within the organization. Decision makers can use this information to examine how prevailing belief systems are influencing performance, and to seek potential employees whose values are most consistent with those of the organization.

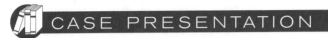

CASE PRESENTATION

Differences in Personal and Organizational Values

Joan has been the nurse manager of her unit for the past ten years and is highly regarded by the hospital's administration. For the past several months, however, she has been feeling more frustrated and less satisfied with her work because of staffing cuts and other institutional decisions related to managed care. Attending to patient needs has always been the most rewarding part of her job. However, recently she feels that she has been forced to overlook these needs and attend more to the needs of the organization. She considers leaving, but she has seniority, good benefits, and two children to support. She is also aware that her distress at work is affecting her family, because she carries a lot of the frustration home with her.

Think About It

How Values Affect Choices

- Identify values evident in this situation. Which of these reflect your personal values?
- What conflicts might arise from these values?
- What do you think Joan should do?
- If you were in Joan's position, what beliefs, ideals, or goals would guide you in making a decision to stay or leave? Identify potential consequences of each choice.

Clarifying Values with Patients

Values of both nurses and patients influence patient care situations. Since patients are the recipients and consumers of health care, it is good to know what they expect or value. Patient and provider perceptions of what constitutes quality of care can be quite different. Great discrepancies in these perceptions may lead to patient dissatisfaction.

This can have a variety of consequences, including affecting a patient's attitude and decisions regarding following recommendations for care and treatment (which may affect recovery), marring the reputation of the agency, or potentiating malpractice litigation. Allanach and Golden (1988) describe the process of a service audit aimed at identifying patient expectations and clarifying their opinions about the level of service. Nursing care behaviors identified as valued by patients in this study relate to the amount of care and time spent with patients and to the technical quality of nursing care. Consider the potential conflict of values when patients expect nurses to spend time with them and the institution puts more emphasis on getting the tasks done.

Ask Yourself

What Would You Do?

- You are busy and two call lights go on at the same time. What factors enter into deciding which one you respond to first?

- Consider that in the above situation one patient is in serious condition and has been verbally abusive to staff, while the other is not quite as serious and is someone you really enjoy being with. Who would you respond to first and why?

- Your patients let you know how much they appreciate the extra care and time you give them compared to the other nurses. At the same time, your evaluation is coming up and your supervisor has indicated that you need to be more efficient with your time. What would you do in this situation and why?

When working with patients regarding health care decisions, nurses need to be aware of personal values and patients' values pertaining to health. When the health values of the nurse and those of the patient are different, the patient may become labeled as uncooperative, self-destructive, noncompliant, ignorant, or unwilling to take responsibility for her or his own health. Attentiveness to cultural and religious values is especially important in this regard. Refer to Chapter 18 for discussion of transcultural and spiritual issues.

Pender (1987; 1996) discusses the role of values in health promotion. She notes that knowing personal values is important, as is the need to avoid imposing our values on patients. Consider, for example, an obese patient with terminal lung cancer and a prognosis of three to six months to live, who continues to smoke and is a confirmed agnostic. If priorities on the care plan include weight loss, smoking cessation, and facilitating the patient's making peace with God, we must consider whether nursing values are being imposed on the patient.

With self-awareness the nurse can be more effective in helping patients to identify their own values. Assisting patients to clearly articulate their values is important because a lack of clarity about values may result in inconsistency, confusion, misunderstanding, and inadequate decision making. The ability to make informed choices, including the process of informed consent, is enhanced by having clarity about our values. "Assisting clients to clarify values; understand the personal and social consequences of acting on current values; achieve greater consistency among values, attitudes, and behaviors; and plan health-related experiences that may result in self-initiated changes in value hierarchies" are key nursing actions (Pender, 1987, p. 161).

Many instruments and processes are available to facilitate exploring values in general and health values in particular. One example is a process that asks people to rank a list of ten health values from most important to least important. The list includes a comfortable life, an exciting life, a sense of accomplishment, freedom, happiness, health, inner harmony, pleasure, self-respect, and social recognition (Pender, 1987, p. 165). Pender notes that if health appears within the top four on the list, the person places a high value on health. However, definitions of health will vary, since each person defines health according to personal beliefs and values.

Another approach to analyzing health values described by Doyle (1994) asks people to identify from a list of ten health-related behaviors, what they do and why they do it. Behaviors include activities such as exercising a minimum of three times per week, talking to a close friend or relative about worries, and practicing sex without using a condom. Doyle notes that the response to why a behavior is practiced provides insight into values surrounding the behavior, such as choosing not to exercise in order to have more time, or choosing to exercise because it helps in weight control.

SUMMARY

This chapter has discussed the importance of self-awareness regarding values and the valuing process. Values are learned and change in response to life situations as a person develops. The process of values clarification enables persons to begin to identify and choose their own values rather than merely act out of prior programming. The interaction between personal values and those of patients and organizations can affect job satisfaction and patient care. The reader is encouraged to explore various processes that facilitate values clarification, both those presented in this chapter and those found in other resources.

CHAPTER HIGHLIGHTS

- Values are highly prized ideals, behaviors, beliefs, or qualities that are shaped by culture, ethnicity, family, environment, and education and are acquired in both conscious and unconscious ways.

- The process of incorporating values begins at an early age and continues throughout life. Some values remain consistent while others change in response to growth and life experiences.

- Awareness of personal values undergirds the ability to make clear and thoughtful decisions and enables us to acknowledge similarities and differences in values when interacting with others, thus promoting more effective communication, care, and facilitation of values clarification with others.

- Values clarification is not intended to instill values; rather, the aim is to facilitate awareness of personal values and the valuing process in order to move toward the point of choosing our own values rather than merely reacting from prior pro-graming.

- The valuing process includes prizing and cherishing, choosing, and acting on beliefs and behaviors.
- Dealing effectively with values conflict requires attention to personal values, the perceived values of others, and the ability to recognize both overt and covert expression of values in a situation.
- Congruence between personal values and those of an institution is an important consideration for a nurse seeking employment.
- Assisting patients to articulate their values and beliefs, an important part of nursing care, may help prevent deleterious consequences related to not addressing differences in values between patients and providers.

DISCUSSION QUESTIONS AND ACTIVITIES

1. A non-nursing classmate asks you what studying values has to do with nursing. How would you respond? Incorporate your understanding of the nature of values and how they become part of us into your response.
2. What values guide your personal life? How did you learn these values? Select something that you consider important in professional nursing practice and trace how you learned this value.
3. Discuss why values clarification is important both personally and professionally.
4. Identify the overt values of your health care agency and identify overt and covert values of nurses and others within the agency. Explain the importance of knowing about both.
5. Describe a situation in which you experienced someone (it could be you) reacting from values that were not conscious at the time. How did this affect the interaction?
6. Determine the health values of three patients or people you do not know well and discuss why nurses need to be attentive to what patients value.
7. Describe a situation in which you experienced values conflict and how you dealt with the conflict.
8. Find current examples of public or professional figures whose personal values seem at odds with their professional or public trust. Discuss your reaction to the discrepancy in values that you identify and the interplay between personal values and professional integrity.

REFERENCES

Adams, K. (1990). *Journal to the self: Two paths to personal growth.* New York: Warner Books.

Allanach, E. J., & Golden, B. M. (1988). Patients' expectations and values clarification: A service audit. *Nursing Administration Quarterly, 12,* 17–22.

Baldwin, C. (1991). *Life's companion: Journal writing as a spiritual quest.* New York: Bantam Books.

Banonis, B. C. (1997). *Principled behavior applied to everyday life*. Charleston, WV: Unpublished manuscript.

Burkhardt, M. A., & Nagai-Jacobson, M. G. (2002). *Spirituality and healing*. Albany, NY: Delmar Publishers.

Chinn, P. L. (1995). *Peace and power: Building communities for the future* (4th ed.). New York: National League of Nursing Press.

Covey, S. R. (1990). *The seven habits of highly effective people*. New York: Simon & Schuster.

Davis, A. J., Aroskar, M. A., Liaschenko, J., & Drought, T. S. (1997). *Ethical dilemmas and nursing practice* (4th ed). Norwalk, CT: Appleton & Lange.

Doyle, E. I. (1994). Recognizing the value-health behavior connection: "What I do and why I do it." *Journal of Health Education, 25*, 116–118.

Edwards, R. B., & Davis, J. W. (1991). *Forms of value and valuation*. Lanham, MD: University Press of America.

Engebretson, J. C. & Headley, J. A. (2000). Cultural diversity and care. In B. M. Dossey, L. Keegan, & C. E. Guzzetta, eds., *Holistic Nursing: A Handbook for Practice* (3rd ed., pp. 283–310). Gaithersburg, MD: Aspen Publishers.

Gaydos, H. L. B. (2000). The art of holistic nursing and the human health experience. In B. M. Dossey, L. Keegan, & C. E. Guzzetta, eds., *Holistic nursing: A handbook for practice* (3rd ed., pp. 51–66). Gaithersburg, MD: Aspen Publishers.

Gingerich, B. S., & Ondeck, D. A. (1993). Values incorporation throughout the organization. *Caring Magazine, 12*, 18–23.

Hartman, R. S. (1967). *The structure of value*. Carbondale, IL: Southern Illinois University Press.

Kahn, S. (1996). *The nurse's meditative journal*. Albany, NY: Delmar Publishers.

Keegan, L. (2000). Holistic ethics. In B. M. Dossey, L. Keegan, & C. E. Guzzetta, eds., *Holistic nursing: A handbook for practice* (3rd ed., pp. 159–170). Gaithersburg, MD: Aspen Publishers.

Kolkmeier, L. G. (1995). Self-reflection: Consulting the truth within. In B. M. Dossey, L. Keegan, C. E. Guzzetta, & L. G. Kolkmeier, eds., *Holistic nursing: A handbook for practice* (2nd ed.). Gaithersburg, MD: Aspen.

Omery, A. (1989). Values, moral reasoning, and ethics. *Nursing Clinics of North America, 24*, 499–507.

Pender, N. J. (1987). *Health promotion in nursing practice* (2nd ed.). Norwalk, CT: Appleton & Lange.

Pender, N. J. (1996). *Health promotion in nursing practice* (3rd ed.). Norwalk, CT: Appleton & Lange.

Progoff, I. (1992). *At a journal workshop*. New York: Tarcher.

Rew, L. (1996). *Awareness in healing*. Albany, NY: Delmar Publishers.

Rew, L. (2000). Self-reflection: Consulting the truth within. In B. M. Dossey, L. Keegean, & C. E. Guzzetta, eds., *Holistic nursing: A handbook for practice* (3rd ed., pp. 407–424). Gaithersburg, MD: Aspen Publishers.

Seroka, A. M. (1994). Values clarification and ethical decision making. *Seminars for Nurse Managers, 2*, 8–15.

Simon, S. B., Howe, L. W., & Kirschenbaum, H. (1995). *Values clarification: A handbook of practical strategies for teachers and students*. New York: Hart.

CHAPTER 5

Values Development

What is firmly established cannot be uprooted.
What is firmly grasped cannot slip away.
It will be honored from generation to generation.
(Lao Tsu, *Tao Te Ching*)

OBJECTIVES

After completing this chapter, the reader should be able to:

1. Discuss influences of culture on values development.

2. Contrast theoretical approaches to moral development.

3. Describe and differentiate the ethic of care and the ethic of justice.

4. Evaluate personal phase of moral development.

5. Discuss gender bias and cultural bias regarding theories of moral development.

INTRODUCTION

Nurses frequently encounter situations that present ethical dilemmas. In some situations the "right" choice seems quite evident, while in other circumstances a considerable lack of clarity about what is "right" may exist. How do we come to know what is right or how to respond in a principled way in a given situation? This chapter reviews factors that influence values formation, theoretical perspectives related to stages of values development, and considerations for nursing regarding moral development.

TRANSCULTURAL CONSIDERATIONS IN VALUES DEVELOPMENT

Human values development, often referred to as **moral development,** is a product of the sociocultural environment in which we live and develop. We learn what is considered right and wrong within the culture in formal ways such as by precept and admonition, through informal processes such as role modeling, and by technical learning in a teacher to student process (Hall, 1973). Norms for etiquette and ethical behavior that are "known" within the culture may be acquired by an outsider through technical learning; however, they are often appreciated by a neophyte only when a transgression has occurred and corrections to, or sanctions for, the behavior have been imposed. There is an innate human capacity for developing an ethical stance to life that emerges through this process.

Leininger (1978; 1984) and Tripp-Reimer (1987) speak of culture in terms of values, beliefs, customs, and behaviors that are learned within and shared by a group of interacting persons. Because values are *learned* within the context of a particular culture, moral values are culturally relative (Gostin, 1995). This suggests that a value such as individual autonomy may be regarded highly in a culture that prizes independence and individualism. However, the same value may be considered contrary to the norm in a society in which persons are defined by their relation to others. Fowler (1981) notes that "we are formed in social communities and that our ways of seeing the world are profoundly shaped by the shared images and constructions of our group or class" (p. 105). Understandings of principles such as justice and care may vary in different cultures. In the ensuing discussion regarding stages of values development, it is important to be aware that the norms described have been derived primarily from Anglo-American and Anglo-European populations. Although significant work has been done, there is a need for further validation of the models within a transcultural context.

Ask Yourself

How Did I Learn My Values?

Think about a professional or personal situation in which you were faced with an ethical dilemma.

- What made it a dilemma for you?

- How did you decide the best course of action?
- What factors did you consider in making your decision?
- What values or principles guided you in this process?
- When and how did you learn these values or principles?

THEORETICAL PERSPECTIVES OF VALUES DEVELOPMENT

Discussions of moral development found in current literature flow primarily from frameworks developed by Kohlberg (1981) and Gilligan (1982). An overview of the work of each of these scholars is presented in this section, followed by discussion of how they contribute to understanding moral reasoning within nursing. Fowler's (1981) work on faith development is briefly discussed regarding insights relative to values development. Kohlberg's theory, which suggests that cognitive development is necessary though not sufficient for moral development, draws upon Piaget's (1963) work on cognitive development in children. Thus, a brief review of Piaget's theory is included here. As you review the models highlighted here, remember that **theory** is a proposed explanation for a class of phenomena. A given theory is not necessarily truth or reality, but it does shed light on truth. Engage critical thinking and intuitive knowing as you read, being attentive to what rings true in your own experience.

Piaget's Stages of Cognitive Development

Piaget's (1963) description of stages of cognitive development addresses how the mind works, that is, the development of intellectual capacities through the time of childhood, from birth to about fifteen years of age. He notes that cognitive development progresses through four stages, provided there is an intact neurological system and appropriate environmental interaction and stimuli. Although Piaget suggests specific ages for each stage, there may be variation due to environmental factors or innate intellectual capacities. Piaget's stages are:

- Sensorimotor (birth to 24 months), includes six substages;
- Preoperational (age 2–7), includes preconceptual and intuitive stages;
- Concrete operations (age 7–11);
- Formal operations (age 11–15).

Piaget believes that there are no further quantifiable changes in cognitive abilities after age fifteen. According to his theory, cognitive development progresses from thought dominated by motor activity and reflex, through development and use of symbolic representations such as language, to logical thought applied to concrete and then to abstract situations.

Kohlberg's Theory of Moral Development

Kohlberg's (1981) theory of moral development was derived initially from interviews conducted with boys distributed in age from early childhood to late adolescence. In these interviews he asked participants to respond to hypothetical ethical dilemmas, such as a man considering stealing a drug to save his dying wife because he cannot afford the drug and has exhausted other possibilities of paying for it. The pattern of the responses that he observed, coupled with inferences about the reasoning behind the responses, suggested a progression in moral reasoning spanning three levels, each of which includes two stages. These levels and stages are summarized as follows:

Level I. The Preconventional Level has an egocentric focus and includes two stages. In Stage 1, *The Stage of Punishment and Obedience*, rules are obeyed in order to avoid punishment. In Stage 2, *The Stage of Individual Instrumental Purpose and Exchange*, conformity to rules is viewed to be in our own interest because it provides for rewards. Fear of punishment is a major motivator at this level.

Level II. The Conventional Level is focused more on social conformity and includes two stages. In Stage 3, *The Stage of Mutual Interpersonal Expectations, Relationships, and Conformity*, concern about the reactions of others is a basis for decisions and behavior, and being good in order to maintain relations, is important. In Stage 4, *The Stage of Social System and Conscience Maintenance*, we conform to laws and to those in authority because of duty, both out of respect for them and in order to avoid censure. For persons in this level, fulfilling our role in society and living up to expectations of others are important, and guilt is more of a motivator than the fear of punishment noted in Level I.

There is a transitional phase between Stages 4 and 5 in which emotions begin to be recognized as a component of moral reasoning. This transition includes an awareness of personal subjectivity in moral decision making and a recognition that social rules can be arbitrary and relative.

Level III. The Post-Conventional and Principled Level has universal moral principles as its focus. It includes two stages. In Stage 5, *The Stage of Prior Rights and Social Contract or Utility*, the relativity of some societal values is recognized, and moral decisions derive from principles that support individual rights and transcend particular societal rules such as equality, liberty, and justice. In Stage 6, *The Stage of Universal Ethical Principles*, internalized rules and conscience reflecting abstract principles of human dignity, mutual respect, and trust guide decisions and behaviors. Persons at this level make judgments based on impartial universal moral principles, even when these conflict with societal standards.

This model proposes a linear movement through hierarchical stages, whereby each stage presupposes having completed the prior stage and is the basis for the subsequent stage. It is the pattern of a person's utilization of a particular level of reasoning that determines the stage, noting that each successive stage requires more advanced levels of moral reasoning. Research utilizing this framework indicates that not everyone moves through all the stages, and that few people actually progress to the postconventional level (Colby & Kohlberg, 1987). Within this framework, women seem to plateau in Stage 3, and most men never move beyond Stage 4. Kohlberg's model is generally considered an **ethic of justice,** because it is an approach to ethical decision making based on objective rules and principles in which choices are made from a stance of separateness.

Gilligan's Study of the Psychological Development of Women

Gilligan (1982; 1987; 1988), a former student of Kohlberg, studied the psychological development of women, arguing that women approach moral decision making from a different perspective than men. In contrast to the justice ethic described by Kohlberg, in which personal liberty and rights are prime, Gilligan noted that women utilize an **ethic of caring,** in which the moral imperative is grounded in relationship with and responsibility for one another. "Women's construction of the moral problem as a problem of care and responsibility in relationship rather than of rights and rules ties the development of their moral thinking to changes in their understanding of responsibility and relationship, just as the conception of morality as justice ties development to the logic of equality and reciprocity" (Gilligan, 1982, p. 73). Gilligan's research did not say that most women think in the care perspective, while most men think in the justice perspective. Rather, as Little (2000) points out, she identified the default perspective that women use, the perspective they feel most comfortable with and that they would turn to first. She noted that many women think in the justice perspective, about one-third of the population are mixed between them, and, when pressed, all people can shift to the other perspective. However, the only ones who start off from the care perspective are women, so if you leave women out of the study, you leave out the care perspective.

Gilligan's research suggests a progression of moral thinking through three phases, each of which reflects greater depth in understanding the relationship of self and others, and two transitions that involve critical reevaluation of the conflict between responsibility and selfishness. The sequence described proceeds from an initial concern with survival, to focusing on goodness, to reflectively understanding care as the most adequate guide for resolving moral dilemmas.

Phase 1. In this phase, *the concern for survival,* the focus is on what is best for the self, and includes selfishness and dependence on others. The *transition* to Phase 2 involves an appreciation of connectedness, and that responsible choices take into account the effect they have on others.

Phase 2. The phase of *focusing on goodness* includes a sense of goodness as self-sacrifice, in which the needs of others are often put ahead of self, and there is a sense of being responsible for others, so that one is regarded positively. This focus on goodness reflects an awareness of relationship with others and may be used to manipulate others through a "see how good I've been to you" attitude. In the *transition* to Phase 3 there is a shifting from concern about the reactions of others to greater honesty about personal motivation and consequences of choices and actions. Responsibility to self is taken into account, along with responding to needs of others.

Phase 3. The phase of *the imperative of care* reflects a deep appreciation of connectedness, including responsibility to self and others as moral equals, and a clear imperative to harm no one. We take responsibility for choices, in which projected consequences and personal intention are the motivation for actions, rather than concern for the reactions of others.

Although Gilligan does not clearly associate particular ages with each phase of development, she suggests a linear process moving from one phase to the next through the transitions. This process may be associated with cognitive and emotional development as they interface with experiences of connectedness. Gilligan's model is generally considered an ethic of care.

Fowler's Stages of Faith Development

Fowler's (1981) discussion of faith development incorporates reflections on the development of values. His insights offer another perspective on the process of moral development. Fowler refers to **faith** as "a generic feature of the human struggle to find and maintain meaning . . . a dynamic existential stance, a way of leaning into and finding or giving meaning to the conditions of our lives" (pp. 91–92). He notes that faith is not synonymous with religion and that it may or may not find religious expression. He suggests that faith development flows from an integration of ways of knowing and valuing. This perspective is different from the work of Piaget and Kohlberg who conceptually separate cognition or knowing from emotion or affection, suggesting that logical knowing is separate from other important modalities of knowing. Fowler writes that "in moral judgments the valuations of actions and their consequences as well as evaluations of self in relation to the expectations of the self and others are difficult to conceive, even in formal and structural terms, apart from inherent affective or emotive elements of knowing" (1981, p. 102).

Fowler (1981) proposes six stages of faith, beginning with an intuitive faith in early childhood and progressing to universalizing faith. He notes that movement through the stages may not be limited to a linear pattern, recognizing that spiraling back to earlier stages may occur in response to various life experiences.

Stage 1. Occurring after the undifferentiated faith of infancy, *Intuitive Projective* faith is image and fantasy filled. The child's understandings and feelings toward the ultimate conditions of life are intuitive and shaped by stories, actions, moods, and examples of those around them.

Stage 2. *Mythic-Literal* faith reflects beliefs and moral rules and attitudes that symbolize belonging within a community or family and that are taken on with literal interpretations. Story provides a major source of meaning, and a world view based on reciprocity and fairness is developed.

Stage 3. *Synthetic-Conventional* faith reflects a movement into a world beyond the family in which values and beliefs derive from experiences in interpersonal relationships. Expectations and judgments of significant others are very influential in determining the values one holds. Although a personal clustering of values and beliefs is emerging in this stage, reliance on those in traditional authority roles or on the consensus of a valued group for validation of beliefs and actions is common. Fowler notes that although this stage arises in adolescence, many adults remain in this stage.

Stage 4.   In the stage of *Individuative-Reflective* faith, persons must begin to take responsibility for their own beliefs, values, and commitments, differentiating personal identity and world view from that of others. In this way one's own values become recognized as factors in judgments on and reactions to actions and decisions of self and others.

Stage 5.   *Conjunctive* faith requires an opening to our inner depths in which we are able to recognize values, beliefs, and myths developed within our particular cultural, social, or religious tradition that separate one from others. This stage requires an attitude of openness to that which formerly might have been perceived as threatening, different, and *other*, appreciating that although our own values provide a framework for ascribing meaning, they are only relative and partial apprehensions of transcendent reality.

Stage 6.   With *Universalizing* faith, the imperatives of absolute love and justice become prime, and we focus energy on transforming the present reality toward a transcendent actuality inclusive of all beings. Fowler notes that persons in Stage 6 are quite rare, frequently being honored more after death than in life.

Ask Yourself

Where Are You in Your Values Development?

- Where do you think you fit in each of the frameworks discussed?
- Where would you place your parents? Classmates? Friends? Government officials? People like Gandhi, Mother Teresa of Calcutta, or Martin Luther King, Jr.?
- Based on your critical thinking and intuitive knowing, which framework rings most true for you?
- What are the implications of a model that suggests that most members of a particular group are morally deficient?

Kohlberg and Gilligan suggest that values development moves from a focus on self and survival, through responding to external forces such as perceived authority or opinions of others, toward being motivated and guided by universal considerations. They also note that it is more common to find adults functioning in the middle phases of relying on external authority as guideposts for moral decisions than to find adults who base their actions and decisions on internalized universal guides that transcend codified rules. Fowler's model acknowledges that both reason and emotional response are factors in moral decision making, and includes the suggestion that development may follow a pattern more spiral than linear. Within this pattern it is conceivable that, in response to life-changing experiences, persons may spiral back to an earlier stage and move through the stages again from a renewed perspective.

CASE PRESENTATION

Three Nursing Students

Pat, Tanya, and Kuan are discussing experiences they had in clinical today. Tanya describes her distress because her dying patient wanted to see her six-year-old granddaughter, which she thought would be very therapeutic, but her preceptor said absolutely not because there were strict rules against children under twelve visiting that unit. Pat notes that she did not have time to even change her patient's bed, but that the sheets were clean so she just straightened them out and the instructor did not even notice. She said the nurses on that unit do that sometimes when they are busy, so it was okay. Kuan says she had gotten behind too, but decided she had better get everything done the right way so she would get a good grade and not get into trouble.

Think About It

Indicators of Values Development

- What insights into the values of each of these students can you glean from this discussion?
- How do you think the theorists noted above would describe the level of development of each of the students?
- How do you think you would have responded in the situations described by the students? What values would guide your response?

SOME NURSING CONSIDERATIONS

Gilligan (1982; 1987) and others (Gilligan, Ward, Taylor, & Bardige, 1988; Kittay & Meyers, 1987; Larrabee, 1993; Noddings, 1984; Little, 2000) have suggested that there are gender differences in approaching moral decision making: women tend to utilize a care or relational perspective, whereas men more frequently use the justice perspective. These authors note that Kohlberg's perspective on moral development tends to portray women's choices as deficiencies in moral capacities. Many authors claim that research related to differences in ethical decision making based on gender is inconclusive and that the justice perspective is used by both women and men (Colby & Kohlberg, 1987; Duckett, Rowan-Boyer, Ryden, Crisham, Savik, & Rest, 1992; Walker, 1993). When considering developmental norms for moral development, nurses must be alert for gender and cultural factors, norms, and bias in order to avoid erroneously classifying particular groups as lacking in moral capabilities.

The literature offers an ongoing deliberation about the ethic of care versus the ethic of justice. A comparison of the two perspectives reveals that the justice framework requires choices to be made from a stance of separateness, based on objective rules and principles. The care perspective arises from natural relatedness with particular others in which the choice is contextually bound and requires responding to others in their terms, developing strategies that maintain connections when possible, and striving to hurt no one. Moral concern within the ethic of justice is with rights and responsibilities; in the ethic of care the concern is with competing needs and responsibility in relationship. Fowler's model suggests that both are important factors in making moral decisions. Although much of the discussion in the literature focuses on the dichotomy between the two, we recognize that, rather than negating each other, the perspectives of justice and care offer different foci from which to examine problems. Offering balance to each other, these perspectives broaden the view from which to see the situation as a whole, and collectively constitute a more comprehensive moral perspective (Cooper, 1989; Little, 2000). Hekman (1995) suggests that a paradigm shift is occurring that requires a reconceptualization of morality and moral language away from the notion of universal morality toward a recognition of a plurality of moral voices.

Because of nursing's concern for relational caring, an ethic of care may more faithfully reflects nursing's experience than a primary focus on justice (Cooper, 1989). Little (2000) notes that one of the lessons the ethic of care offers to health care professionals is the directive to meet the needs of *particular* others, recognizing that these needs are not always clear. This means caring about persons as individuals, and developing processes to help them figure out what they need. Part of this process, she suggests, is developing a caring heart, recognizing that emotions are a constitutive part of the moral life. Considering the politics of caring she speaks to the need of restructuring our health care systems to value caring through supporting and justly compensating those who do the sometimes emotional and taxing caring work.

It has also been suggested that nursing move beyond current models of biomedical ethics to a model that encompasses at least the concepts of care and justice (Cooper, 1990). One study exploring whether nurses deal with moral decisions using the justice or the care perspective found that both perspectives were utilized, with care being predominant overall (Chally, 1992). In this study, older nurses with more professional experience were more likely to utilize the care perspective than younger nurses with less experience. The author proposed a possible developmental process through which growth in experience leads from a reliance on rules to guide one's choices to a focus on the needs of patients and families, which is reflective of the care perspective. In their research exploring holistic ethics, Victoria Slater and colleagues (personal communication November 13, 2000) discovered that holistic nurses blend the justice and care ethics. She notes that the pure justice ethic is about autonomy, whereas the pure care ethic is about relationships and nonviolence. The way holistic nurses blended them is seen in their sense that violating a person's autonomy (justice) means doing violence (care) to that person. They came to their ethical decision based on experience and intuition. They fit their ethical decision to the situation with a focus of maintaining the patient's autonomy, which, for these nurses, was a form of nonviolence.

We need to understand that there are different perspectives from which moral decisions are made, so that we can better appreciate our own and our patients' approaches to ethical dilemmas. We need to identify honestly our own phases of values development and ethical perspective in order to better understand personal responses to situations and to recognize more effectively how our approaches may differ from those of colleagues or patients. Acknowledging differences and similarities may prevent making inappropriate judgments about another's moral capabilities, and make possible better communication and collaboration in care.

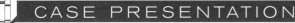

CASE PRESENTATION

A Difficult Decision

Reba's eighty-two-year-old father has been hospitalized with a stroke that has left him severely incapacitated, requiring total care. She has been informed that her father is ready for discharge, and the physician is suggesting that he go to a nursing home. Reba feels that she should take him home with her because her faith says to care for her parents, but the house is small and would need a bathroom added to the first floor. She also has concerns about performing her father's care because she works full time and has three small children. She has considered quitting her job, but the family needs her income because her husband's work is seasonal. When visiting her father, she tells the nurse, Moira, that she does not know what is best for him, noting that her sister in another state told her it is her duty to care for their father, but her husband says it is too much to take on with all her other family responsibilities. She asks Moira what she should do.

Think About It

Justice or Care—Is One Way Better?

- What factors and forces do you think weigh most heavily in this situation?
- How would you respond if you were Moira?
- How would you approach this situation from the perspective of justice? From the perspective of care? Do you think one approach is better than the other? Explain.
- How would you describe Reba's phase of moral development? Her husband's? Her sister's?

SUMMARY

This chapter has presented an overview of theoretical perspectives related to values development, the importance of recognizing that values and beliefs are culturally relative, and nursing considerations related to moral development. Students are encouraged to explore and critique each model of values development in order to formulate a personal knowledge base to guide their own processes of development. Each perspective provides insight into what is true.

CHAPTER HIGHLIGHTS

- Human values development, which is a product of our sociocultural environment, reflects the content and process of learning what is right and wrong within the culture.
- Values development moves from a focus on self, through responding to external forces, toward being guided by universal considerations.
- Moral values are culturally relative.
- Current models of values development need further transcultural and transgender validation.
- Kohlberg's model, often referred to as an ethic of justice, suggests that choices are based on objective rules and principles and are made from a stance of separateness.
- In Gilligan's model, often referred to as an ethic of care, the moral imperative is grounded in relationship and mutual responsibility. Choices are contextually bound, requiring strategies that maintain connections and a striving to hurt no one.
- The notion of a plurality of moral voices, which recognizes that perspectives of both justice and care are factors in moral decision making, is an important consideration for nursing.
- Understanding varying perspectives from which moral decisions are made enables nurses to appreciate their own and their patients' approaches to ethical dilemmas and to avoid making inappropriate judgments about another's moral capabilities.

DISCUSSION QUESTIONS AND ACTIVITIES

1. What does it mean to say that moral values are culturally relative?
2. What factors would you consider in determining a person's phase of moral development?
3. Explore the model that you think best reflects the process of values development. Discuss it with classmates, giving rationale for your choice.
4. Identify stages of values development of three patients of different ages.
5. Compare and contrast the ethic of care and the ethic of justice, and discuss this topic with classmates. Which perspective do you think is most appropriate for nursing? Why?
6. Why is it useful for nurses to be aware of phases of values development for themselves, patients, and colleagues?

REFERENCES

Chally, P. S. (1992). Moral decision making in neonatal intensive care. *Journal of Obstetrics, Gynecology, and Neonatal Nursing, 21*(6), 475–482.

Colby, A., & Kohlberg, L. (1987). *The measurement of moral judgment volume I: Theoretical foundations and research validation.* Cambridge, MA: Cambridge University Press.

Cooper, M. C. (1989). Gilligan's different voice: A perspective for nursing. *Journal of Professional Nursing, 5*(1), 10–16.

Cooper, M. C. (1990). Reconceptualizing nursing ethics. *Scholarly Inquiry for Nursing Practice, 4*(3), 209–221.

Duckett, L., Rowan-Boyer, M., Ryden, M. B., Crisham, P., Savik, K., & Rest, J. R. (1992). Challenging misperceptions about nurses' moral reasoning. *Nursing Research, 41*(6), 324–331.

Fowler, J. W. (1981). *Stages of faith: The psychology of human development and the quest for meaning.* San Francisco: Harper & Row.

Gilligan, C. (1982). *In a different voice: Psychological theory and women's development.* Cambridge, MA: Harvard University Press.

Gilligan, C. (1987). Moral orientation and moral development. In E. F. Kittay & D. T. Meyers, eds., *Women and moral theory* (pp. 19–33). Savage, MD: Rowman & Littlefield.

Gilligan, C., Ward, J. V., Taylor, J. M., & Bardige, B. (1988). *Mapping the moral domain.* Cambridge, MA: Harvard University Press.

Gostin, L. O. (1995). Informed consent, cultural sensitivity, and respect for persons. *Journal of the American Medical Association, 274*(10), 844–855.

Hall, E. T. (1973). *The silent language.* Garden City, NY: Anchor Press.

Hekman, S. J. (1995). *Moral voices, moral selves.* University Park, PA: Pennsylvania State University Press.

Kittay, E. F., & Meyers, D. T. (1987). *Women and moral theory.* Savage, MD: Rowman & Littlefield.

Kohlberg, L. (1981). *The philosophy of moral development.* New York: Harper & Row.

Lao Tsu. (1972). *Tao Te Ching* (Gia-fu Feng & Jane English, trans.). New York: Vintage Books.

Larrabee, M. J., ed. (1993). *An ethic of care.* New York: Routledge.

Leininger, M. (1978). *Transcultural nursing: Concepts, theories and practice.* New York: John Wiley & Sons.

Leininger, M. (1984). *Transcultural care diversity and universality: A theory of nursing.* Thorofare, NJ: Slack.

Little, M. (2000). Introduction to the ethics of care. Presentation at *New century, new challenges: Intensive bioethics course XXVI*, Kennedy Institute of Ethics, Georgetown University, Washington, DC, June 10, 2000.

Noddings, N. (1984). *Caring: A feminine approach to ethics and moral education.* Berkeley, CA: University of California Press.

Piaget, J. (1963). *The origins of intelligence in children* (M. Cook, trans.). New York: Norton.

Tripp-Reimer, T. (1987). Cultural assessment. In J. P. Bellack, & P. A. Bamford, eds., *Nursing assessment: A multidimensional approach* (pp. 226–246). Boston: Jones & Bartlett.

Walker, L. J. (1993). Sex differences in the development of moral reasoning: A critical review. In M. J. Larrabee, ed., *An ethic of care* (pp. 157–176). New York: Routledge.

CHAPTER 6

Ethical Decision Making

Peace requires that you do what in your heart you know-that your chosen values guide your actions.

(Chinn, 1995)

OBJECTIVES

After completing this chapter, the reader should be able to:

1. Describe and differentiate ethical dilemmas, moral uncertainty, practical dilemmas, moral distress, and moral outrage.

2. Describe the process of making thoughtful decisions.

3. Discuss the nursing process as a decision making model.

4. Discuss similarities between scientific process and ethical decision making.

5. Describe the role of emotions in ethical decisions.

6. Examine the process of ethical decision making.

7. Apply the ethical decision making process to clinical case situations.

INTRODUCTION

Everyone makes decisions as part of everyday living. Some decisions seem routine, such as what to have for lunch or what to wear to work. Other decisions, like where to go to college, which job to accept, or whether to marry, call for more deliberation. Nurses constantly make decisions. We decide matters related to management of care, institutional policy, or when to collaborate or initiate referrals. Often we make decisions without conscious awareness of the process but have an innate sense of *knowing* what to do.

Ethical decision making may not seem as clear-cut as decisions made in other areas of life. How do we decide whether to remove life support measures for a parent or whether to cut funding for childhood immunizations in lieu of other, equally important programs? What factors are involved in an ethical dilemma that makes "the right choice" either evident or obscure? This chapter defines the concept of ethical dilemma, relates ethical decision making to nursing process, and presents a guide for ethical decision making.

MORAL/ETHICAL PROBLEMS

Jameton (1984) describes three different types of moral problems: *moral uncertainty*, which occurs when the nurse identifies a moral problem but is unsure of the morally correct action; *moral dilemma*, which occurs when two or more mutually exclusive moral claims clearly apply and both seem to have equal weight; and *moral distress*, which arises when the nurse knows the morally correct action and feels a responsibility to the patient, but institutional or other restraints make it nearly impossible to follow through with appropriate action (p. 6). Wilkinson (1987–88) added another category to Jameton's typology: *moral outrage*, which occurs when someone else in the health care setting performs an act the nurse believes to be immoral.

Moral Uncertainty

Moral uncertainty occurs when we sense that there is a moral problem, but are not sure of the morally correct action, when we are unsure what the moral principles or values apply, or when we are unable to define the moral problems (Jameton, 1984). This happens to us when we have a sense that something is not quite right. We are uncomfortable with a situation, but can't figure out the problem. Jameton (1984) offers the example of a nurse caring for an older patient who is somewhat neglected, with little attention being given to the patient's problem. The nurse feels dissatisfied with the patient's treatment, but is unable to pinpoint the nature and cause of the inadequacy.

Moral/Ethical Dilemmas

A dilemma exists when a difficult problem seems to have no satisfactory solution or when all solutions to a problem appear to be equally favorable (Davis, Aroskar, Liaschenko, & Drought, 1997). An **ethical dilemma** occurs when there are conflicting moral claims. Dilemmas present in at least two ways. According to Beauchamp and

Childress (1994), a conflict can be experienced when there is evidence to indicate that a certain act is morally right and evidence to indicate that the act is morally wrong, but no evidence is conclusive. An example of this can be seen in the example of a terminally ill patient. While most would think it is morally right to preserve life, many would believe it is morally wrong to prolong suffering. A dilemma may also occur when the agent believes that one or more moral norms exist to support one course of action, and one or more moral norms exist to support another course of action, and the two actions are mutually exclusive. Health care providers face this type of dilemma, for example, when they must decide who gets the critical care bed. Should they make the decision relative to who is most deserving, who arrives first, who can pay, or who has the best chance of survival? Different people perceive or conceptualize conflicts in different ways. Conflicting moral claims can be said to occur, for example, between obligations, principles, duties, rights, loyalties, and so forth.

Let us examine different perceptions of conflicting moral claims. The nurse might perceive a conflict between adherence to two different principles, such as wishing to avoid the suffering a patient experiences as a result of hearing a bad prognosis, while at the same time respecting the patient's right to know. In this instance, the nurse might perceive a direct conflict between the principles of nonmaleficence (the wish to do no harm) and autonomy (assuring that the patient is self-governing). In another instance, the nurse might perceive a conflict of duties. This type of conflict can occur, for example, when nurse managers must make decisions regarding staffing patterns. The nurse manager will recognize a duty to the institution, but will also feel a duty to meet the needs of individual patients and nurses. This will often result in a conflict, when the needs of the institution do not allow for meeting the needs of individuals.

There are instances in which the nurse might feel conflicting loyalties. For example, in caring for a promiscuous patient with AIDS, the nurse might experience a conflict between being loyal to the patient and being loyal to society. In this instance, the nurse could experience a conflict between doing that which seems morally right and avoiding that which carries legal consequences. This situation can also be conceptualized as a conflict between the nurse's duty to maintain confidentiality and the duty to warn those at risk. All of these examples portray ethical dilemmas that nurses commonly experience. These moral problems offer conflicting moral claims, however conceptualized, and solutions that appear to be equally unfavorable.

? Think About It

Facing Ethical Dilemmas

Put yourself in the position of the nurse in each of the examples noted in the discussion of ethical dilemmas above.

- How would the situation present a conflict for you?
- How do you think you would respond in each situation?
- Why would you respond in that manner?
- Think about a personal experience of a moral dilemma and describe why it was a dilemma for you.

Practical Dilemmas

One must be careful to differentiate between moral and **practical dilemmas.** Occasionally, situations present themselves in which moral claims compete with nonmoral claims. Nonmoral claims can often be identified as claims of self-interest (Beauchamp & Childress, 1994). Consider, for example, the nurse who must to work overtime, caring for a gravely ill patient. The nurse might perceive a dilemma because she made a promise to take her children to the circus. Though the nurse might say that her duty to the children conflicts with her duty to care for the patient, it can be argued that the duties are not of equal moral weight. The duty to keep the promise to her children is a practical duty that is grounded in self-interest rather than having a moral claim. In decisions that involve practical dilemmas, moral claims have greater weight than nonmoral claims. Differentiating moral and practical dilemmas is an important facet of decision making.

Moral Distress

Occasionally, nurses face situations that present moral problems which seem to have clear solutions, yet they are unable to follow their moral beliefs because of institutional or other restraints. Nurses in these predicaments are said to experience **moral distress** (Jameton, 1984). These situations can be differentiated from those that present moral dilemmas. When moral distress occurs, there are no conflicting moral claims. The *right* action is clear, yet institutional or other restraints make it nearly impossible to pursue this course of action. It is important to note that nurses who experience moral distress feel a personal responsibility to the patient. The distress occurs when the nurse violates a personal moral value and fails to fulfill perceived responsibility. For example, nurses in the hurried atmosphere of a particular hospital's same-day surgery report that they are expected to have sedated patients sign consent forms, recognizing that the physicians have often neglected to explain the scheduled procedures fully. The nurses know that this practice is one that does not respect patients' rights to informed consent, yet feel they have neither personal authority nor access to decision-making channels, and therefore believe themselves to be powerless to make the necessary changes. Jameton points out that in situations of this sort, it can be personally risky for staff to criticize a practice that helps the hospital make ends meet.

Situations in which nurses feel moral distress represent practical, rather than ethical, dilemmas. Nurses may face the choice of continuing to participate in a system that they feel is ethically flawed, resigning, or acting in a manner that they believe is correct but that could jeopardize employment. Moral distress will undermine integrity if it is easier for the nurse to comply with policies that are believed to be morally wrong than to pursue the ethically correct action.

Though moral problems of all types are difficult, situations involving moral distress may be the most difficult moral problems facing nurses (Nathaniel, 2000). Reports of the number of nurses who experience moral distress vary. Nearly fifty percent of nurses in one study report that they had acted against their consciences in providing care to the terminally ill (Rushton, 1995). Studies have shown that as many as 30 percent to 50 percent of nurses either leave their units or leave nursing altogether as a result of moral distress (Wilkinson, 1987–88; Millette, 1994; Redman & Fry, 2000).

Other studies show that moral distress causes nurses to have physical and psychological problems, sometimes for many years. Some relate "burnout" to their experience of moral distress, and suggest that many nurses leave the profession as a result. More important, there is anecdotal evidence that nurses' moral distress affects quality of patient care and subsequent health outcomes (Nathaniel, 2000).

The consequences of moral distress may be profound. There is evidence that, as a result of moral distress, some nurses loose their capacity for caring, avoid patient contact, and fail to give good physical care. Hamric (2000) calls moral distress, "a powerful impediment to nursing practice" (p. 201). Nurses may physically withdraw from the bedside, barely meeting the patient's basic physical needs, or may leave the profession altogether (Fenton, 1988; Hefferman & Helig, 1999; Kelly, 1998). Loss of nurses from the workforce is an indirect but strong threat to patient care. The nursing shortage is compounded by a health care system in which increasingly complex technology is used to care for patients who are very old, very young, or very sick. Those in society with the greatest need may be the ones who suffer more acutely when nursing care is affected (Nathaniel, 2000).

Unrelieved moral distress over a period of time can erode the nurse's values and affect confidence and self-esteem. Unfortunately, there is no assurance that following the morally correct course of action will mean employer or legal support. Nurses should view these situations as practical dilemmas. Ethical decision making assures that moral claims hold greater weight than nonmoral claims. Thus, in the example offered above, the moral claim of respecting the right to informed consent constitutes greater weight than the nonmoral claim of system efficiency. The decision making guide described in this chapter can be used to help nurses make practical decisions when facing moral distress.

Ask Yourself

Have You Experienced Moral Distress?

Moral distress occurs in situations that present moral problems which seem to have clear solutions, yet institutional or other restraints prohibit morally correct action. Consider a situation in which you experienced moral distress.

- What were the circumstances?
- How did you feel?
- How did you resolve the distress?

Moral Outrage

Moral distress and moral outrage share the common element of feelings of powerlessness (Jameton, 1993). **Moral outrage** occurs when someone else in the health care setting performs an act the nurse believes to be immoral (Wilkinson, 1987–88). In cases of moral outrage, nurses do not participate in the act, and therefore do not believe they are responsible for wrong, but perceive that they are powerless to prevent it. The nurse is more likely to be on the fringes of the moral situation rather than directly involved. For example, the charge nurse on a medical/surgical floor on the evening shift is working at the desk when the nursing supervisor comes to the floor to use the telephone to call a hospital administrator. The charge nurse overhears the supervisor describing a situation in which a patient was endangered when a physician insisted on performing a surgical procedure in the patient's room. The surgeon was in a hurry and felt the patient would be safe, even though there were violations of patient privacy, informed consent, and safety. The charge nurse has no involvement in the situation, but recognizes a grave moral problem. Whistleblowing may be a response to moral outrage.

MAKING DECISIONS

The process of making thoughtful decisions follows a similar pattern in most circumstances. This pattern includes gathering data, comparing options, using some criteria for weighing the merit of each option, and making a choice. Evaluation of outcomes or circumstances surrounding the choice provides more data regarding the *rightness* of the choice. A simple example of this process is how you choose what clothes to wear today. The data you gather includes such things as where you are going, what you will be doing, the weather, what is clean or handy, your mood, the colors you prefer, and the style of clothing you anticipate others will be wearing. You may narrow choices down to several options that would be acceptable or appropriate, and you compare these based on some criteria. The criteria may be what is least wrinkled, or feels most comfortable, or makes you look or feel more confident, or is more appropriate for weather conditions, or a combination of such considerations. Using the criteria, you narrow down options and make a choice. As you move through the day, you gather more data about the *rightness* of your decision. For example, are you comfortable? Do you feel dressed appropriately for the meeting? Are you warm enough? Does the color seem to make you stand out? Your evaluation of whether you made the right decision provides information about the strength or validity of the criteria you used to guide your decision, and whether to use these same criteria to guide similar decisions in the future.

Nursing Process and Ethical Decision Making

As nurses we commonly use the **nursing process** model for decision making. Utilizing both logical thinking and intuitive knowing, the nursing process is a deliberate activity that provides a systematic method for nursing practice. The nursing process directs nursing practice, standardizes nursing care, and unifies nurses (Christensen & Kenney, 1990). Familiar to most nurses and endorsed by the American Nurses Association, the process generally includes the following interactive and sequential steps: problem identification based on assessment of subjective and objective data; development of a plan for care, guided by desired outcomes; implementation of interventions; evaluation of the outcomes; and revision of the plan over time. Criteria used in making nursing care decisions derive from areas such as knowledge of normal anatomy, physiology, psychology, pathophysiology, therapeutic communication, family dynamics, pharmacology, microbiology, nursing and other theories, human energy fields, familiarity with standards of care and protocols, experience related to what has worked in similar situations, and intuitive knowing. The process is systematic and involves both logical thinking and intuitive knowing.

Scientific Process and Ethical Decision Making

The process of decision making in ethics follows a procedure that is similar to the scientific process. "A comparison between the giving of good reasons in science, which is called 'explanation,' and the giving of good reasons in ethics, which is called 'moral justification,' reveals striking procedural similarities bordering on identity" (Gibson, 1991, p. 3). Gibson notes similarities between the scientific process of explanation, which moves from *observation → hypothesis → law → theory*, and the moral justification process of ethics, which moves from *assessed ethical dilemma → rule → principle → theory*. A strong knowledge base regarding societal rules, ethical principles and theories, and professional codes and standards is as important to making ethical decisions as knowledge of principles related to physical, psychological, social, and human science is to other nursing judgments.

ETHICAL DECISION MAKING

We often approach ethical problems with a problem-solving frame of reference. Similar to both nursing process and scientific inquiry, the ethical problem solving process generally includes the following steps: (1) defining the problem, (2) identifying objectives to be achieved, (3) listing alternatives for meeting objectives, (4) evaluating each objective, and (5) choosing the best alternative.

Differences of culture or values among the various participants involved in ethical decision making often become an important issue. In this regard, defining the problem includes both determining the ethical issue at hand and identifying the value systems of those involved. Consider, for instance, parents who wish to terminate life support for a seriously injured child hospitalized with no hope of recovery. The parents believe that life support is causing harm by interfering with the natural process of death which they believe should be in God's hands, while the physician feels that removing life support constitutes murder. The problem includes both the issue of terminating life support and the conflicting values between physician and family. Although both parties might identify what is best for and least harmful to the child as the ultimate objective, the list of potential options would be different for the family and the physician. Determining which principles and theories guide the people involved enables the nurse to help clarify the issue and facilitate the process of coming to an ethical decision.

Emotions and Ethical Decisions

Many approaches to ethical decision making describe a primarily cognitive process in which emotions are subordinated to reason. In a holistic view of people, however, both thinking and feeling are credible ways of knowing, each having a legitimate role in ethical decision making. Callahan (1995) suggests that heart and mind should not be viewed as antagonistic in the moral arena; rather, both reason and emotion should be active and in accord as we come to an ethical decision. Noting that emotions should influence reason while reason is monitoring emotions, she describes emotions as personal signals providing information regarding both inner processes and interactions with the environment.

It is important to appreciate not only what you *think* about what is right or wrong in a situation, but also what you *feel* in relation to the circumstances and decision to be made. If you are feeling discomfort, even though reason is pointing in a particular direction, it is wise to further explore both the arguments posed through reason and your reactions to them. Callahan (1995) writes:

> In our technological culture perhaps the greatest moral danger arises not from sentimentality, but from devaluing feeling and not attending to or nurturing moral emotions. Numbness, apathy, isolated disassociations between thinking and feeling are also moral warning signals . . . the absence of emotional responses of empathy and sympathy become critical bioethical issues. (pp. 30–31)

The goal is to have head and heart in harmony as the decision is made.

In the same way that people may approach an issue with differing moral reasoning, their emotional responses might be quite different from your own. In such situations you might see validity in the other's response and broaden your own view. On the other hand, you may recognize that the chasm between the two is too deep to bridge. Callahan suggests that such social conflicts and challenges present new ethical problems that may require dealing with the consequences of an ethical decision by repeating the decision making process.

❓ Think About It

The Role of Emotions in Decision Making

Consider your emotional response to the following situations and how it would affect your dealing with and caring for the people involved.

- You work in a clinic primarily serving an indigent immigrant population, and you hear one of your coworkers comment that "it's a waste of time trying to do health education, because these people are all so stupid, and just a drain on the system."

- You just started working for a group of gynecologists, and discover that the physician you are assigned to work with asks all his young patients about their sexual fantasies.

- You are working in an emergency department at the local hospital, where a two-year-old child dies as a result of injuries sustained while being "disciplined" by the mother's boyfriend. The child had previously been placed in foster care due to neglect, and had been returned to the mother's care only a week prior to this event.

PROCESS OF ETHICAL DECISION MAKING

The nature of the ethical problem requires a decision-making process in which key facets are revisited from evolving perspectives, even as you move toward a decision or resolution. Many models for decision making describe step-by-step processes that are linear in nature, not reflecting the potential for an evolving perspective. The guidelines presented here provide a framework for entering a decision making process that requires an ongoing evaluation and assimilation of information. This decision making process is spiral in nature, with each step being revisited as often as is required and molded by the dynamics of changing facts, evolving beliefs, unexpected consequences, and participants who move in and out of the process. The following text describes the steps involved in the process of ethical decision making.

Gather Data and Identify Conflicting Moral Claims

When an ethical problem occurs, gather information or facts in order to clarify issues. Identification of the conflicting moral claims that constitute the ethical dilemma is the first part of the process. You should examine the situation for evidence of conflicting obligations, principles, duties, rights, loyalties, values, or beliefs. Additionally, data provide an understanding of the ethical components, principles of concern, and the various perceptions of issues and principles by those involved in the situation. You must pay attention to societal, religious, and cultural values and beliefs. Often, a situation you initially think constitutes an ethical dilemma will actually turn out to be a practical dilemma. This recognition allows the participants to appropriately weigh choices and expedite decision making.

Identify Key Participants

Identify the key persons involved in the decision-making process and delineate each person's role. Determining rights, duties, authority, context, and capabilities of decision makers is a critical component of the process (Curtin & Flaherty, 1982; Husted & Husted, 1995). The focal question is, "Whose decision is this to make?" Identification of the principal decision maker is sometimes all that is needed to facilitate the process. Recognition that one has the legitimate authority to make an important decision is an empowering event. Once the principal decision maker is identified, the roles of the other participants can be explicitly outlined. For example, nurses often feel the burden of difficult ethical decisions, even though the responsibility for the decision lies with the patient or the nearest relative. In these instances, the nurse serves as a resource for information, a source of emotional support for those making the difficult decision, and a facilitator of the decision making process.

Determine Moral Perspective and Phase of Moral Development of Key Participants

Knowledge of moral development and ethical theory may provide a helpful framework for understanding participants and their perspectives and responses in the process. Assess how those involved fit into paradigms of moral development. It is valuable to recognize, for instance, whether the principal decision maker is at a developmental level in which choices reflect a desire to please others, thus susceptible to choosing an alternative solely on the basis of seeking approval. (See Chapter 5 for an in-depth discussion of moral development.)

It is also crucial to identify the participants' ethical perspectives. For example, if one of the major participants involved in discussions relative to discontinuing life support believes that it is always wrong to take a life (see discussion of deontology in Chapter 2), the process of negotiation with those who believe differently is likely to be frustrating. It would be more beneficial under those circumstances to begin the discussion by defining the point at which death actually occurs, thus finding common ground. When those involved present with diverse values, your role may be to facilitate their coming to a consensus around goals and understanding principles.

Determine Desired Outcomes

Identifying the desired outcomes and their potential consequences is a substantial step in the decision-making process. At this point, participants will exclude those outcomes that are totally unacceptable. As with the nursing process, implementation of a plan of action cannot logically occur without explicit knowledge of the desired outcome. Likewise, evaluation of the success or failure of the plan is measured by the degree to which the outcome is met. Clarifying the outcomes and their anticipated consequences enhances the understanding of options and alternatives.

Identify Options

Having determined the desired outcomes, participants should identify possible options for action. Various options begin to emerge through the assessment process. Participants must consider legal and other consequences. They must also determine which alternatives best meet the identified outcomes and fit their basic beliefs, lifestyles, and values. This process helps to narrow the list of acceptable alternatives. It is critical to eliminate all unacceptable alternatives and begin the process of listing, weighing, ranking, and prioritizing those that are found to be acceptable. Participants must make a choice among options with both head and heart; taking time to dwell with remaining alternatives, recognizing that there is rarely a good solution. Once the selection is made, the decision makers must be willing to act upon the choice.

Act on the Choice

Taking action is a major goal of the process, but can be one of the most difficult parts. It can stir numerous emotions laced with both certainty and doubt about the rightness of the decision. Participants must be empowered to make a difficult decision, setting aside less acceptable alternatives. Chapters 19 and 20 discuss empowerment in more depth. It is important to be attentive to the emotions involved at this point of the process.

Evaluate Outcomes of Action

After acting upon the decision, participants begin a process of response and evaluation. As in all decision making, reflective evaluation sheds light on the effectiveness
and validity of the process. Evaluate the action in terms of the effects upon those
involved. Ask, "Has the original ethical problem been resolved?" and "Have other problems emerged related to the action?" As the situation changes and new data emerge,
participants must identify subsequent moral problems and adjust the course of action
based upon both new information and responses to the previous decision.

Figure 6–1 is a guide for ethical decision making. Questions may need to be revisited several times and may emerge at various points as the process unfolds and new
data are presented. For example, information about options may begin to emerge before
all the parties involved are identified, and data regarding ethical perspectives of the various parties may be clarified only at the point when options are being discussed. No
matter how much information the participants gather, they may make the decision with
an awareness that they would like to have still more data, although having a long list
of viable options may actually make it more difficult to come to a decision.

Figure 6–1 **A Guide for Decision Making**

Gather Data and Identify Conflicting Moral Claims

- What makes this situation an ethical problem? Are there conflicting
  obligations, duties, principles, rights, loyalties, values, or beliefs?
- What are the issues?
- What facts seem most important?
- What emotions have an impact?
- What are the gaps in information at this time?

Identify Key Participants

- Who is legitimately empowered to make this decision?
- Who is affected and how?
- What is the level of competence of the person most affected in relation to
  the decision to be made?
- What are the rights, duties, authority, context, and capabilities of
  participants?

Determine Moral Perspective and Phase
of Moral Development of Key Participants

- Do participants think in terms of duties or rights?
- Do the parties involved exhibit similar or different moral perspectives?
- Where is the common ground? The differences?
- What principles are important to each person involved?
- What emotions are evident within the interaction and with each person
  involved?

- What is the level of moral development of the participants?

Determine Desired Outcomes

- How does each party describe the circumstances of the outcome?
- What are the consequences of the desired outcomes?
- What outcomes are unacceptable to one or all involved?

Identify Options

- What options emerge through the assessment process?
- How do the alternatives fit the lifestyle and values of the person(s) affected?
- What are legal considerations of the various options?
- What alternatives are unacceptable to one or all involved?
- How are alternatives weighed, ranked, and prioritized?

Act on the Choice

- Be empowered to make a difficult decision.
- Give yourself permission to set aside less acceptable alternatives.
- Be attentive to the emotions involved in this process.

Evaluate Outcomes of Action

- Has the ethical dilemma been resolved?
- Have other dilemmas emerged related to the action?
- How has the process affected those involved?
- Are further actions required?

APPLYING THE DECISION-MAKING PROCESS

Application of the decision-making guide in clinical situations is illustrated in the following case and discussion:

> A couple is pregnant with their second child after numerous unsuccessful attempts with artificial insemination. During a routine ultrasound at 28 weeks gestation, the physician discovers that the fetus is anencephalic. The life expectancy of an anencephalic baby is only a few days to weeks after birth. The couple struggles with the choice to terminate the pregnancy at this time or to carry the child to term.

Gathering Data and Identifying Conflicting Moral Claims

One conflict relates to the principle of nonmaleficence (the wish to do no harm). Terminating the pregnancy can be perceived as harmful to the baby, while carrying it to term may result in emotional or physical harm to the mother. Another conflict relates to the duty to preserve life, allowing the pregnancy, birth, and death of the baby to take its natural course, versus the duty to alleviate the suffering that carrying the pregnancy to term might impose on the mother. Some of the important facts in this situation include knowing the life expectancy of a baby born with anencephaly, knowing the parents' attitudes toward abortion, appreciating the feelings that this news bring forth, and knowing the meaning of this pregnancy to the parents.

Identifying Key Participants

Valuing input from the physician and others, both parents have the moral and legal right and the responsibility to make the decision. They may want to consult religious ministers, family, or friends, and they may request a second opinion. Though mentally competent, the parents may have difficulty making a decision soon after receiving the painful news. Since this is not an emergency, the nurse and others should allow time and provide support, while the parents process the information and deal with emotions. If, for example, one parent wants the pregnancy terminated and the other is strongly opposed, participants should further explore who has the right to make the ultimate decision.

Determining Moral Perspective and Phase of Moral Development of Key Participants

It is important to consider whether the stance of both parents is the same. Are they thinking about the rights of the infant versus the rights of the mother, or the duty to preserve the family integrity? If one parent thinks the pregnancy should be terminated and the other feels that the baby has a right to life, no matter how short it may be, can a common ground be reached? Do the parents seek guidance from those in authority, or from beliefs regarding right and wrong in this situation? Do they talk of a relationship with the baby in utero and the impact of choosing to end its life—on the baby, its sibling, or their relationship?

Determining Desired Outcomes

Through discussion of outcomes, more insight into ethical theory may emerge. In this situation, participants could describe the desired outcome as prevention of unnecessary suffering for the mother and the baby. Further exploration might reveal the sense that carrying the baby to term would create such anguish for the mother that her emotional health, and even family integrity, would be threatened. In that instance, terminating the pregnancy would be more compassionate than prolonging the suffering of the mother and allowing the inevitable, yet slow, natural death of the baby. Legal considerations would include laws related to abortion.

Identifying Options

In this case, the physician presented the options at the outset: the parents could terminate the pregnancy, or allow it to go to term. One might well look at the risks for the mother involved in both choices. Participants need to clarify beliefs regarding life, abortion, family responsibility, duties, and the like. If carrying the pregnancy to term presents a health risk for the mother, an additional dilemma would arise regarding responsibility to the older sibling and family integrity versus responsibility to the baby.

If either carrying the pregnancy to term or terminating it now is acceptable, participants have the task of determining factors that may weigh one alternative more strongly than the other. They may decide that the grieving process of the baby's death has already begun and would only be intensified if the pregnancy were carried to term. With this in mind, they might decide to end the pregnancy.

Acting on the Choice

Deciding to terminate the pregnancy, the parents move toward action. As logistics of scheduling and preparing for the termination proceed, it is important to attend to the parents' emotional response and to ensure that they have other needed support.

Evaluating Outcomes of Action

The parents resolved the dilemma of whether to terminate the pregnancy or carry it to term by choosing to proceed with termination. Reactions to the choice may emerge in the forms of guilt, depression, acceptance, or always wondering how things might have been different if the other path had been chosen. If the parents have long-term reactions, such as deep guilt or depression, they might come to a point of saying that, faced with such a situation again, they should decide to carry the pregnancy to term. On the other hand, they may examine issues surrounding the emotions with the awareness that the decision to terminate the pregnancy helped them deal with these issues and that, in spite of the pain, they made the best decision at the time.

Think About It

Various Responses to Terminating Pregnancy

Consider which areas of the "Guide for Decision Making" in Figure 6–1 may have to be revisited in the following variations of the case presented above.

- The mother indicates that she thinks she will "go crazy" if she carries the pregnancy to term, and the father says "no one is going to kill my child."
- This is a young single mother from another culture who believes she has been "witched" and that the baby will be normal if she has the proper ceremony.
- The local hospital has a religious affiliation that does not permit abortions. The parents feel that terminating the pregnancy is the better decision, but they have no transportation to the hospital, a two-hour drive away, where the procedure can be done.

SUMMARY

Ethical decision making requires knowledge and attention to many factors. Determining the existence of an ethical dilemma is the beginning step in the process which includes defining the problem, identifying desired objectives, listing and evaluating alternatives, choosing the best course of action based on one's knowledge and the current circumstances, and evaluating the outcomes of the action taken. One must consider both reason and emotion in making ethical decisions. Nurses are encouraged to utilize the decision making process described in this chapter as a guide in dealing with dilemmas encountered in clinical settings. As with every other nursing skill, comfort and competency with ethical decision making comes with repeated practice.

CHAPTER HIGHLIGHTS

- Dilemmas exist when difficult problems have no satisfactory solutions or when all the solutions appear equally favorable.
- In decisions involving practical dilemmas, moral claims hold greater weight than nonmoral claims.
- Making thoughtful decisions in any arena follows a pattern that includes gathering data, comparing options based on particular criteria, making and acting on a choice, and evaluating outcomes or circumstances surrounding the choice.
- One's value system affects how one defines and deals with an ethical issue; thus, resolution of ethical dilemmas requires determining the ethical issue at hand and identifying the value systems of those involved.
- Both emotion and reason have legitimate roles in ethical decision making.
- Ethical decision making requires ongoing evaluation and assimilation of information, with revisiting of various steps in the process as often as required by the dynamics of changing facts, evolving beliefs, unexpected consequences, and participants moving in and out of the process.
- Familiarity with and practice in applying ethical decision making enables the nurse to develop competence and confidence with the process.

DISCUSSION QUESTIONS AND ACTIVITIES

1. Search an on-line database for full-text articles related to nurses' ethical decision making. How do other models compare to the one presented in this text?
2. Working in small groups, discuss ethical and practical dilemmas that you have experienced, then choose an example of each type of dilemma to illustrate for the class.
3. Describe a situation in which you or someone you know experienced moral distress, noting moral and nonmoral claims in the situation.
4. Talk with practicing nurses about their experiences of ethical dilemmas. Identify their approaches to dealing with such dilemmas, including their processes of ethical decision making.

5. Debate the role of reason and emotion in ethical decisions with classmates.

6. Use the ethical decision-making process to revisit an ethical dilemma that you have encountered in the past, or to guide you through a current dilemma. Examine your sense of comfort with each part of the process, noting areas of strength and areas needing more practice.

7. Discuss the interaction among moral development, moral perspective, and ethical decision making.

8. How would you approach an ethical dilemma in which the parties involved exhibit different moral perspectives?

9. How might legal considerations affect the process of making ethical decisions?

REFERENCES

Beauchamp, T. L., & Childress, J. F. (1994). *Principles of biomedical ethics* (4th ed.). New York: Oxford University Press.

Callahan, S. (1995). The role of emotions in ethical decision making. In J. H. Howell & W. F. Sale, eds., *Life choices: A Hastings Center introduction to bioethics.* Washington, DC: Georgetown University Press.

Chinn, P. L. (1995). *Peace and power: Building communities for the future* (4th ed.). New York: National League of Nursing Press.

Christensen, P. J., & Kenney, J. W. (1990). *Nursing process: Application of conceptual models* (3rd ed.). St. Louis, MO: Mosby.

Curtin, L., & Flaherty, M. J. (1982). *Nursing ethics: Theories and pragmatics.* Bowie, MD: Brady.

Davis, A. J., Aroskar, M. A., Liaschenko, J., & Drought, T. S. (1997). *Ethical dilemmas and nursing practice* (4th ed.). Norwalk, CT: Appleton & Lange.

Fenton, M. (1988). Moral distress in clinical practice: Implications for the nurse administrator. *Canadian Journal of Nursing Administration, 1,* 8–11.

Gibson, J. (1991). An introduction to the study of ethics and ethical theories. In B. R. Furrow, S. H. Johnson, T. S. Jost, & R. L. Schwartz, eds., *Bioethics: Health care, law, and ethics* (pp. 1–6). St. Paul, MN: West.

Hamric, A. B. (2000). Moral distress in everyday ethics. *Nursing Outlook, 48,* 199–201.

Hefferman, P., & Heilig, S. (1999). Giving "moral distress" a voice: Ethical concerns among neonatal intensive care unit personnel. *Cambridge Quarterly of Healthcare Ethics, 8,* 173–178.

Husted, G. L., & Husted, J. H. (1995). *Ethical decision making in nursing.* St. Louis, MO: Mosby.

Jameton, A. (1984). *Nursing practice: The ethical issues.* Englewood Cliffs, NJ: Prentice-Hall.

Kelly, B. (1998). Preserving moral integrity: A follow-up study with new graduate nurses. *Journal of Advanced Nursing, 28,* 1134–1145.

Millette, B. E. (1994). Using Gilligan's framework to anlayze nurses' stories of moral choices. *Western Journal of Nursing Research, 16*(6), 660–674.

Nathaniel, A. K. (2000). A concept analysis of moral distress. Unpublished Manuscript.

Redman, B., & Fry, S. T. (2000). Nurses' ethical conflicts: What is really known about them? *Nursing Ethics, 7*(4), 360–366.

Rushton, C. H. (1995). The Baby K case: Ethical challenges of preserving professional intgegrity. *Pediatric Nursing, 23*(1), 16–29.

Wilkinson, J. M. (1987–88). Moral distress in nursing practice: Experience and effect. *Nursing Forum, 23*(1), 16–29.

PRINCIPLED BEHAVIOR IN THE PROFESSIONAL DOMAIN

Part III examines various categories of issues that affect the profession of nursing and the everyday practice of individual nurses. Recognizing nursing as a profession, the chapters describe nurses' responsibility related to ethical, legal, professional, and practice issues. These issues are examined in light of ethics and contemporary nursing. This part includes chapters discussing legal issues affecting nurses; professional issues such as autonomy, authority, and accountability; issues related to the relationship between nurses and the health care system; issues related to technology and self-determination; and scholarship issues.

CHAPTER 7

Legal Issues

We are caught in an inescapable network of mutuality, tied in a single garment of destiny. Whatever affects one directly, affects all indirectly.

(Martin Luther King, Jr.)

OBJECTIVES

After completing this chapter, the reader should be able to:

1. Recognize the difference between ethics and the law, and discuss the relationship of each to the other.
2. Describe sources of law.
3. Distinguish between constitutional law, statutory law, administrative law, and common law.
4. Describe the difference between public and private law.
5. Discuss instances in which nurses might be accused of breaches of public law.
6. Define tort, and distinguish between unintentional and intentional torts.
7. Discuss recent legal trends in health care.
8. Discuss methods that nurses can use to limit liability.
9. Describe the role of the expert nurse witness.

INTRODUCTION

Up to this point, the focus of this book has been upon values, morals, and ethics. You will recall from Chapter 2 that moral thinking, though influenced in great measure by prevailing cultural tradition, is essentially an individual enterprise. Ethics are rules of behavior produced by moral thinking and may be either informal or formal rules of actions. Professional organizations, such as the American Nurses Association, the Canadian Nurses Association, and the International Council of Nurses, provide documents outlining a formal set of ethical guidelines. These guidelines offer some general rules that are intended for use as a tool to guide professional behavior but are not, in themselves, fully enforceable. Laws, on the other hand, consist of enforced rules under which a society is governed. Many laws either directly or indirectly affect the practice of nursing. Highly publicized issues such as termination of life support and "no code" status indicate a recent trend toward involving the legal system in issues that were previously thought to be ethical in nature. This chapter discusses the relationship between ethics and the law, general legal concepts, areas of potential liability for nurses, and recent legal trends. The legal regulation of nursing is addressed in Chapter 8.

RELATIONSHIP BETWEEN ETHICS AND THE LAW

Law is the system of binding rules of action or conduct that governs the behavior of people in respect to relationships with others and with the government (Guido, 1997; Rhodes & Miller, 1984). Laws, meant to reflect the moral beliefs of a given population, are devised by groups of individuals serving in official capacity. There are four basic functions of the law in society: (1) to define relationships among members of society, and to declare which actions are and are not permitted; (2) to describe what constraints may be applied to maintain rules, and by whom they may be applied; (3) to furnish solutions to problems; and, (4) to redefine relationships between people and groups when circumstances of life change (Kozier & Erb, 1992).

The law establishes rules that define our rights and obligations, and sets penalties for people who violate them. Laws also describe how government will enforce the rules and penalties. In the United States and Canada, there are thousands of state, provincial, federal, and local laws. Among others, these laws ensure the safety of citizens, protect property, promote nondiscrimination, regulate the professions, provide for the distribution of public goods and services, and protect the economic and environmental interests of society.

How are ethics and laws related? Laws are intended to reflect popular belief about the "rightness or wrongness" of particular acts and are, like ethics, built upon a moral foundation. In most countries laws represent an attempt to codify ethics. Law can serve as the public's instrument for converting morality into clear-cut social guidelines, and for stipulating punishments for offenses (Beauchamp, 2001). One would expect that laws would be congruent with the prevailing moral values of a society; indeed, they usually are. For example, most people would agree that the murder of an innocent person is an immoral act. Laws that prohibit murder reflect this ethical standard. Murder of the innocent is both ethically and legally prohibited in every culture. As society's needs and attitudes evolve, laws emerge to reflect these changes. Occasionally, however, governments create and enforce laws that many people believe to be unjust or immoral. In a democratic society, constitutional law provides mechanisms to change or abolish unjust or unpopular laws.

Some authors of nursing ethics texts take the view that professional ethical standards are congruent with the law, that is, that which is legal is also ethical, and vice versa. These authors imply that following a set of ethical guidelines, such as those provided by the American Nurses Association, the Canadian Nurses Association, and the International Council of Nurses, provides nurses a legal safety net. This is usually, but not necessarily, true. Laws exist that can be considered (by some at least) to be unethical. Some illegal acts are considered by many to be ethical.

What are some reasons for the possible discrepancy between that which is legal and that which is ethical? First, there are differences between ethical points of view. Deontology and utilitarianism, for example, offer quite opposite answers to some basic ethical questions. While the utilitarian perspective would allow consideration of abortion or euthanasia, for example, to provide for the good of many, deontological views might require that life be protected regardless of circumstance. Thus, a law thought to be ethical by the utilitarian might be considered unethical by the deontologist. Second, human behavior and motivation are more complex than can be fairly reflected in law. Think back to Chapter 4. Individuals may consider the same act either right or wrong, depending to some extent on their stage or level of moral development. For example, acts of civil disobedience, such as those committed by Mahatma Gandhi and Martin Luther King, Jr., although unquestionably illegal, are generally considered to be motivated by high ethical standards. In his letter from the Birmingham Jail, Martin Luther King, Jr., wrote, "there are two types of laws: just and unjust. I would be the first to advocate obeying just laws. One has not only a legal but a moral responsibility to obey just laws. Conversely, one has a moral responsibility to disobey unjust laws" (1996, p. 574). Third, the legal system judges action rather than motivation. For example, nurses following personal moral convictions or professional ethical codes can find themselves at odds with policies or practices of employing institutions. In certain instances, the legal system may determine that an employing institution has the right to dismiss or discipline a nurse for laying aside institutional policy in favor of ethical considerations. Fourth, depending upon the political climate and other variables, laws change. Recent examples of laws that have changed include those related to expanded roles of nurses, abortion, fetal tissue use, organ transplantation, self-determination, confidentiality for AIDS patients, informed consent, and legal definitions of death. As defined in Chapter 3, integrity is fidelity in adherence to moral norms sustained over time. One should be able to predict that nurses with integrity will not alter their basic moral beliefs in response to changes in the law. Thus, there are several valid circumstances in which there may be a discrepancy between that which is legal and that which is considered ethical.

GENERAL LEGAL CONCEPTS

Nurses need to familiarize themselves with the law and legal system for several reasons. First, the law authorizes and regulates nursing practice. Nurse practice acts of the individual states describe both the activity of nurses and the boundaries of nursing. Chapter 8 discusses the legal regulation of nursing in greater depth. Second, the legal system scrutinizes nursing actions and omissions. The profession is in a dynamic state of change: advanced practice nurses are expanding the traditional boundaries; critical care nurses are performing complex and vital tasks; staff nurses are caring for older and sicker patients; and many nurses are practicing in new settings. Recognizing that health care is experiencing a storm of litigation, we must have basic knowledge about law and the legal process. This knowledge will help ensure that our actions are consistent with legal principles, and will help to protect us from liability. Third, knowledge of legal principles is a necessary component of ethical decision making. In order to make informed choices, nurses, physicians, patients, and families must be able to identify potential or real legal implications.

Sources of Law

There are at least four different sources of law that affect the practice of nursing: constitutional law, statutory (legislative) law, administrative law, and common law. Additionally, law can be divided into two main branches—private law and public law. Some laws are made by legislation, some by rule-making bodies, and some by judicial precedent. Adding to an already confusing mix, there is frequent overlap between the sources and branches of the law.

Constitutional Law. A constitution is a formal set of rules and principles that describe the powers of a government and the rights of the people. The principles laid out in a constitution, coupled with a description of how these principles are to be interpreted and carried out, form the basis of **constitutional law.** The Constitution of the United States is the preeminent source of this country's law. Ensuring legal rights and responsibilities of citizens and establishing the general organization of the federal government, constitutional law in the United States supersedes all other laws.

Nurses must be aware that the Bill of Rights of the United States Constitution and subsequent amendments guarantees each citizen the rights, among others, of equal protection, due process, freedom of speech, and freedom of religion. Nursing actions must take into account these basic rights. Rights guaranteed in the Bill of Rights are consistent with the ethical principles of autonomy, confidentiality, respect for persons, and veracity. The same rights that apply to patients also apply to nurses. As participants in the health care system, we cannot be forced to forfeit any constitutionally-guaranteed rights.

Statutory/Legislative Law. Formal laws written and enacted by federal, state, or local legislatures are known as **statutory** or **legislative laws.** Congress and the state legislatures pass thousands of laws each year; these are added to the hundreds of volumes of federal and state statutes already in force. Because many people think that every problem in society can be solved by passing a law, legislatures make more and more laws to satisfy the demands of society and special-interest groups. Changes in Medicare and Medicaid laws, statutory recognition of nurses in advanced practice (including prescriptive authority), and proposed health care reform legislation are all examples of statutory or legislative law.

Administrative Law. **Administrative law** involves the operation of government agencies. National, state, and local governments set up administrative agencies to do the work of government. These agencies regulate such activities as education, public health, social welfare programs, and the professions. Administrative law consists mainly of the legal powers granted to administrative agencies by legislative bodies and the rules that the agencies make to carry out their powers. State boards of nursing are examples of this type of agency. These boards are granted the authority to execute the intent of state statutes by creating, implementing, and enforcing comprehensive and appropriate rules and regulations. As administrative bodies, the role of boards of nursing is to protect the public, rather than advocate for nurses. Rules promulgated by the individual states' boards of nursing carry the same weight as other law.

Common Law. The United States (except Louisiana), Canada (except Quebec), Great Britain, and other English-speaking countries have a **common law** system. Constituting the basis of the judicial system, this type of law is also known as case law. In the common law system, decisions are based upon earlier court rulings in similar cases. These are also known as **precedents.** Over time, precedents take on the force of law.

Types of Law

Law can be divided into two different types: public and private. Recall that law is a system of enforceable principles and processes that governs the behavior of people in respect to relationships with others and with the government. In general, legal problems related to the relationship between people and the government are the domain of public law, and problems occurring as a result of relationships between people are the domain of private law.

Public Law. **Public law** defines a person's rights and obligations in relation to the government and describes the various divisions of government and their powers. One important branch of public law is **criminal law.** Criminal law deals with crimes— that is, actions considered harmful to society. Even though a crime might be committed against a particular person, the government considers the commission of a serious act, such as murder, to be harmful to all of society. In the United States, each state, as well as the federal government, has its own set of criminal laws. Nevertheless, the criminal laws of each state must protect the rights and freedoms guaranteed by the federal constitution. Crimes range in seriousness, from public drunkenness to murder. Criminal law defines these offenses and sets the rules for the arrest, the appropriate procedures to ensure due process, and the punishment of offenders.

In the course of practice, nurses can be accused of a variety of criminal offenses.

For example, nurses can be accused of directly injuring a patient, either intentionally or unintentionally. Nurses can also be accused of crimes related to their actual relationship with the government. These include such actions as falsifying narcotic records, failure to renew licenses, and fraudulent billing. Crimes are delineated according to seriousness as either felonies or misdemeanors.

Felonies are serious crimes that carry significant fines and jail sentences. Examples of felonies include first- and second-degree murder, arson, burglary, extortion, kidnaping, rape, and robbery. These crimes are punishable by jail terms. Nurses are rarely accused of felonies in the course of practice. However, this can occur. For example, it is possible that those participating in the unauthorized removal of life support from a terminally ill patient could be accused of first-degree murder, because of the intentional nature of the act which resulted in death. This could occur even though the act might be viewed as beneficent by a majority of people. A nurse who unintentionally causes the death of a patient by administering a medication to which a patient is allergic could be charged with second-degree murder (manslaughter).

A **misdemeanor** is a less serious crime, usually punishable by a fine, a short jail sentence, or both. Examples of misdemeanors include disturbing the peace, solicitation, assault, and battery (assault and battery are also considered intentional torts and can be decided by private or civil law). A nurse slapping a patient or giving an injection without consent can be accused of the misdemeanor of battery.

Think About It

Institutional Versus Individual Negligence

Occasionally, nurses find themselves in situations in which institutional policies and practices are inconsistent with public law. In these instances, nurses and other staff members can be accused of crimes. In 1986, members of the staff of a nursing home in Louisiana were charged with cruelty, neglect, and mistreatment of the infirm. In the *State of Louisiana v. Brenner* (1986), the staff was charged for the following reasons:

1. Failure to feed and care for the patients adequately

2. Failure to train the staff properly

3. Failure to provide adequate medical supplies

4. Failure to supply adequate staff

5. Failure to maintain a sanitary nursing home

6. Failure to maintain patients' records

7. Failure to see that the appropriate and necessary health services were performed.

   - Ethics and the law are usually, but not always, consistent. Think about each of the seven accusations listed above in terms of breaches of ethical principles. What is the relationship between the accusations and ethical principles?

- Imagining that you live in a small community and are employed by a nursing home with similar problems. How do you think you would deal with the problems in a manner that is both legal and ethical? How do you think you would deal with the situation if you feel compelled to maintain your employment at the nursing home?
- Do you believe that individual nurses should be punished for actions that are clearly caused by institutional negligence? Substantiate your answer with ethical arguments.

Private Law.   **Private law** is also called **civil law.** It determines a person's legal rights and obligations in many kinds of activities that involve other people. These activities include everything from borrowing or lending money to buying a home or signing a job contract. More than a million civil suits are tried in the United States courts each year. There are six branches of private law: contract and commercial law, tort law, property law, inheritance law, family law, and corporation law. The branches of private law that are most applicable to nursing practice are contract law and tort law. Noncompliance with private law generally leads to monetary compensation granted the injured or complaining party (**plaintiff**).

Contract Law.   **Contract law** deals with the rights and obligations of people who make contracts. A **contract** is an agreement between two or more people that can be enforced by law. Contracts may be either written or oral; however, in the presence of both a written and oral contract, the written contract takes precedence. In health care, contracts may be either expressed or implied. Expressed contracts occur when the two parties agree explicitly to its terms, as in an employment contract. Implied contracts occur when there has been no discussion between the parties, but the law considers that a contract exists (Kozier & Erb, 1992). The nurse-patient relationship is essentially an implied contract with which the nurse agrees to give competent care.

Tort Law.   A **tort** is a wrong or injury that a person suffers because of someone else's action, either intentional or unintentional. The tortious action may cause bodily harm; invade another's privacy; damage a person's property, business, or reputation; or make unauthorized use of a person's property. The victim may sue the person or persons responsible. Tort law deals with the rights and obligations of the persons involved in such cases. Many torts are unintentional, such as damages that occur as a result of accidents. But if a tort is deliberate and involves serious harm, it may also be treated as a crime. The purpose of tort law is to make the person whole again, primarily through the award of monetary damages. Because it involves negligence and malpractice, tort law is the branch of law with which nurses are most familiar.

   Unintentional torts occur when an act or omission causes unintended injury or harm to another person. Nurses are familiar with the unintentional torts of negligence and malpractice. **Negligence** is "the omission to do something that a reasonable person, guided by those ordinary considerations which ordinarily regulate human affairs, would do, or doing something which a reasonable and prudent person would not do" (Creighton, 1986, p. 141).

As part of ensuring the safety of citizens, the law requires that every person is accountable for behaving in a reasonable way, particularly if the welfare of others is jeopardized. For example, there is certainly no law against throwing rocks into the air. However, within a crowd of people, this is not the act of a reasonable person. Although the person throwing rocks may enjoy the beauty of the arc or the distance of the throw and has no intention of harming others, a resultant injury would be the outcome of negligence. A nurse who pours liquid on the floor in a patient's room would be held to the same standard: that is, a reasonable person would recognize that wet floors often cause falls, and would immediately clean the floor and warn people who may be walking in the vicinity.

Negligence can also occur as a result of an omission. The nurse in the situation above may have walked into the room and found that the patient had spilled water. Had she ignored the spill, the nurse would be responsible for the results of her negligence in omitting to remove the danger, even though she did not actually cause the spill. Acts of negligence in nursing can be judged upon the criteria of the knowledge and abilities expected of a reasonable and prudent nurse, as opposed to a reasonable and prudent person. Because the knowledge base of nursing is broad, technical, and specific to the profession, these criteria go far beyond those required of the ordinary person.

Malpractice is a type or sub-set of negligence, committed by a person in professional capacity. Over and above simple negligence, malpractice is the form of negligence in which any professional misconduct, unreasonable lack of professional skill, or nonadherence to the accepted standard of care causes injury to a patient or client. Creighton (1986) also includes lack of fidelity, evil practice, and illegal or immoral conduct in the definition of malpractice. Malpractice is the segment of the tort law of negligence specifically reserved for the professional person. To be held liable for malpractice, the nurse must fail to act as other reasonable and prudent professional nurses who have the same knowledge and education would have acted under similar circumstances (Catalano, 1991, p. 69). There are four components that are required to prove liability for malpractice: (1) it must be established that the nurse has a duty owed to the patient; (2) there must be a breach of standards of care or failure to carry out that duty; (3) actual harm or injury must be suffered by the patient; and, (4) there must be a causal relationship between the breach of duty and the injury suffered (O'Keefe, 2000).

Figure 7–1 **Components of Malpractice**

1. Duty owed to the patient
2. Breach of standards of care or failure to carry out duty
3. Actual harm or injury suffered by the patient
4. Causal relationship between the breach of standards of care or duty and the injury

Accurate data about nurses' malpractice suits are difficult to obtain. Miller-Slade (1997) cites a study of malpractice claims against nurses that led to verdicts for the patients. Of 219 patient deaths, inadequate communication with the doctor led to seventy-six; inadequate nursing assessment, forty-six; medication errors, forty-two; inadequate nursing intervention, seventeen; inadequate care, twenty-one; unsafe environment, seven; inadequate infection control, three; and improper use of equipment, seven. Another study found that the most common causes of malpractice lawsuits, in order of frequency, are medication and treatment errors; lack of observation and timely reporting about the patient; defective technology; infections caused by or made worse by poor nursing care; poor communication of important information; and failure to intervene to protect the patient from poor medical care (Physician Insurers Association of America, 1993); O'Keefe (2000) suggests that nursing malpractice settlements can be viewed in terms of the nursing process, identified as a standard of care by the American Nurses Association and many state boards of nursing. Nurses can be accused of malpractice if they fail to assess, plan, implement, or evaluate the patient condition or response to treatment. Because the two actions are similar, and the process is iterative, assessment and evaluation are considered together.

Assessment and evaluation are fundamental nursing duties. Because these basic nursing functions have a long history as standards of nursing care, failure to assess and evaluate may lead to malpractice judgments. O'Keefe (2000) identifies requirements in the duty to assess and evaluate.

1. The nurse must possess the knowledge and skill to properly assess and/or monitor a significant condition or change in the patient. There is a duty to know what the patient's condition should be, what it has been and what is is now.
2. The nurse must actually carry out the assessment, monitoring, and evaluation.
3. The nurse must notify the physician if assessment, evaluation, or monitoring reveals a condition that should be reported. The nurse must report the patient's status and must thoroughly document the patient's condition and details of when and to whom the condition was reported.
4. The nurse must skillfully carry out appropriate nursing and medical interventions in an effort to correct the problem.
5. The nurse must continue to assess and monitor until the patient is stable. (p. 137)

The nursing standard of care is breached if each of these requirements are not met. If harm comes to the patient as a result of the nurse's failure to assess, the nurse could be held liable. *Ferrs vs. County of Kennebec* (1998) offers an example of a nurse's failure to assess so extreme as to be labeled "deliberate indifference." In the summer of 1996, a woman was arrested and placed in the county jail. When she was admitted, the woman told the jail officials that she was pregnant. Two days later she began having vaginal bleeding and pelvic pain. The woman complained to the nurse that she was having a miscarriage. The nurse took the woman's pulse, told her she was menstruating, instructed her to lie down, and refused to give her sanitary napkins. The woman was unable to continue to lie down because of her pain, but the nurse made no further attempt to assess her condition, telling her that she would be transferred to another cell if she continued to refuse to lie down and follow orders. Continuing to complain of severe pain, the woman was transferred to a smaller cell, and had no further contact with the nurse. A few hours later she had a miscarriage in her jail cell. After release, the woman filed a lawsuit. Finding in favor of the woman, the court determined that it was obvious that the woman was complaining of a serious condition that was ignored and untreated by the nurse. The nurse made no effort to assess or treat the woman beyond taking her pulse.

Because it is an integral part of the nursing care plan, a recognized standard of care, and a requirement of many federal program regulations, failure to plan may also result in accusations of malpractice. Though injury to the patient would directly result through the actions or omissions of the nurse, failure to record a plan of care stands as evidence that the nurse is negligent. In *Smith v. Juneau* (1997), nurses were found negligent for failing to develop a plan of care. Caring for an orthopedic patient in traction, the nurses failed to develop a plan of care to protect the patient's skin. There was no plan to reposition the patient or to assess the patient's skin under the traction sling. The court held that, because the nurses failed to plan and implement care to protect the skin, serious ulcers developed.

The essence of nursing care, nursing interventions both include and extend beyond actions taken personally by the nurse (O'Keefe, 2000). Implementation is the embodiment of the ethical principle of beneficence. The nurse has a duty to do or promote good, to prevent harm, and to remove evil or harm. This includes such things as maintaining expertise in practice and reporting the dangerous practice of others. Medication errors are examples of failure to implement properly.

Accounting for approximately seven thousand deaths a year, the most common area for nursing liability relates to medication errors (Lee, 2000). There are many ways that nurses can make errors of medication preparation and administration. The nurse can give the wrong medication, in the wrong dose, by the wrong route, at the wrong time, or to the wrong patient. Because of the frequency and likelihood of medication error and the potentially serious consequences that can result, nurses need to be especially careful in administering medications. Nurses are responsible for safe and appropriate administration of medication, regardless of physician orders, workload, unusual circumstance, or institutional policy. There are many examples of medication errors cited in the literature. It is not unusual for damages to be awarded to victims or families when medication errors occur. Creighton (1986) discusses a particular case in which a nurse, in an attempt to assist on a busy pediatric unit, administered a lethal dose of digitalis to an infant. This nurse did not usually work with pediatric patients, and was unfamiliar with pediatric doses. Even though the nurse thought the dose ordered seemed high, she did not check the literature, discuss the dose with a pharmacist, or question the physician. The parents in this case recovered substantial damages because the nurse's actions were determined to constitute malpractice.

Another area of frequent liability related to failue to implement nursing care is neglecting to remove foreign objects (Eskreis, 1998). Sponges and other small items can inadvertently be left in patients' body cavities. This can be a cause for serious post-operative complications. The nurse responsible for counting the sponges is often held liable for malpractice. Creighton (1986) discusses a particular case of a sponge being overlooked:

> Out of an award of $36,000, a scrub nurse and a circulating nurse had to pay $4,000 apiece in a case in which a laparotomy sponge was left in a patient during abdominal surgery although they had reported the sponge count correct. Since the surgeon had ordered the metal rings removed from the sponges, which was a safeguard provided by the employer, he became the nurses' special employer during the surgery and was liable with them. (p. 144)

In a similar case, a surgeon left a large surgical sponge in a patient's abdomen after a hysterectomy. The jury in the initial trial found both the hospital and the physician to be negligent, and further, that the nurses involved were agents of the hospital and not the physician. On appeal, the court found that it was a reasonable inference from the evidence that the sponge count done before surgery was performed negligently or that the procedure for counting sponges was below the standard of care. The court ordered a new trial, unless the physician agreed to a $125,000 damage award divided between the defendants (*Truhitte v. French Hospital,* 1982).

Since nursing care focuses on the psycho-social-spiritual realms as well as the physical, failure to implement care in these areas may result in nursing malpractice. Intentional infliction of emotional distress is an extreme example of this. There are certain contractual relationships, such as in the transmission and delivery of telegrams announcing the death of a close relative and services incident to a funeral and burial, that carry with them deeply emotional responses. Legal claims have been recognized that require a duty to exercise ordinary care to avoid causing emotional harm in such situations. Furrow, Johnson, Jost, & Schwartz (1991) argue that this duty also applies to the delivery of medical and nursing services. They describe an interesting and complex case involving several instances in which nurses and other health care workers contributed to the emotional distress of Larry and Susan Oswald. In *Oswald v. LeGrand* (1990), the plaintiffs described a sequence of events that preceded the premature birth of their third child. Just prior to her five-month checkup, Susan began experiencing bleeding and painful cramping. Her physician, Dr. Smith, ordered an ultrasound, subsequent to which Susan was examined by Dr. Smith's associate, Dr. LeGrand. Finding no explanation for the problems, Dr. LeGrand instructed Susan to go home and stay off her feet. Later the same day, Susan began bleeding heavily and was taken by ambulance to Mercy Health Center. The bleeding having spontaneously stopped, Dr. Smith discharged Susan with instructions to take it easy. The following day, with symptoms worsening, and fearing a miscarriage, Larry drove Susan to the Mercy emergency room. Another associate of Smith and LeGrand, Dr. Clark, examined Susan and advised her that there was nothing to be done and she should go home. Larry insisted that Susan be admitted and Dr. Clark honored the request. Susan was transferred to the labor and delivery ward where her first contact was with a nurse who said, "'What are you doing here? The doctor told you to stay home and rest.'" Later, another nurse told Susan that if she miscarried there would not be a baby but rather a "big blob of blood'" (Furrow et al., p. 166). Susan reports that she was scared. The next morning Susan overheard a loud argument outside her door, in which Dr. Clark was heard to yell, "'I don't want to take that patient. She's not my patient and I am sick and tired of Dr. Smith dumping his case load on me'" (p. 166). Urged by Larry, Dr. Clark apologized and assured Susan that he would care for her until he left for vacation at noon that day, at which time Dr. LeGrand would take over. Susan began experiencing a great deal of pain at around 9:00 A.M., and Dr. Clark instructed the staff to schedule her for an ultrasound and amniocentesis. After viewing the ultrasound, Dr. Clark told the Oswalds that the situation was unusual and left without further explanation one-half hour before his scheduled off-time. Confused, distressed, in extreme pain, and still in the hallway outside the x-ray lab, Susan began giving birth. Summoned by Larry, two nurses delivered a one-pound baby girl, whom they determined to have no pulse or respiratory activity. They wrapped the baby in a towel, placed her on an instrument tray, and told the parents she was stillborn. After having called relatives to break the sad news, Larry touched the baby's hand and was startled when his grasp was returned. The nurses rushed the infant to the neonatal intensive care unit where she died several hours later.

Ask Yourself

Emotional Harm

- In the above case, do you think there was negligence on the part of any of the health care providers? If so, explain your thinking.

- If you believe there was negligence, do you think the premature birth or death of the infant was directly caused by the negligence?

- Larry and Susan contend that they have suffered severe emotional distress as a result of alleged breaches of professional conduct. Think about the several instances in which either the physicians or nurses may have contributed to the Oswalds' emotional distress.

- Do you feel there should be a duty to exercise ordinary care to avoid causing emotional harm? Was that duty breached in this instance?

- What are the ethical implications of the nurses' behavior?

Patient burns may also be considered a failure to implement nursing care. Burns can occur as a result of fires, baths, showers, hot water bottles, or heating pads. Patients who are comatose or have diminished sensitivity are especially prone to burns. In one case a three-month-old infant suffered second- and third-degree burns on his buttocks after an operating room nurse placed him on a heating pad at the instruction of the anesthesiologist. The purpose of the heating pad was to help the child maintain body temperature during surgery. Though neither the nurses nor the surgeon noted anything unusual after surgery, arriving at home, the parents found the infant to have blisters draining bloody fluid. The child required subsequent skin grafting. Although admitting liability in this case, the defendants attempted to exclude from evidence the manufacturer's warning to avoid use of the heating pad on an infant, invalid, or sleeping or unconscious person. The manufacturers warned that burns could result from improper use (*Smelko v. Brinton*, 1987). In another case, a patient received a judgment against a hospital after he was seriously burned. The patient was paralyzed and had a speech impediment. He was left alone while smoking his pipe. The pipe fell from his mouth and set the bed on fire (Creighton, 1986, p. 145). Clearly a reasonable and prudent nurse would not leave a paralyzed person alone with a lit pipe in his mouth.

Intentional torts are "willful or intentional acts that violate another person's rights or property" (Catalano, 1991, p. 69). A tort must include three elements to be considered intentional: the act must be intended to interfere with the plaintiff or his property; there must be intent to bring about the consequences of the act; and the act must substantially cause the consequences. There is no legal requirement that damages or injury actually result from the act; proof of the defendant's intention is sufficient (Catalano). (See Figure 7–2.) Examples of intentional torts include fraud, invasion of privacy, assault, battery, false imprisonment, slander, and libel.

Figure 7–2 **Components of Intentional Torts**

---

1. The defendant's act must be intended to interfere with the plaintiff or his property.
2. The defendant must intend to bring about the consequences of the act.
3. The act must substantially cause the consequences.
4. There is no legal requirement that the act causes damages or injury—proof of intention is sufficient.

Fraud is a deliberate deception for the purpose of securing an unfair or unlawful gain. Although nurses are seldom accused of fraud, when this occurs it is usually prosecuted as a crime. Examples of potential areas of nurses' fraud include falsification of information on employment applications, untruthful billing procedures, false representation of a patient's physical condition in order to induce contracts for services, and falsification of patient records to cover up an error or avoid legal action. As is true with some other intentional torts, fraud can lead to both civil and criminal proceedings. Because of the deliberate nature and potential harm of fraudulent acts, court decisions tend to be harsh. Advanced practice nurses' (APN) third-party billing procedures are an area of potential fraud. Identified as one of the top priorities of the U.S. Department of Justice, fraudulent medical service billing can be intentional or unintentional. Complex billing procedures and inequality of reimbursement set the stage for errors in billing and "upcoding" for APN visits. Complicated "incident to" codes and reimbursement levels for APNs at 15 percent less than physicians lead some medical practices to try to find ways to bill for APN services at the physician rate. This practice can lead to charges of fraud against both nurses and physicians. Each incident of fraud can result in up to five years imprisonment, up to $25,000 fine, and exclusion from Medicare and Medicaid reimbursement for at least five years (Mazzocco, 2000).

The **right to privacy** is the right to be left alone or to be free from unwanted publicity. Individuals have the right to withhold themselves and their lives from public scrutiny. The intentional tort of **invasion of privacy** occurs when a person's privacy is invaded. Fiesta (1988) outlines four types of invasions of privacy: intrusion on the patient's physical and mental solitude or seclusion; public disclosure of private facts; publicity that places the patient in a false light in the public eye; and appropriation of the patient's name or likeness for the defendant's benefit or advantage (p. 160). There are many cases involving invasions of privacy. In *Bethiaume v. Pratt*, a dying patient being treated for cancer of the larynx was repeatedly photographed at the direction of his surgeon. On the day of his death the patient asked not to be photographed, but nevertheless the physician photographed him after lifting his head to place a pillow under it. A court decided that the physician be held liable for invasion of privacy (Fiesta, 1988, p. 160).

In another invasion of privacy case, Earl Spring, a senile seventy-eight-year-old man, was residing in a nursing home where he was undergoing kidney dialysis. In an attempt to discontinue dialysis treatments, his legal guardians, his wife and son, were involved in a prolonged court battle. In opposition to the family's position, and without their consent, the nursing home staff permitted right-to-life advocates to interview the senile man. Interviews with the patient and four nurses were published. After winning a Superior Court ruling regarding discontinuing the dialysis, Mrs. Spring sued the nursing home and the four nurses for $80 million in damages. She claimed that her husband's right to privacy had been violated. Although the attorney for the nursing home maintained that the patient had become a "public figure," the jury found in favor of Mrs. Spring, awarding her $2.5 million.

The terms *assault* and *battery*, though usually used together, have different legal meanings. Both are intentional torts. **Assault** is defined as the unjustifiable attempt or threat to touch a person without consent that results in fear of immediately harmful or threatening contact (Bernzweig, 1990). Touching need not actually occur. **Battery** is the unlawful, harmful, or unwarranted touching of another or the carrying out of threatened physical harm. Battery includes any willful, angry, violent, or negligent touching of a person's body or clothes, or anything held by or attached to the person (Creighton, 1986, p. 185; Guido, 1997). In the course of everyday activities, nurses have been accused of both assault and battery. For example, if a nurse threatens to give an injection to an unruly or noncompliant adult patient without consent, actionable assault has occurred. Battery is often thought of as such actions as slapping, shoving, or pinching, but the courts have upheld battery charges in actions that were much more subtle. Regardless of intent or outcome, touching without consent is considered battery. Even when the intention is beneficent and the outcome is positive, if the act is committed without permission, the nurse can be charged with battery. Surgical procedures that are performed without informed consent are the most common example of battery occurring in the hospital setting.

The case of *Robertson v. Provident House* (1991) illustrates an example of battery involving nurses. Although having an order for an "as needed" indwelling catheter, a quadriplegic patient objected when nurses tried to insert one. He had experienced pain and complications with indwelling catheters in the past. The nurse reportedly told the patient to "shut up" and then proceeded to insert the catheter. The catheter was removed after repeated requests from the patient and family. Subsequently, ignoring the patient's objections, the nurse reinserted the catheter. Injury occurred when a nurse forcefully pulled the catheter out. The family eventually sued for damages and recovered $25,000. The Louisiana Supreme Court found that battery occurs when a nurse ignores the objections of the patient and performs an invasive procedure, like the insertion of an indwelling catheter.

Fiesta (1988) cites a case in which a patient was involuntarily committed to a mental hospital. A practicing Christian Scientist, the patient refused medications and other treatment. The patient was apparently forced to take medication. Not having been shown to be a danger to herself or others, mentally ill, or incompetent, the court allowed her to recover for both assault and battery.

Creighton (1986) offers an exception to the requirement of consent from competent adults. In some states, nurses are permitted to obtain blood and other specimens, without consent, at police request from persons under arrest.

False imprisonment is the unjustifiable detention of a person within fixed boundaries, or an act intended to result in such confinement, without consent and without authority of law (Creighton, 1986; O'Keefe, 2000). Such acts can include physical restraint of the person, or acts intended to accomplish confinement, such as refusing the patient clothing or car keys. If false imprisonment is accompanied by forcible restraint or the threat of restraint, assault and battery may also be charged. However, each state has legal procedures granting authorization to detain, for a limited period of time, specific categories of persons who are disoriented, mentally ill, or substance abusers or who have contagious diseases. Generally, these persons can be held without consent while the hospital reports them to authorities and obtains commitment or custody orders (Rhodes & Miller, 1984).

Nurses have been accused of false imprisonment for restraining patients, locking patients in rooms, and detaining patients for payment of bills. An example of false imprisonment is seen in the case of *Big Town Nursing Home, Inc. v. Newman* (1970), in which a sixty-seven-year-old man was kept against his will for nearly two months. Having been brought to the nursing home by his nephew, the man attempted to leave several times and was forcibly detained. The staff of the nursing home restrained him in a chair and denied him the use of a telephone and his clothing. The court found that the staff of the nursing home acted recklessly, willfully, and maliciously in unlawfully detaining him. In the case of *Blackman for Blackman v. Rifkin* (1988), the court held that some circumstances justify detainment. In this instance, the court upheld the hospital's duty to prevent further harm by detaining a highly intoxicated patient with a head injury, despite her insistence that she be allowed to leave. The court ruled that the hospital could assume that the patient would have consented to the treatment had she not been intoxicated.

Defamation occurs when one harms a person's reputation and good name, diminishes others' value or esteem, or arouses negative feelings toward the person in others by the communication of false, malicious, unprivileged, or harmful words. Only those remarks or statements that might arouse derogatory opinions about a person are considered defamation. Additionally, defamation only occurs when the words are communicated to a third person—two persons directing remarks and epithets to each other are not liable for defamation. In most states there are two distinct forms of defamation, slander and libel. **Slander** occurs when one defames or damages the reputation of another by speaking unprivileged or false words. Slander can occur in nursing practice when nurses make cruel, false, or unsubstantiated claims against patients. By making value judgments or voicing the opinion that a patient is uncooperative, malingering, unintelligent, or drug-seeking, a nurse may be committing actionable slander. Nurses may also be accused of slander as a result of inappropriate defamatory remarks voiced against another professional. **Libel** consists of printed defamation by written words and images that injure a person's reputation or cause others to avoid, ridicule, or view the person with contempt. Nurses risk accusations of libel, for example, when writing information in patients' charts that can be damaging. Judgmental, critical, or speculative statements made in patients' charts such as, "The patient is drug-seeking," or "The patient is rude," can lead to charges of libel, particularly if the patient has reason to believe that the words adversely affect care given by others.

If the defamatory remarks have the potential of harming the business prospects of the person, proof of damage is not needed. An example of this can be seen in the case of *Schessler v. Keck* (1954). In this case, an unmarried female caterer had a false positive test for syphilis. Though the patient had never had the disease, a nurse seeing her catering at a party told the hostess that the woman was being treated for syphilis. This resulted in destroying the patient's business. The appeals court found that there was a valid basis for her claim of slander.

Nurses have also been the object of defamatory remarks. A physician accused his office nurse of having mixed up reports on a patient's chart and lying about it. He fired her the next day and called a meeting of his office employees. He told his staff that he couldn't work with anyone who was a liar, untrustworthy, and disloyal. A jury awarded the nurse $125,000 in damages (Creighton, 1986).

In certain instances, derogatory remarks may not constitute defamation. Two defenses to defamation include truth and privilege. In fact, there may be a legal or moral duty to pass on defamatory information in certain circumstances. For instance, a nurse has the duty to report suspected child abuse, a director of nursing service has a duty to report truthfully the character and qualifications of nurses to potential employers, and peer review groups are required to discuss privileged information for the purpose of improving services, disciplining providers, and so forth. Additionally, nurses are ethically obligated to report the illegal or incompetent practice of others. To avoid charges of defamation, prudent nurses will take care to observe appropriate channels of communication when making reports of this nature. In the absence of privileged communication, truth is a good defense for defamation.

RECENT LEGAL TRENDS

The combination of an evolving health care delivery system, increased public awareness, and a vigorous legal system have led to changes in the delivery of care, exposure to potential sources of liability, and changing legal trends. The public has begun to subject both the individual provider and the health care system to intense legal scrutiny. Litigation involving managed care organizations, increasing numbers of malpractice claims against nurses, and movement toward criminalization of negligence are three recent legal trends. Legal implications of confidentiality and telenursing are also mentioned here because of recent laws and potential of both civil and criminal penalties for breaching patients' confidentiality.

Legal Trends Involving Managed Care Organizations

Promising efficiency and economy of health care delivery, managed care organizations (MCOs) are replacing traditional fee-for-service providers. As a result of policies that encourage restrictions of expensive services, MCOs are experiencing significant financial corporate liability losses (Fiesta, 1996b). Being both the insurer and provider of care, MCOs have a vested interest in providing the most cost-efficient services. This can sometimes lead to diminution of the quality of care and liability. Managed care liability may be direct or indirect.

Direct liability occurs when negative patient outcomes result from the MCO's actions that are unduly influenced by cost-containment measures. Such actions may include improper denial of care, or financial incentives to providers that result in a denial (O'Keefe, 2000). Fiesta cites a case in Georgia in which a jury awarded $45 million to a family whose son had his hands amputated as a result of Kaiser Permanente's efforts to minimize health care costs. The malpractice occurred when the child's mother called the MCO's emergency line to report that her infant son was lethargic and had a temperature of 104 degrees. The nurse on duty first told the mother to place the child in a tepid bath and, after checking with a physician, instructed her to take the child to an approved Kaiser Permanente affiliate, even though there was a closer hospital. The child's heart stopped en route to the hospital and gangrene resulted from lack of circulation to his extremities. The family's lawyer argued that this was an example of what happens when cost-conscious managed care providers try to cut corners.

A MCO may be held indirectly liable because of its relationship with the physician or provider of care (O'Keefe, 2000). They choose the clinicians who provide care to members. Having a duty to investigate provider credentials and expertise and to offer competent and qualified providers, MCOs take on potential liability under the corporate negligence doctrine (Fiesta, 1996b). Courts have concluded that by limiting members' choice of providers to a select group, there is an unreasonable risk of harm if the clinicians are unqualified or incompetent. MCOs must be careful that decisions regarding quality and availability of care are not negatively affected by financial considerations.

Malpractice Claims Against Nurses

As the health care system changes, nurses are the target of a growing number of malpractice charges. According to Fiesta (1996a), though many of the current issues point toward examples of corporate liability, cases involving the actions of individual nurses are also increasing. Traditional errors such as burns, falls, and medication errors seem to be more common than in the past. This leads to the speculation that negligent actions are a direct result of increased stress in the workplace and decreased morale, which together lead to the overall effect of distracting nurses from focusing clearly on individual patients. "As the health care delivery system undergoes monumental change, it is apparent that the traditional areas of liability exposure continue to exist while simultaneously new areas of risk exposure are evolving" (1996a, p. 22). Validated trends in malpractice litigation include the following:

1. Nurses continue to appear as named defendants, emphasizing the fact that nurses are professionally accountable for their own actions.

2. Telephone call situations continue to indicate high levels of liability exposure, because of the potential for miscommunication and the lack of documentation supporting the defendant's version of the conversation.

3. Failure to communicate and to access the chain of command continues to be a major liability risk for nurses.

4. Obstetrical cases continue to present high monetary losses when negligence is established. (Fiesta, 1996a, pp. 22–24)

Criminalization of Nurses' Professional Negligence

Traditionally, nurses who make errors that cause harm to patients have been charged with the unintentional tort of professional negligence (malpractice). Either heard in civil court or settled out of court, charges of negligence against nurses have not resulted in criminal prosecution. It appears, however, that there may be a disturbing legal trend toward charging nurses with criminal negligence in particular cases. Cathy A. Klein, a nurse practitioner and practicing defense attorney, reports on one such case:

> Until recently, the risk of criminal prosecution for nursing practice was non-existent unless nursing action arose to the level of criminal intent, such as the case of euthanasia leading to murder charges. However, in April, 1997, three nurses were indicted by a Colorado grand jury for criminally negligent homicide in the death of a newborn. Public records show that one nurse was assigned to care for the baby. A second nurse offered to assist her colleague in caring for the baby. A third nurse was a nurse practitioner working in the hospital nursery. Because the baby was at risk for congenital syphilis, the physician ordered that the nurses give 150,000 units of intramuscular penicillin-which would have required five separate injections. In relation to other problems the same day, the baby was subjected to a lumbar puncture which required six painful attempts. To avoid inflicting further pain, Nurse Two asked the nurse practitioner if there was another route available for administration of the penicillin. Nurse Two and the nurse practitioner searched recognized pharmacology references and determined that IV administration would be acceptable. The nurse practitioner had the authority to change the route and directed Nurse Two to administer the medication intravenously rather than intramuscularly. Unrecognized by the nurses, the pharmacy

erroneously delivered the medication prepared and ready to administer in a dose ten times greater than was ordered—1.5 million units. As Nurse Two was administering the medication intravenously, the baby died. The Colorado Board of Nursing initiated disciplinary proceedings against Nurse Two and the nurse practitioner, but not against Nurse One. The grand jury indicted all three nurses on charges of criminally negligent homicide, but did not indict the pharmacist. (C. A. Klein, personal communication, May, 14, 1997)

This case is an ominous reminder of the days of witch hunts, when bad outcomes of childbirth led to the execution of nurse midwives. It is a frightening example of the devastating and unpredictable consequences that can occur when a nurse makes a serious error.

Ask Yourself

Criminal Negligence Versus Malpractice

- What feelings are evoked as you consider the example above?
- Should the courts take into consideration the fact that the nurses' error occurred because they wanted to avoid causing the baby unnecessary pain? Discuss your thinking.
- Can you think of other occupations in which the consequences of unintentional errors have greater legal implications? Discuss your answer with classmates.
- How should the profession respond to this frightening new legal threat?

Confidentiality of Electronic Communications

This is the age of electronic communication. We use electronic media every day: telephone, wireless phone, cell phone, fax machine, voice mail, pager, intranet, Internet, videotape, satellite and microwave transmission, and radio communication. We discuss patient care over telephones, send records via fax or e-mail, and participate in video conferencing. Regardless of the media, we still have a duty to protect patient privacy and confidentiality. Interception of electronic confidential material can occur in a variety of ways, either unintentional or intentional. For example, unauthorized personnel may have access to electronic information on an institution's computer network; wireless or cordless telephone communications may be inadvertently intercepted; and Internet communications pass through a number of non-secure operator computers. Nurses' use of electronic communications raises a number of legal and ethical questions. What are the legal implications of electronic communications? What is our responsibility of maintaining patient confidentiality? How does electronic communication affect the regulation of nursing practice?

Telenursing is the provision of nursing care utilizing any form of electronic media. In addition to confidentiality issues stipulated in codes of ethics and state nursing regulations, telenursing is regulated by other laws, such as the Uniform Health Care Information Act (UHCIA) and federal wiretap statutes. Any information transmitted over wire, cable, or like connection are subject to federal wiretap statutes. These statutes prohibit intercepting and recording of information and preclude its use in legal proceedings. Although there are no reported legal cases involving telenursing practice, in general case law supports the patient's right to confidentiality regardless of the type of media. Currently under revision, the UHCIA identifes some legal implications of telenursing. These implications include identification of standards for disclosure, the nurse's potential for civil and criminal liability, and elements necessary for valid disclosure authorization from the patient (O'Keefe, 2000). In general, the nurse must follow the standard of reasonableness to protect the confidentiality of health care information. In other words, the nurse must reasonably believe that health care information is secure, or that authorization for its disclosure is authentic. The nurse may legally disclose health care information if there is valid authorization. Authorization must be written, dated, and signed by the patient; specify the type or nature of information to be disclosed; and identify the person to whom the health care information will be disclosed. Failure to use reasonable safeguards to secure the confidentiality of health information may result in criminal and/or civil liability. Criminal liability may include conviction of a misdemeanor, with a fine not exceeding $10,000 and/or imprisonment of no more than one year. Civil remedies include recovery of damages, particularly if the nurse is found to have obtained or disclosed information with malice or gross negligence (O'Keefe, 2000).

Different types of electronic media have different risks of unintentional disclosure. For example, wireless telephone communications are more likely to be intercepted than either land-based or cellular telephone communications and non-encrypted Internet e-mail is more susceptible to interception than encrypted (O'Keefe, 2000). Nurses can be reasonably assured that institutional network communications systems provide privacy of information. Although many health care personnel have access to institutions' intranet computer network systems, employees are bound by a duty of confidentiality as required by the institution.

Telenursing also raises questions about the regulation of nursing practice. Many of these questions are yet to be fully addressed. What are the implications for nurses who staff telephone advice lines for hospital networks or managed care organizations with multistate networks? Can nurses offer advice to patients in states in which they are not licensed? If the purpose of a telecommunications system is to help to provide access to providers or specialists, what is the nurse's role in implementing orders from out-of-state physicians? Although there are no standards governing telenursing, both the American Nurses Association and the National Council of State Boards of Nursing are studying the issues. We must recognize that we are at the cusp of a new era of health care information. Without the guidance of regulations and standards, we must be sensitive to the legal and ethical implications of telenursing, carefully safeguarding patients' rights to privacy and confidentiality.

RISK MANAGEMENT

Recognizing the litigious state of today's society, how can nurses limit the risk of lawsuits? Much of today's litigation occurs as a result of events over which nurses have little control. Unfortunate outcomes can result from institutional circumstances, errors or incompetence of other professionals, or unpredictable or intractable physical phenomena. Other litigation occurs as a result of thoughtless or negligent actions on the part of nurses or other professionals. Though it is impossible to completely eliminate the risk of litigation, attention to a number of critical factors may reduce the threat of malpractice suits. Critical factors include maintaining open communication with patients, conscientious practice, and autonomy. (See Figure 7–3.)

Figure 7–3 **Reducing the Risk of Malpractice Litigation**

I. Maintain Good Communication
- Be courteous, show respect, and take time to listen attentively
- Do not belittle patients or make value judgments
- Involve patients in decision making
- Assess patients' level of understanding
- Explain in language that patients can understand
- Clarify and verify telephone orders; whenever possible, avoid accepting telephone orders or giving advice over the telephone

II. Maintain Expertise in Practice
- Keep up-to-date in both knowledge and skills
- Do not attempt any task or give any medication that is unfamiliar
- Practice within the professional and statutory scope of practice
- Be familiar with and follow institutional and professional standards of care
- Be attentive to patients' changing health status
- Pay close attention to detail, avoiding distraction
- Document objectively, thoroughly, and in a timely fashion

III. Maintain Autonomy and Empowerment
- Challenge questionable physician orders
- Seek attention for patients with changing health status
- Challenge bureaucratic structures that threaten patient welfare
- Avoid institutional settings that produce systematic and persistent threats to patient welfare

Maintaining Communication with Patients

On many occasions, nurses could have prevented malpractice lawsuits had they paid careful attention to interpersonal relationships and good communication techniques. Patients tend to become angry if they believe they are not being taken seriously, are not being listened to, are being belittled, or are denied involvement in the decision making process. Regardless of the professional's knowledge or ability, angry patients are more likely to file lawsuits. One of the most important factors in reducing the risk of litigation is a genuine regard for others. This quality produces nurses who are courteous, honest, and caring. They maintain open lines of communication, spend the time that is required to show respect, have genuine interest and patience, and listen to understand. The value of untiring listening cannot be overemphasized. Anecdotal information reveals that a professional's lack of listening is a key element for patients who are inclined to file lawsuits. In addition to the psychosocial benefits, listening with a discerning ear can lead to clues of health status that might otherwise have gone undetected. Good communicators listen objectively, avoid making value judgments, and include patients in health care decisions.

Patients may also sue when there are negative outcomes resulting from a lack of understanding of self-care, treatment options, potential outcomes of treatments, side effects of drugs, and so forth. In addition to listening skills, good communication techniques include assessing patients' level of understanding and finding ways to help patients to understand important information. Nurses with a genuine regard for others are more likely to be aware of patients' level of understanding. They will teach and explain, being respectful, yet using language that patients understand. They will ensure that informed consent is truly informed. They will continue to check and recheck patients' level of understanding, involving other family members when appropriate. Because lawsuits are frequent, and it is particularly difficult to assess patients' level of understanding, nurses need to be especially careful about giving advice or patient teaching over the telephone.

Maintaining Conscientious Practice

There are many factors related to conscientious practice. Recall that expertise in practice is not only one hallmark of a professional but is also a legal and ethical imperative. There have been monumental advances in knowledge and technology in the past several years. With the advent of health insurance in the post–World War II era and malpractice litigation in recent years, standards of care have become very stringent. Society's expectations of nurses' knowledge and abilities are high. Consequently, nurses must strive to maintain up-to-date knowledge and technical skills. Lack of knowledge is no defense in a court of law. It is, in fact, tantamount to an admission of negligence. It is important that nurses know and uphold institutional, professional, and legal standards of practice and work within their scope of practice, never attempting to perform any task or administer any medication that is unfamiliar. Nurses' actions are examined in light of current information, professional or statutory scope of practice, and institutional and professional practice standards. Statements such as "Everyone does it that way," "That is what I learned in school 20 years ago," or "I did the best I could" will not protect a nurse from being found negligent.

Conscientious practice also includes close attention to detail. Nurses make serious errors when they become overly tired or distracted, are called away from tasks, are inattentive to patients' changing health status, or do not take the time to document thoroughly. Attention to detail will eliminate many errors that result in charges of negligence. Ethics and the law are closely related in regard to attention to detail. Recall from Chapter 2 that deontological ethics requires that each person is seen as an end and not as a means only, and that one is compelled to fulfill one's duty to others, thus implying that nurses must focus clearly upon each patient and each task. Attention to detail will serve to improve patient outcomes and protect the nurse against lawsuits.

Maintaining Autonomy and Empowerment

As the examples in this chapter have illustrated, the courts demand that nurses practice autonomously. Time and again, court decisions have indicated that society expects nurses to be courageous in questioning physicians' orders (particularly those given over the telephone), vigorous in seeking attention for patients with changing health status, and active in challenging bureaucratic structures that threaten patient welfare. The courts know that nurses have in-depth knowledge in areas such as pharmacology and pathophysiology, and expect nurses to protect patients from harm. Facing institutional situations that systematically present threats to patient safety and welfare, and being unable to bring about change, nurses may find they can protect themselves from liability only by leaving the situation.

Liability Insurance

Despite efforts to reduce the risk of liability, nurses are increasingly vulnerable to claims of malpractice. Regardless of nurses' level of expertise, patients can be injured. Even if a claim has no merit, the process of defense is time consuming, emotionally exhausting, and costly. Liability insurance is an important risk management strategy that protects assets and income and affords nurses peace of mind. Professional liability insurance provides for payment of lawyer fees and settlement or jury awards. It also provides nurses a mechanism of accountability in that they have the ability to pay should their actions cause injury (Guido, 1997). Nurses should never be without liability coverage.

Choosing a particular type of malpractice policy can be confusing and intimidating. How much coverage is appropriate? Are occurrence-based or claims-made policies better? Do nurses need individual policies if they have employer-sponsored coverage? Is it important that nurses be knowledgeable about their unique malpractice risks?

There are two basic types of insurance coverage. Occurrence-based policies provide broad coverage. These policies cover the nurse for claims arising from incidents that occur during the period of time that the policy is in effect. Occurrence-based policies protect the nurse when lawsuits are filed after the policy has expired, even if the policy was not renewed. In particular, nurses who work with children or infants run the risk of lawsuits being filed many years after an injury occurs. Claims-made policies provide coverage only in instances in which both the injury and the claim are made during the time in which the policy is in effect. This type of coverage is adequate if the nurse maintains continuous coverage and purchases a tail to provide uninterrupted extension for a period of time after the policy period. Occurrence-based policies are preferable for most nurses.

Another distinction is made between malpractice policies and professional liability policies. Generally speaking, *malpractice policies* offer coverage exclusively for claims of malpractice. Though specific coverage differs from policy to policy, *professional liability* insurance offers protection against various injuries that are not directly related to malpractice (Mitchell & Grippando, 1993).

Nurses also question whether they need individual coverage if their group or employer provides insurance. *Individual coverage* is purchased by the individual and offers the policy holder twenty-four-hour protection against liability claims for actions that fall within the scope of professional nursing practice, either paid or volunteer services (Guido, 1997). Individual coverage pays lawyer fees and monetary damages (in relation to limits of the specific policy) and offers the nurse some control over details of the defense strategy. Infrequently used by nurses, *group coverage* is purchased by professionals who have essentially the same job descriptions and covers only those activities performed during office hours. This is particularly attractive as a less expensive choice for nurse practitioners in group practice. *Employer-sponsored coverage* is purchased by the employing agency for the purpose of protecting business concerns. Coverage under employer-sponsored policies limits the protection to activities performed within the scope of employment. Though employers may claim that employer-sponsored coverage is adequate, it is actually the most limited type of liability insurance. In fact, if found negligent, nurses may be required to repay the employer a portion of the loss. Guido (1997) reports that nurses who rely solely on hospital policies have a greater chance of inadequate monetary protection and legal counsel.

NURSES AS EXPERT WITNESSES

The role of expert witness is relatively new to the nursing profession. Because of the complex and highly technical nature of nursing, attorneys require the assistance of knowledgeable and experienced expert witnesses. These witnesses may be hired by either the plaintiff or the defendant. Serving the legal system, expert witnesses are neither parties to the dispute nor patient advocates. Ideally, they remain honest and give objective opinions to the court.

Serving as an expert witness involves a complex and extensive process of examining evidence, reviewing pertinent nursing literature, giving depositions, and testifying in court. The expert witness is expected to be familiar with the following: all medical records of the patient during the time of the incident; pertinent written policies and procedures of the institution; the nursing care plan, including nursing assessment, diagnosis, plan, interventions, and evaluation; the state nurse practice act; the Joint Commission on Accreditation of Healthcare Organizations manual; applicable nursing standards; current professional literature outlining accepted practice at the time of the incident; and opinions from the state board of nursing (Dyke, 1989). The witness must describe the standards of care to the court, evaluate the nurse's actions against them, and discuss conclusions relative to the accusation of malpractice. Effectiveness of the expert witness is influenced by the breadth of experience, degree of preparation, depth of knowledge, and confident delivery.

The use of expert witnesses gives strength to the argument that nursing is a true profession. It supports the autonomy of nursing in that no other professional can appropriately judge the practice of nurses. Strickland and Fishman (1994) suggest that nursing leaders should collaborate with members of the legal profession to establish professional standards for the role, and develop educational programs for interested and qualified nurses.

SUMMARY

As the enforceable system of principles and processes that govern the behavior of people, laws reflect moral and ethical tradition. Though there is sometimes disagreement regarding the rightness or wrongness of certain laws, the laws are generally consistent with popular beliefs.

Laws in the United States are either constitutional, statutory, or administrative, and are divided into public and private realms. Public law deals with the relationship between persons and the government, and private law deals with the relationship between people. Nurses and other health care providers are more likely to be involved in liability cases related to tort law, a division of private law. Tort law includes unintentional torts, such as negligence and malpractice, and intentional torts, such as fraud, invasion of privacy, assault, battery, false imprisonment, and defamation.

Recent trends in health care delivery systems have both created new areas of liability and increased instances of traditional negligence. Managed care organizations, while assuming the roles of both insurer and provider of health care, are frequently charged with corporate negligence. Perhaps because of increased stressors in the workplace, nurses are experiencing an increasing number of malpractice claims related to the traditional kinds of errors.

With the increase in malpractice litigation, nurses are wise to take certain precautions to limit the risk of lawsuits. Critical factors include maintaining open lines of communication with patients through the use of good listening techniques, accepting demeanor, and attention to patients' level of understanding; maintaining conscientious practice, including retaining expertise and ensuring attention to detail; maintaining autonomy through courageous and vigorous patient advocacy; and maintaining continuous professional liability insurance. When patients charge nurses with malpractice, expert nurse witnesses can serve the court by describing standards of care, evaluating the nurse's action against standards, and discussing conclusions relative to the accusation of malpractice.

CHAPTER HIGHLIGHTS

- Ethics is the foundation of law; however, because laws are created by individuals and there are differences in beliefs among people, ethics and the law are not always congruent.

- Constitutional law is based upon the Constitution and supersedes all other law.

- Statutory law is created through the lawmaking process in state or federal legislatures; it is also called legislative law.

- Administrative law consists mainly of the legal powers granted to administrative agencies by the legislature, and the rules that the agencies make to carry out their powers.

- Common law, also known as case law, is a system of law based largely on previous court decisions.
- Public law defines a person's rights and obligations in relation to government, and describes the various divisions of government and their powers.
- Private law, also called civil law, determines a person's legal rights and obligations in many kinds of activities that involve other people.
- A tort is a wrong or injury that a person suffers because of someone else's action, either intentional (willful or intentional acts that violate another person's rights or property) or unintentional (an act or omission that causes unintended injury or harm to another person).
- Changes in health care financing and delivery have caused litigation related to corporate liability.
- Nurses can limit the risk of liability through maintaining open communication with patients, expertise in practice, attention to details, and autonomy.
- Supporting the autonomous nature of nursing, expert nurse witnesses serve the court through the process of examining evidence, applying nursing standards, reviewing pertinent nursing literature, and explaining conclusions.

DISCUSSION QUESTIONS AND ACTIVITIES

1. Search the World Wide Web for references to recent court decisions. You may begin by visiting the site www.npg.com/npg/1999/index.html. Find examples of recent court cases related to issues such as termination of life support, fetal tissue use, genetic engineering, and patient self-determination. Discuss your ethical beliefs related to the court decisions. What ethical principles are applicable?

2. Discuss with classmates their opinions about the courts becoming involved in issues that have traditionally been considered ethical in nature.

3. Read the Bill of Rights of the United States Constitution. How do the rights guaranteed in the Bill of Rights relate to patient care? How do they relate to nurses' employment?

4. Discuss recent examples of state or federal legislation that create changes in the health care delivery system or in the practice of nursing.

5. In the common law system, how do previous court decisions affect the outcome of current cases?

6. Discuss instances in which nurses can be charged with crimes of public law, even though acts were committed without malice in the process of giving nursing care.

7. Discuss specific examples of unintentional torts of which nurses have been accused.

8. How can you protect yourself from being accused of an unintentional tort?

9. In what instances can nurses be charged with intentional torts, even though they follow a professional code of ethics?

10. Discuss areas of potential liability for nurses and the present health care delivery system.

REFERENCES

Beauchamp, T. L. (2001). *Philosophical ethics: An introduction to moral philosophy* (3rd ed.). Boston: McGraw-Hill.

Bernzweig, E. P. (1990). *The nurse's liability for malpractice* (5th ed.). St. Louis, MO: Mosby.

Big Town Nursing Home, Inc. v. Newman, 461 S.W.2d 195 (Tex. Civ. App. 1970).

Blackman for Blackman v. Rifkin, 759 P.2d 54 (Colo. App. 1988), *cert. denied* (1989).

Catalano, J. T. (1991). *Ethical and legal aspects of nursing*. Springhouse, PA: Springhouse.

Creighton, H. (1986). *Law every nurse should know* (5th ed.). Philadelphia: Saunders.

Dyke, R. M. (1989). The nurse expert witness: Professional implications. *Neonatal Network, 8*(3), 3–39.

Erskeris, T. R. (1998). Seven common legal pitfalls in nursing. *American Journal of Nursing, 98*(4), 34–44.

Ferris vs. County of Kennebec, 44F. Supp. 2d 62—ME (1998)

Fiesta, J. (1988). *The law and liability: A guide for nurses* (2nd ed.). New York: John Wiley & Sons.

Fiesta, J. (1996a). Legal update, 1995: Part 1. *Nursing Management, 27*(5), 22–24.

Fiesta, J. (1996b). Legal update, 1995: Part 2. *Nursing Management, 27*(6), 24–25.

Furrow, B. R., Johnson, S. H., Jost, T. S., & Schwartz, R. L. (1991). *Liability and quality issues in health care*. St. Paul, MN: West.

Guido, G. W. (1997). *Legal issues in nursing* (2nd ed.). Norwalk, CT: Appleton & Lange.

King, M. L., Jr. (1996). Letter from the Birmingham jail. In J. Feinberg, ed., *Reason and responsibility: Readings in some basic problems of philosophy* (9th ed., pp. 572–580). Belmont, CA: Wadsworth. (Reprinted from M. King, Jr., *Why we can't wait*, 1963, John Davis Agency).

Kozier, B., & Erb., G. (1992). *Concepts and issues in nursing practice* (2nd ed.). Menlo Park, CA: Addison-Wesley.

Lee, G. (2000). Legal issues: Proving nursing negligence. *American Journal of Nursing, 100*(11), 55–56

Mazzocco, W. J. (2000). "Mixed" billing raises questions. *Advance for Nurse Practitioners,* 24–25.

Miller-Slade, D. (1997, May). Liability theories in nursing negligence cases. *Trial,* 52–57.

Mitchell, P., & Grippando, G. (1993). *Nursing perspectives and issues.* (5th ed.). Albany, NY: Delmar.

O'Keefe, M. E. (2000). *Nursing practice and the law: Avoiding malpractice and other legal risks.* Philadelphia: F. A. Davis.

Oswald v. LeGrand, 453 N.W.2d 634 (Iowa 1990).

Physician Insurers Association of America. (1993). *Medication Error Study.* Rockville, JD: Author.

Rhodes, A. M., & Miller, R. D. (1984). *Nursing and the law* (4th ed.). Rockville, MD: Aspen Systems.

Robertson v. Provident House, 576 So. 2d 992 (La. 1991).

Schessler v. Keck, 271 P.2d 588 (Cal. Ct. App. 1954).

Smelko v. Brinton, 740 P.2d 591 (Kan. 1987).

Smith v. Juneau, 692 So. 2d 1365 (1997).

State of Louisiana v. Brenner, 486 So. 2d 101 (La. 1986).

Strickland, O., & Fishman, D. (1994). *Nursing issues in the 1990s.* Albany, NY: Delmar.

Truhitte v. French Hospital, 180 Cal. Rptr. 152 (Cal. Ct. App. 1982).

CHAPTER 8

Professional Issues

[A]s we stand on the threshold of a historic event in nursing, let us repeat that we join to accomplish for nursing those objectives impossible to do so singularly. We are living in a very complicated world and with the pressures of science, technology, and societal demands, nursing must foster its image, determine its goals, and plan its direction, or the outside forces will indeed obliterate this profession.

(Zschoche, 1983)

OBJECTIVES

After completing this chapter, the reader should be able to:

1. Discuss the meaning of the term professional, including traits commonly associated with professional status and the historical debate regarding the professional status of nursing.
2. Relate codes of ethics to professional status.
3. Discuss the relationships among the concepts of expertise, ethics, and professional status.
4. Discuss autonomy in terms of both the individual nurse and the profession of nursing.
5. Discuss the relationship between professional autonomy and ethics.
6. Discuss the concept of *accountability*, including various mechanisms of nursing accountability.
7. Explain the relationship between accountability and professional status.
8. Define the concept of *authority*, differentiating between professional and personal authority.
9. Discuss the concept of unity and its relationship to professional status in nursing.

INTRODUCTION

An examination of ethics in nursing inevitably leads us to questions about whether nursing is a profession. Is nursing a profession? What are the criteria that define a profession? Who decides? This chapter begins by examining the meaning and historical context of the term profession, and then discusses the professional status of nursing and the selected characteristics of expertise, autonomy, accountability, authority, and unity in nursing.

PROFESSIONAL STATUS

Professions exist for the purpose of meeting the needs of society. The larger society determines its needs, and authorizes certain people to meet those needs. There is a uniform process by which professionals develop the values that lead to a type of social responsibility and desire to meet the needs of society (Aydelotte, 1990). Professionals contract with society by promising to meet a set of identified needs better than any other group of people. In turn, society grants the profession a monopoly over these particular services. Historically, professions have attempted to instill in their members a somber recognition of the profound nature of their responsibility through the recitation of pledges and oaths, such as the Hippocratic Oath for physicians and the Nightingale Pledge for nurses.

Since before the turn of the twentieth century, nurses and others have debated the professional status of nursing. Professions have been described in a number of ways. Gruending (1985) describes a **profession** as a complex, organized occupation preceded by a long training program. Professional education is geared toward the acquisition of exclusive knowledge necessary to provide a service that is either essential or desired by society. These attributes lead to a monopoly that provides autonomy, public recognition, prestige, power, and authority for the practitioner. Many other distinguishing attributes of professions have been proposed over the years. Among others, these include expertise, accountability, the presence of systematic theory, ethical codes, a professional culture, an altruistic service orientation, competence testing, licensure, high income, credentialing, the description of a scope of practice, and the establishment of standards.

Ask Yourself

Is Nursing a Profession?

Most nursing programs have course content that is geared toward identifying the professional status of nursing through the use of identified traits or functions.

- Do you recall discussions in earlier courses about the professional status of nursing? If so, what do you recall from those discussions?

- What (or whose) criteria were used to judge professional status?

- Based upon what you recall, would you identify nursing as a profession, an emerging profession, a quasi-profession, or an occupation struggling to become a profession?

A classic source describing the criteria of professionals is Abraham Flexner. An educator, Flexner was well known for his 1910 evaluation of the professional status of medical schools. In 1915, Flexner listed traits that he observed in the established professions of medicine, law, and the clergy. He then proposed that in order to be recognized as professions, all occupations must meet these criteria. Following are six criteria that he utilized to identify professions:

1. professions involve essentially intellectual operations;
2. they derive their raw materials from science and learning;
3. this material they work up to a practical and definite end;
4. they possess an educationally communicable technique;
5. they tend to self-organization;
6. they are becoming increasingly altruistic in motivation. (Flexner, 1915, pp. 901–912)

Unsolicited by the nursing community, Flexner evaluated nursing according to his criteria. He judged that nursing was not a profession. Optimistically, he proposed that occupations could alter their status by developing these traits.

Subsequently, in 1945 and 1959, two educators, Genevieve and Roy Bixler, published landmark articles in the *American Journal of Nursing* (AJN) evaluating the professional status of nursing. These articles utilized criteria similar to those proposed by Flexner. They listed the following seven criteria of a profession:

1. A profession utilizes in its practice a well-defined and well-organized body of specialized knowledge which is on the intellectual level of the higher learning;
2. A profession constantly enlarges the body of knowledge it uses and improves its techniques of education and service by the use of the scientific method;
3. A profession entrusts the education of its practitioners to institutions of higher education;
4. A profession applies its body of knowledge in practical services which are vital to human and social welfare;
5. A profession functions autonomously in the formulation of professional policy and in the control of professional activity, thereby;
6. A profession attracts individuals of intellectual and personal qualities who exalt service above personal gain and who recognize their chosen occupation as a life work; and
7. A profession strives to compensate its practitioners by providing freedom of action, opportunity for continuous professional growth, and economic security. (Bixler & Bixler, 1959, pp. 1142–1147)

Predictably, the Bixler evaluations came to the same conclusion as Flexner: Nursing was deficient as a true profession.

Though both Flexner and the Bixlers had a tremendous lasting impact on nursing, none were nurses. Even though their lists of traits seem to have been chosen arbitrarily, their approach assumes that true professions will demonstrate all of the essential attributes. Fowler (1990) calls their lists of characteristics "an untidy aggregation of overlapping, arbitrarily chosen, or undifferentiated elements, lacking a unifying theoretical framework that explains their interrelationship" (p. 24).

Prior to the Flexner report, American nurses were secure in their identity as professionals. Even physicians and the judicial system recognized nursing as a profession. However, following the Flexner report and the subsequent Bixler articles, nurses began to question their status as professionals (Parsons, 1986). Like sixteenth-century women who came to believe the myth that women were intrinsically evil, nurses accepted the idea that nursing was not a true profession (Newman, 1990; Sleicher, 1981). The process of examining and evaluating, though, resulted in many positive changes for nursing. Striving to meet the criteria set by Flexner and the Bixlers, nurses became involved in research to create a unique body of knowledge for nursing, to move "professional" nursing education to the university setting, to become politically involved, to increase the autonomy of nursing, and to extend practice boundaries.

There are those who argue that the process used to identify traits of professions was flawed from the inception (Achterberg, 1990; Ehrenreich & English, 1973; Parsons, 1986). There are even those who suggest that the term *professional* is sexist, elitist, and racist. At the turn of the century, the three "professions" that were said to be universally accepted as such—medicine, law, and the clergy—were overwhelmingly male and Caucasian. As a result of the cultural and religious influences discussed in Chapter 1, by the time Flexner wrote his report, women had been systematically purged from both professional education and practice. Examining and describing traits of the male-dominated "professions," and subsequently using those findings as criteria to judge the professional status of other occupations, may have effectively excluded all predominately female groups.

Nurses as Professionals

For lack of a better word, nurses continue to discuss their occupation in terms of a profession. Recognizing that there are a myriad of sources claiming to define the term professional by describing traits, attributes, functions, or characteristics, there will likely never be agreement about the professional status of nursing. Even though these discussions are important, for the purposes of this chapter, we make the assumption that nursing is a true profession.

In many ways nurses, as professionals, are connected to each other and set apart from others. Professionals are connected to each other by common experiences, language, and body of knowledge. We are set apart from others by virtue of the prestige and mystique offered members of a profession, and by the knowledge that comes from personal, intimate, and spiritual experiences surrounding the beginning and the end of life (Nathaniel, 1994).

Beletz describes a professional as "one bound by values and standards other than those of his or her employing organization, setting one's own rules, seeking to promote standards of excellence, and being evaluated and looking for approval from one's own professional peers" (1990, p. 18). Jameton further suggests that being a professional is similar to having a calling. He describes a calling as "something one feels called upon to do, perhaps by God, by some deep need in one's being, or by the demands of historical circumstance. A calling is central to one's life and gives it meaning" (1984, p. 18). Moving the discussion further, Reed (2000) declares that nursing is a spiritual discipline. She argues that regarding a discipline as spiritual enhances the meaning of a profession. Reed writes that there is a pragmatic and normative call to action which is freely chosen by its members—one in which the person is said to be "called" or "launched outward to others" (p. 132).

EXPERTISE

Expertise relates to the characteristic of having a high level of specialized skill and knowledge. It is a "composite of a knowledge base, gained through long years of study in an academic setting, and superior skill. Expertise is the primary distinguishing difference between professionals and nonprofessionals" (Beletz, 1990, p. 17). Professionals must have the knowledge and functional skills required to meet the needs of society and thereby fulfill the purpose of the profession. Regarding expertise, Jameton writes:

> Professions maintain their autonomy partly through their claim to maximal competence [expertise]. So long as people believe that the professionals are the only ones who fully understand their work, it is very hard to supervise or criticize them. (1984, p. 21)

We gain expertise in a variety of ways. Extensive educational requirements, intense guided practice, examination for licensure, certification, and mandatory continuing education are ways that we either attain, maintain, or assert expertise. Florence Nightingale recognized the importance of an education consisting of depth and breadth of general knowledge, combined with a very specific nursing focus. Today we have a knowledge base that is continually expanded through research. Having completed basic nursing education and successfully demonstrated a minimum level of competence through licensure examination, we are further required (either ethically or legally) to continue the learning process and maintain up-to-date knowledge and technical proficiency. Continuing education programs assist us in this process. Our expertise is also advanced through graduate nursing education, specialty preparation, and the certification process.

Merely claiming expertise is not enough. Through the various mechanisms of accountability, we must prove to society that we are faithful to the promise the profession makes. In response, society grants us the authority to practice with a certain measure of autonomy. Thus, the professional realms of expertise, accountability, autonomy, and authority are interrelated.

Ask Yourself

When the Bottom Line Becomes Personal

Imagine that one of your loved ones becomes gravely ill and needs to be hospitalized. Your third-party payer determines the hospital and provider you must use. Because of your background, you are familiar with the nursing skills and knowledge needed to care adequately for your loved one. The nurses demonstrate poor knowledge and lack of basic skills, potentially leading to threats to the well-being of your family member.

- How would you feel in this circumstance?
- What do you think nurses' responsibilities are regarding their ability to care adequately for your loved one?
- Discuss your beliefs concerning an ethical requirement to maintain expertise in the area of practice.
- Does the profession have an obligation to society in this regard?

AUTONOMY

The word **autonomy** literally means "self-governing." The concept of nursing autonomy can be discussed on two levels: autonomy of the profession and autonomy of the individual practitioner. Self-regulation is the mark of collective professional autonomy. Individual autonomy involves self-determination, responsibility, accountability, independence, and a willingness to take risks. Autonomy is generally considered to be an important criterion in judging professional status of an occupation. People who are considered to be professionals have the power and authority to control various aspects of their work, including goals toward which to work, whether to work and with whom, details of how the work is to be done, choice of clientele, and so forth (Jameton, 1984). We continue to debate whether nurses have autonomy.

Since the profession of nursing is self-regulating, it can be said to be autonomous. Unlike the early years of this century, most state boards of nursing are now predominately made up of nurses. Given their authority granted by statutory law, boards of nursing enforce the individual states' nurse practice acts. This ensures the autonomy of the profession in each state. Among other tasks, boards of nursing oversee the schools of nursing within the states, control licensure, and discipline nurses.

Jameton (1984) implies that the profession of nursing maintains autonomy through the combination of a claim to maximal competence and a continuing monopoly over their work. He writes:

> Professions also maintain their autonomy by means of monopoly over their work. In our competitive culture, people do not achieve autonomy simply by declaring it or believing in it. Professions maintain their control over their work partly by keeping people with other skills and

other ideas from doing the same work. Only nurses may legally practice nursing. Licensure, educational requirements, certification of
schools, and the like help nurses maintain control over nursing practice. This control is strengthened when nurses—rather than physicians and nonprofessionals—control the processes of licensure and
certification. (p. 21)

No other group has the ability to do the work of nurses; consequently, there is a legal
restriction barring non-nurses from practicing nursing. This legally sanctioned monopoly helps to establish autonomy.

In recent years, non-nurse groups and organizations have attempted to undermine
the autonomy of the profession of nursing in various ways. The American Medical
Association's effort in the 1980s to institute a new category of bedside health care
provider, the Registered Care Technician (RCT), can be viewed as an attempt to gain
access into the domain of nursing, and thereby threaten the autonomy of the profession. Recognizing the implications of this proposal, in an unprecedented joint effort,
a number of disparate nursing organizations successfully banded together to oppose
this plan.

In the mid-1990s, hospital associations moved to gain some control over the profession of nursing. These groups targeted specific states in which to attempt drastic
changes in nurse practice acts (*State Scan,* 1996). These efforts included proposals to
legislate changes in the membership and the responsibilities of the state boards. In at
least one state, this effort included replacing an essentially all-nurse board with a new
board consisting of physicians, hospital administrators, consumers, and nurses. Recognizing a threat to the integrity of the profession, nurses in various states continue
to work to defend against opening of nurse practice acts by non-nursing groups. As
competition for health care dollars becomes more fierce, nurses will be acutely aware
of outside efforts that threaten the autonomy of the profession.

Nurses are both legally and ethically required to practice autonomously.
Autonomous practice serves as a safeguard for the patient, nurse, physician, and institution. Nursing codes of ethics support the nurse's autonomous decision making and
responsibility. Both the American Nurses Association (ANA) *Code for Nurses with Interpretive Statements* (1985) and the subsequent ANA *Code of Ethics for Nurses* (2001)
explicitly and implicitly call for autonomous action of nurses, particularly in relation
to assuming responsibility and accountability for individual nursing judgments and
actions and in regard to protecting the safety of patients. Similarly, the Canadian Nurses
Association *Code of Ethics for Registered Nurses* (1997) and the International Council
of Nurses *ICN Code of Ethics for Nurses* (2000) implicitly and explicitly reflect nursing
autonomy and responsibility. The purpose of autonomy as described in these codes
is to protect the patient from harm, and allow for the full benefit of professional nursing care.

We often hear questions about the autonomy of individual nurses. As a nurse, do
you really have autonomy? Can you say that you are autonomous, even though you
are required to follow physicians' orders? Are you autonomous, even though you can't
get to know the patients because you have too many patients and too much work to

do? Lyon defines autonomous nursing practice as "the diagnosis and treatment of phenomena that nurses have the self-directed authority to treat" (1990, p. 270). Furthermore, she writes that nursing has a social mandate for two different scopes of practice: the medical scope that requires physician authorization to initiate treatment, and the autonomous nursing scope that requires no authorization.

As a practical necessity, hospitals and other health care institutions, having physicians as their clients, must provide qualified staff to carry out physicians' orders. Combined with the provision of nursing care, carrying out of the medical plan of care is an essential service of many institutions. When we seek employment at these institutions, we are implicitly agreeing to perform the functions for which we are hired. Accepting a position implies this contract. Nevertheless, we are legally and ethically required to use independent judgment in making nursing decisions. We are required to be autonomous when we make these independent nursing judgments. The exercise of independent nursing judgment should be welcomed by institutions because of the safeguards that are afforded. It is not unusual to hear about a nurse who refuses to carry out a physician's order that is later found to be incorrect. Such actions protect patients from physician negligence, and thus prevent litigation against the nurse, the physician, and the institution. The fact that nurses are often found legally negligent for following questionable physicians' orders, or failing to follow through with the hierarchical chain of command when questioning or disagreeing with acts or omissions of physicians or others, proves that the courts not only recognize, but expect, nursing autonomy.

Ask Yourself

Judgments About Physicians' Orders

Nurses are frequently asked to give medication with which they are not familiar. Unable to quickly determine the appropriateness or safety of a given drug, nurses may decide to refuse to administer a particular drug.

- What feelings, emotions, and values are involved in the nurse's decision to refuse to follow a physician's order?
- What are some predictable reactions of the nurse's coworkers, supervisors, and physicians when a nurse refuses to follow a physician's order?
- What ethical principles can be used to guide such decisions?
- How is the nurse empowered in these types of situations?
- How would it affect the nurse if the drug in question is later found to be safe and appropriate? How should this affect future decisions?

Autonomy does not mean that we have absolute control of every facet of practice. Accepted as one of the three prototype professions, medicine, for example, no longer retains the measure of control it once enjoyed. Government regulations now guide such facets of medical care as reimbursement levels and length of hospital stays. Managed care organizations limit expensive procedures, referral networks, and formulary medications. Consequently, physicians, though continuing to maintain professional status, are experiencing less absolute control over patient care than ever before. In the past, some (including Abraham Flexner) based the argument that nurses were not autonomous on comparisons between the independent decision-making capacities of medicine and nursing. That comparison no longer illustrates a great degree of distinction.

It is clear that nurses do not always feel autonomous, and, in fact, some may not practice autonomously. Certainly there are nurses who spend each workday complying with physicians' orders and completing various nonautonomous tasks, never exercising independent nursing functions, nor making nursing diagnoses and initiating self-directed treatment. In the truest sense, these nurses are only marginally practicing professional nursing and cannot be said to be autonomous. When we practice in this manner, we fail our ethical duty to make independent nursing judgments.

ACCOUNTABILITY

According to the American Nurses Association (1985), "**Accountability** refers to being answerable to someone for something one has done. [It is] grounded in the moral principles of fidelity and respect for the dignity, worth, and self-determination of clients" (p. 8). Safe, autonomous practice is ensured through various processes of nursing accountability. Accountability is related to both responsibility and answerability. Because of the trust accorded nurses by society (gained through recognition of nurses' expertise) and the right given the profession to regulate practice (autonomy), individual practitioners and the profession must be both responsible and accountable.

Related to the concepts of autonomy and authority, accountability is an inherent part of everyday nursing practice. Each nurse is responsible for all individual actions and omissions. The ANA *Code for Nurses with Interpretive Statements* and the subsequent *Code of Ethics for Nurses* (2001) makes it clear that each nurse has the responsibility to maintain ethical and competent practice regardless of circumstances, stating that "neither physicians' orders nor the employing agency's policies relieve the nurse of accountability for actions taken and judgments made" (1985, p. 9). As has been previously noted, the courts have tended to support this claim.

Mechanisms of Accountability

Accountability is based upon the implicit contract between nursing and the larger society. Donabedian (1976) writes that self-regulation to ensure quality in performance is at the heart of the relationship between society and the professions—in fact, accountability is the "hallmark of a mature profession" (p. 8). The profession of nursing has developed several mechanisms through which this relationship between nursing and society is made explicit, thereby acknowledging to both the professional and the public the areas of nursing accountability. These mechanisms include codes of nursing ethics, standards of nursing practice, nurse practice acts, nursing theory and practice derived from nursing research, educational requirements for practice, advanced certification, and mechanisms for evaluating the effectiveness of nurses' performance of nursing responsibilities (ANA, 1985). In both a professional and a legal sense, it is necessary that we are familiar with various mechanisms of accountability.

Codes of Nursing Ethics. Nearly universally accepted as one criterion of a profession, a code of ethics is profoundly important to nursing. A **code of nursing ethics** is an explicit declaration of the primary goals and values of the profession that indicates the "profession's acceptance of the responsibility and trust with which it has been invested by society" (ANA, 1985, p. iii). Like other professions, nursing has developed and enforces specific obligations to ensure that members of society will find them to be competent and trustworthy. These obligations are correlative to the rights of individual patients and society as a whole (Beauchamp & Childress, 1994). Upon entrance into the profession, nurses make an implicit moral commitment to uphold the values and moral obligations expressed in their code. Nurses are called upon to base professional judgment upon consideration of consequences and the universal moral principles of respect for persons, autonomy, beneficence, nonmaleficence, veracity, confidentiality, fidelity, and justice (ANA, 1985). Examples of professional codes of ethics for nurses include the American Nurses Association *Code of Ethics for Nurses* (2001), the International Council of Nurses *Code for Nurses* (2000), and the Canadian Nurses Association *Code of Ethics for Registered Nurses* (1997) (see Appendices).

Standards of Nursing Practice. **Standards of nursing practice** are written documents outlining minimum expectations for safe nursing care. Standards may describe in detail specific acts performed by nurses or may outline the expected process of nursing care. We use standards to guide and evaluate nursing care. Courts look to standards of nursing practice for guidance when malpractice cases are deliberated. The two basic types of standards of nursing practice are internal and external standards (Fiesta, 1988).

Internal standards of nursing practice are those developed within the profession of nursing for the purpose of establishing the minimum level of nursing care. They help to ensure that nurses are competent and safe to practice. These documents guide us in giving nursing care, and can be used as a yardstick to measure the practice of individual nurses. Like other types of standards, internal standards can be used to determine whether the actions of nurses accused of malpractice are consistent with reasonable minimum expectations. An example of internal standards is the American Nurses Association *Standards of Nursing Practice*. These comprehensive standards utilize the nursing process. They make nurses accountable for ensuring that each step of the process is followed in the delivery of nursing care. The ANA also publishes standards of care for nurses in advanced or specialty roles, such as nurse practitioners, maternal-child nurses, geriatric nurses, psychiatric nurses, community health nurses, and others.

External standards of nursing practice consist of guides for nursing care that are developed by non-nurses, the government, or institutions. These standards describe the specific expectations of agencies or groups that utilize the services of nurses. They serve the same function as internal standards—guidance and evaluation. Examples of external standards include such documents as the nurse practice act of each state, guidelines by the Joint Commission on Accreditation of Healthcare Organizations, and formal policies and procedures for individual agencies. Nurses are responsible and accountable to know and follow the standards of care for the profession, the specialty (if applicable), the geographic area, and the institution.

Nurses in administrative or advisory capacities are often responsible for developing institutional standards. These nurses sometimes develop standards that describe ideal nursing care. This type of standard may actually create a risk by placing both practicing nurses and the employing institution in jeopardy of malpractice litigation. Because standards are used to judge nursing actions, they should reflect reasonable expectations for safe nursing care, rather than optimal or ideal care. While ensuring safe patient care, nursing standards must be practical and reasonable.

CASE PRESENTATION

When Standards Are Difficult to Meet

Linda is a registered nurse in charge of a large psychiatric unit. At any given time her unit houses an average of twenty-two patients with a variety of diagnoses, ranging from drug dependence to acute psychoses. The unit is usually staffed by one registered nurse, two licensed practical nurses, and two attendants. Hospital policy requires that the registered nurse evaluate each patient's physical and mental status at least twice per shift, supervise the administration of all psychotropic medication, participate in group activities, supervise the implementation of each patient's plan of care, and be available to individual patients for one-to-one interaction. There are additional standards that describe the appropriate care for patients who are potentially suicidal: "Patients who are identified as suicidal will be isolated in private rooms and continuously monitored by a registered nurse." On one particular day two of the patients are identified as potentially suicidal, six geriatric patients with dementia need to be fed and ambulated, one patient is exhibiting violent behavior, and all the patients need individual assessment. Linda calls the supervisor for assistance but is told that there is no one available to help her. The reader will no doubt have noticed that in addition to the other duties, Linda is required to simultaneously and continuously monitor two patients in separate rooms—a physical impossibility. Linda tries to meet all of her obligations under these very strict standards, yet while she is answering a question raised by one of her staff members, one of the suicidal patients manages to injure herself attempting to jump out of a window.

Think About It

Problems Posed by Unreasonable Institutional Standards

- What dilemmas are posed by these standards?
- What were Linda's alternatives?

- What is the purpose of the standards that Linda is required to follow?
- What do you see as the legal liability created by the standards?
- Do you think the institution shares the legal blame for the situation?
- What is the effect of the standards on Linda's practice?
- Is there any way that Linda can meet the standards?
- What do you think you would do in similar circumstances?
- What are the ethical implications for the institution and for Linda?

Nurse Practice Acts.   As the foremost legal statute regulating nursing, the **nurse practice act** of each state protects the public, defines nursing practice, describes the boundaries of practice, establishes standards for nurses, and protects the domain of nursing. Nurse practice acts are considered a form of nursing standard. Utilized by courts in determining the appropriateness of nursing actions, violations can result in either civil or criminal prosecution.

Each of the fifty states independently develops, updates, and interprets their own nurse practice act. Though both the ANA and the National Council of State Boards of Nursing, Inc., have developed model nurse practice acts in the past, the laws continue to be different in each state. Some nurse practice acts are very general and somewhat vague in describing parameters of the professional role. These laws are considered to be permissive, allowing nursing practice to change and grow in a dynamic way. Others list each act that nurses are permitted to perform. As nursing continues to evolve, these very specific nurse practice acts, while originally applauded as recognizing nurses' legitimate authority to perform certain advanced tasks, have become restrictive. Murphy says, "Specificity in the statute is not without its costs. Specifically worded statutes tend to freeze the status quo rather than accommodate evolving roles" (1990, p. 33). With nurses continually expanding the domain of nursing, very specific, restrictive nurse practice acts have become a barrier to advanced nursing practice. Reflecting this concept, the ANA document *Nursing's Social Policy Statement* states:

> Nursing's scope of practice is dynamic and evolves with changes in the phenomena of concern, in knowledge about various interventions' effects on patient or group outcomes, or in the political environment, legal conditions, and cultural demographic patterns in society. (1996, p. 12)

Because we are legally accountable to follow the standards set by the nurse practice acts within our states, we must be particularly attentive to the language describing the definition of nursing and the scope of nursing practice. Nurses are accountable to know and follow their states' nurse practice acts. Because legislatures meet and pass laws regularly, nurse practice acts can be changed often. We are responsible for knowing even the most recent changes in our states' nurse practice acts and for implementing these changes in practice.

Moreover, we are called upon to be active in promoting needed changes in nurse practice acts. The codes of ethics for both the ANA (1985, 2001) and the International Council of Nurses (2000) speak specifically about the nurse's responsibility to participate in the profession's efforts to implement and improve nursing standards. Recent changes in the health care delivery system, financing mechanisms, and roles of other health care professionals require careful study of existing nurse practice acts and judicious implementation of well-considered changes.

It is the job of state boards of nursing to interpret and carry out the provisions of the various states' nurse practice acts. Initially established by state governments nearly one hundred years ago, there are now state boards of nursing in all fifty states, the District of Columbia, and five United States territories: Guam, the Virgin Islands, Puerto Rico, American Samoa, and the Northern Mariana Islands. Their goal is to promote and protect public health, safety, and welfare through ensuring the safe practice of nursing. The boards accomplish this by establishing standards for safe nursing care, issuing licenses to practice nursing, monitoring the practice of nurses, and disciplining nurses as needed. State boards of nursing vary in their composition. Some consist almost exclusively of registered nurses, while others have a mix of registered nurses, licensed practical nurses, advanced practice nurses, and consumers (National Council of Boards of Nursing, 2000).

Nursing Theory and Practice Derived from Research. A frequently cited characteristic of professions is the existence of a unique body of knowledge derived from research. Recall that Genevieve and Roy Bixler's first two characteristics of a profession relate to a unique body of knowledge. The Bixlers' second characteristic actually calls for professions to constantly enlarge the body of knowledge by use of the scientific method (1959). In the past, authorities debated whether nursing's body of knowledge was unique to the profession, or was borrowed from behavioral and physical sciences and medicine. It seemed clear to some that nursing knowledge had been derived from the combination of experience and intuition, and by borrowing from other disciplines (Leddy & Pepper, 1989). Responding to arguments that nursing was not a true profession because of this lack of a clearly unique body of knowledge, nurses in academic and clinical settings began gathering data and doing legitimate research. The process of theory building and research in nursing continues to increase the unique body of nursing knowledge. The benefit of this process is twofold. First, the expanded knowledge base allows nurses to respond to the needs of society more knowledgeably and skillfully. Second, the presence of a clearly unique body of knowledge aids in validating nursing as a true profession.

AUTHORITY

The term **authority** relates to the state of having legitimate power and sovereignty. The authority to practice nursing is granted by statute, based upon the contract the profession has with society. The granting of authority acknowledges the professional's rights and responsibilities, and in turn requires that there be mechanisms for public accountability (ANA, 1996). Authority assumes a certain measure of autonomy. Donabedian relates authority to both autonomy and accountability:

Society grants the professions authority over functions vital to itself and permits them considerable autonomy in the conduct of their affairs. In return, the professions are expected to act responsibly, always mindful of the public trust. Self-regulation to assure quality in performance is at the heart of this relationship. It is the authentic hallmark of a mature profession. (1976, p. 8)

In a practical sense, authority is granted by society in the form of the permission for the profession to exist, coupled with the privilege granted to individuals to practice the profession. Thus, as with autonomy, authority for nurses is two-tiered. State legislatures create laws designed to protect the public's health and safety. The establishment of nurse practice acts is the exercise of this type of power. Nurse practice acts define nursing, describe the scope of practice, and grant the state boards of nursing the power to oversee the licensure of nurses and the practice of nursing in the states. Thus, the state boards of nursing have the legitimate authority to regulate the practice of nursing within each state.

Having specified requirements for entry into practice, defined nursing, and described the scope of nursing practice, nurse practice acts empower state boards of nursing to grant individual nurses the authority to practice. This authority is granted through the process of examination and licensure. Licensure benefits both the public and the professional. It protects the public from the unqualified, and it protects professionals' job territory by establishing a monopoly. The legal protection afforded by licensure enhances our status by authenticating the profession (Beletz, 1990). After meeting all requirements for entry into practice, we are granted the legal authority to practice nursing.

The authority given each nurse to practice is contingent upon the nurse continuing to uphold the established standards of nursing. State boards of nursing have the power and responsibility to discipline nurses who do not follow established standards or who violate provisions of licensure law. Discipline can take several forms, including suspension or revocation of license.

UNITY

There is general agreement that one of the defining characteristics of a profession is a sense of unity among its members. This unity is multifaceted and based on what Aydelotte (1990) calls moral uniformity and class ideology among its practitioners. Unity relates to the ability of nurses to organize for the purpose of fulfilling the profession's promises and the relationships that nurses have with one another.

It is only through unity that nursing is able to coherently standardize the professional characteristics of competence, autonomy, authority, and accountability. Through political and policy processes, we work together to meet the health care needs of society and to improve the status of the profession. The structural component of a professional community is realized through a professional association. The professional association provides a collective identity and serves as the voice of the profession to both the profession and society (Beletz, 1990). It fulfills four basic functions: to standardize services provided by its members, to provide a professional hub for members, to assist with educational needs of members, and to perform political, advisory, and policy functions. There is an expectation that professionals will be active members of their professional association.

Although systematic organization of professional groups is necessary in fulfilling the professions' responsibilities, we also need unity among individual members. Unity involves showing sympathy, care, and reciprocity to those with whom one appropriately identifies, working closely with others toward shared goals, keeping promises, making mutual concerns a priority, sacrificing personal interests to the relationship, and attending to these over a period of time (Jameton, 1984). Beletz eloquently describes this type of unity:

> The professional's bond with colleagues emanates from relationships established by shared mysteries of a common technical language, educational background, rites of passage, styles of work, attire, and a consciousness of being set apart and insisting on being set apart from other occupational categories. Colleague relationships are expected to be cooperative, equalitarian, and supportive vis-à-vis clientele and peers. (1990, p. 19)

Though loyalty is a virtue, there are certain risks when we experience a strong sense of loyalty to each other. Jameton (1984) warns that nurses must be careful that their loyalty to each other does not supersede loyalty to patients. For example, mistakes that nurses or doctors make should be reported to patients. Because of a sense of loyalty and friendship that exists between coworkers, there is a risk that our duty to patients will be neglected. We are required to examine and prioritize conflicting loyalties closely. Jameton identifies nurses' main priorities as: patients, nurses and the nursing profession, physicians, hospitals, other health professions, and society. Questioning which of these priorities should be central and which should be peripheral, he suggests that the best choices for first priority are patient, nursing, and society.

Ask Yourself

Are Nurses Loyal to Nursing?

Nurses who are politically active in a particular state nurses' association report an incident that led them to question nurses' loyalty to the profession. At the prompting of hospital and physicians' lobbying groups, a number of nurse administrators participated in writing proposed legislation that would dismantle the all-nurse board of nursing in favor of one composed of hospital administrators and physicians.

- How would you characterize the loyalty of these nurses to the profession and to other nurses?

- What circumstances could justify prioritizing employer loyalty above loyalty to patients or to other nurses?

- What are the ethical implications of the actions of the nurses described in this situation?

- What should the role of nurses' associations be in these situations?

SUMMARY

Because ethics is a commonly cited criterion for judging the professional status of an occupation, the study of ethics must include a discussion of nursing's professional status. In order to discuss professional issues in nursing rationally, one must examine the meaning and historical context of the term professional. Beginning with Abraham Flexner's 1915 opinion that nursing did not meet his criteria for professional status, there has been continuing debate about this topic. Striving to create professional status for nursing, nurses have worked to solve the deficiencies that were identified by Flexner and others. There are those who believe that the original methods of determining professional status were flawed by a cultural background of sexism, racism, and elitism. Though this debate will continue, there are a number of traits that are nearly universally accepted as belonging to professional groups. Expertise, autonomy, accountability, authority, and unity were discussed as professional characteristics of nursing.

CHAPTER HIGHLIGHTS

- Acknowledgment of professional status is dependent upon meeting particular criteria that include, but are not restricted to, expertise, autonomy, authority, accountability, and unity.
- Historical and cultural influences have affected the trait definitions commonly used for the term professional.
- A system or code of ethics is generally accepted as one trait of professions.
- Because society allows professionals a monopoly over the services they provide, ethics demands that those services must be provided with expertise.
- Because it is self-regulating, the profession of nursing can be said to be autonomous.
- There are legal and ethical imperatives for individual nurses to practice autonomously.
- Autonomy does not mean full and absolute control over every aspect of practice.
- Grounded in the moral principle of fidelity, accountability refers to being answerable to someone for something one has done.
- Mechanisms of accountability include, but are not restricted to, codes of nursing ethics, standards of nursing practice, nurse practice acts, and nursing theory and practice derived from nursing research.
- Authority for nurses to practice is granted through the legal processes of society.
- Nursing unity relates to the profession's ability to organize for the purpose of fulfilling the promises made to society.

DISCUSSION QUESTIONS AND ACTIVITIES

1. Write your own definition of the term professional.
2. List ten different occupations and compare their common characteristics. Which occupations meet your criteria for professional status?

3. Discuss the relationship between historical and cultural influences and Flexner's method of identifying professions.

4. Discuss the relationship between the concepts of fidelity, professionalism, and expertise.

5. Discuss the statement, "To be less than maximally competent is unethical."

6. Find recent examples of case law that relate to court opinions regarding autonomy in nursing.

7. Observe a registered nurse at work. List tasks that the nurse performs and categorize them as autonomous or dependent.

8. Read the nurse practice act in your state. Evaluate your state's law in terms of its usefulness as a mechanism of accountability.

REFERENCES

Achterberg, J. (1990). *Woman as healer*. Boston: Shambhala.

American Nurses Association. (1985). *Code for nurses with interpretive statements*. Washington, DC: Author.

American Nurses Association. (1996). *Nursing's social policy statement*. Washington, DC: Author.

American Nurses Association. (2001). *Code of ethics for nurses*. Washington, DC: Author.

Aydelotte, M. (1990). The evolving profession: The role of the professional organization. In N. L. Chaska, ed., *The nursing profession: A time to speak* (pp. 16–23). St. Louis, MO: Mosby.

Beauchamp, T., & Childress, J. (1994). *Principles of biomedical ethics* (4th ed.). New York: Oxford University Press.

Beletz, E. (1990). Professionalization: A license is not enough. In N. L. Chaska, ed., *The nursing profession: Turning points* (pp. 16–23). St. Louis, MO: Mosby.

Bixler, G. K., & Bixler, R. W. (1959). The professional status of nursing. *American Journal of Nursing, 59*(8), 1142–1147.

Canadian Nursing Association (1997). *Code of ethics for registered nurses*. Author.

Donabedian, A. (1976). Foreword in M. Phaneuf, Ed., *The nursing audit: Self-regulation in nursing practice* (2nd ed.). Norwalk, CT: Appleton & Lange.

Ehrenreich, B., & English, D. (1973). *Witches, midwives, and nurses: A history of women healers*. New York: The Feminist Press.

Fiesta, J. (1988). *The law and liability: A guide for nurses*. New York: John Wiley & Sons.

Flexner, A. (1915). Is social work a profession? *School Society, 1*(26), 901–911.

Fowler, M. (1990). Social ethics and nursing. In N. L. Chaska, ed., *The nursing profession: A time to speak* (pp. 24–31). St. Louis, MO: Mosby.

Gruending, D. L. (1985). Nursing theory: A vehicle of professionalization. *Journal of Advanced Nursing, 10*, 553–558.

International Council of Nurses (2000). *The ICN code of ethics for nurses*. International Council of Nurses, Geneva Switzerland. Retrieved January 23, 2001 from the World Wide Web: http://icn.ch/index.html/

Jameton, A. (1984). *Nursing practice: The ethical issues*. Englewood Cliffs, NJ: Prentice-Hall.

Kozier, B., & Erb, G. (1994). *Concepts and issues in nursing practice* (2nd ed.). Menlo Park, CA: Addison-Wesley.

Leddy, S., & Pepper, J. M. (1989). *Conceptual bases of professional nursing* (2nd ed.). Philadelphia: Lippincott.

Lyon, B. (1990). Getting back on track; nursing's autonomous scope of practice. In N. L. Chaska, ed., *The nursing profession: A time to speak* (pp. 267–274). St. Louis, MO: Mosby.

Murphy, J. D. (1990). The legal perspective of nurse autonomy. In N. L. Chaska, ed., *The nursing profession: A time to speak* (pp. 32–39). St. Louis, MO: Mosby.

National Council of Boards of Nursing. (2000). *What are boards of nursing.* Chicago: Author. Retrieved January 31, 2001 from the World Wide Web http://www.ncsbn.org/

Newman, M. A. (1990). Professionalism: Myth or reality. In N. L. Chaska, ed., *The nursing profession: A time to speak* (pp. 49–52). St. Louis, MO: Mosby.

Parsons, M. (1986). The profession in a class by itself. *Nursing Outlook, 34,* 270–275.

Reed, P. G. (2000). Nursing reformation: Historical reflections and philosophic foundations. *Nursing Science Quarterly, 13*(2), 129–136.

Sleicher, M. N. (1981, April). Nursing is not a profession. *Nursing & Health Care,* 186–218.

State Scan. (1996, March/April). *Nurse Practitioner World News, 1,* 22–23.

Zschoche, D. (1983). Letter calling for a national nurses' congress. In M. M. Styles, The anatomy of a profession. *Issues in Critical Care, 12,* 570–575. (Original letter December 29, 1972).

CHAPTER 9

Professional Relationship Issues

*These virtues we acquire by first exercising them . . .
Whatever we learn to do, we learn by actually doing
it . . . By doing just acts we come to be just; by doing
self-controlled acts, we come to be self-controlled;
and by doing brave acts, we become brave.*
(Aristotle, *Nicomachean Ethics*)

OBJECTIVES

After completing this chapter, the reader should be able to:

1. Identify relationships and potential conflicts that nurses face in the professional realm.
2. Characterize the nature of various conflicts.
3. Examine beliefs about the relative strength of various obligations.
4. Identify nurses' primary obligation.
5. Discuss issues related to nurses' relationships with other nurses, institutions, physicians, and subordinates.
6. Discuss issues related to racial discrimination, sexual harassment, and discrimination against persons with disabilities.

INTRODUCTION

Armed with knowledge about the physical, psychological, social, and spiritual realms of nursing care, and proudly possessing a wide range of coveted technical and professional skills, new nurses expectantly enter the workforce. Anticipating respect for our opinions and encouragement to focus our efforts on giving excellent care, we soon realize that our attention must be divided between giving patient care and dealing with problems among providers and within the institutional system. This dichotomy can present a confusing and frustrating challenge, forcing us to examine conflicting loyalties, question previously held values, make decisions based upon both practical and moral considerations, and test skills of negotiation.

The nurse continually affirms that each person is a moral agent, an autonomous being worthy of respect having the duty to pursue solutions to problems of a moral nature. It is important that solutions consistently honor the uniqueness and value of each person and faithfully adhere to ethical principles. This process requires us to critically examine our own particular values and determine an ethically sound method of conflict resolution, even before conflict arises.

Recognizing that the profession of nursing struggles to overcome contextual barriers with cultural and historic overtones, we must enter professional relationships with attentiveness and skill. Rather than attempting to offer solutions to a comprehensive list of system-related problems, this chapter provides the opportunity to examine critically selected problems related to nurses' relationships within the health care delivery system. We suggest that students further prepare themselves to deal with conflict by learning morally sound skills of negotiation and conflict management.

PROBLEM SOLVING IN THE PROFESSIONAL REALM

Practical and ethical dilemmas are part and parcel of everyday nursing practice. Though many dilemmas involve patient centered issues such as self-determination, confidentiality, and the like, we frequently encounter troubling moral questions related to professional relationships, conflicting role expectations, and patterns of interaction within the institutional setting. In the long run, problems of this nature can affect patient well-being both directly and indirectly and are, therefore, important to us on a professional level. These problems are often more troubling to us than problems directly involving patients. Recognizing that dilemmas of this sort are frequent and troubling, we must consider rational methods of solving problems before they occur. If we fail to try to solve conflict, we may add to the problem.

Although there is no absolute formula with which to solve conflicts, there are some general guidelines that can be helpful. First, we must maintain attentiveness to personal values and beliefs. Firm and consistent adherence to personal values allows us to approach problems with integrity. Second, we should construct a hierarchy of loyalty or obligation based upon both personal and professional values and beliefs. For example, do you owe a primary obligation to the physician, the institution, or the patient? Third, when conflicts arise, we should determine the nature of the problem.

Is the dilemma ethical, or practical in nature? Is it a conflict of loyalty, obligation, duty, values, principles? Fourth, it is important to consider and weigh alternatives thoughtfully, including the degree of immediate harm or potential for harm, as well as the long-range effects that could occur with any given alternative. Although some alternatives may seem attractive initially, there may be long-term effects that are undesirable. Fifth, it is imperative to develop solutions that recognize each person as an autonomous being, worthy of respect. Utilization of these steps will help us resolve most professional conflicts.

Maintain Attentiveness to Personal Values

Prior to other considerations, we must maintain our own personal values and beliefs. This attention to integrity is unrelated to self-interest and predicates action based upon coherent and integrated moral values. Integrity ultimately leads to trustworthiness and the respect of others. Beyond questions of loyalty or duty, we are compelled to maintain integrity in seeking to do the right thing. This is sometimes referred to as attention to matters of conscience. Childress (1978) distinguishes between **appeals to conscience** and appeals to self-interest or convenience in that appeals to conscience are personal and subjective beliefs, founded on a prior judgment of rightness or wrongness. These are motivated by personal sanction, rather than external authority. Institutions, in turn, must recognize the nurse as a person and encourage ethical autonomy. This enables us to act in ways that are rational, free from coercion or manipulation, and consistent with personally held values and principles (Benjamin & Curtis, 1986).

In addition to enhancing professional relationships, the nurses' integrity aids patient well-being. Gadow (1980) asserts that only nurses who act out of self-unity can truly assist patients in reaching decisions that express their complex totality as individuals. Integrity is required of us since the welfare of patients is our primary obligation.

Clarify Obligation

Even nurses who possess a high level of integrity do not escape a sense of conflicting loyalty on occasion. When this happens, how do we determine the best course of action? We can be prepared by examining **obligations,** and devising a rational and consistent hierarchy. An obligation signifies being required to do something by virtue of a moral rule, a duty, or some other binding demand. Some obligations derive from a particular role or relationship (Honderich, 1995). We may believe an obligation is owed to any of the following: the patient, other patients who may be affected in the future by problems that occur in the present, the employer with which the nurse has an implied or expressed contract, the profession of nursing, peers and other coworkers, physicians, the broader society, family, and self.

Obligation to Patients.   As a part of professional nursing practice, we have an obligation to patients above all others. Because nurses are professionals, we have a moral obligation to maintain fidelity—we must be faithful to the promises made to society, and thus give priority to meeting the needs of each patient. The International Council of Nurses *Code of Ethics for Nurses* (2000) makes clear that the nurse's primary responsibility is to the patient. By following established professional codes of ethics and maintaining integrity and loyalty to patients, we also fulfill related obligations to the broader society, the profession, and ourselves.

Obligation to the Institution. Our secondary obligation is to the institution. By accepting and maintaining terms of employment and payment for services, we have both a legal and moral obligation to the institution. This obligation, however strong, does not suggest that we should jeopardize personal integrity or subordinate loyalty to the patient. To succeed in the age of technological advancement, competition, and litigation, institutions need the services of nurses who express the professional characteristics of autonomy, integrity, and ethically-based practice. Conflicts arise when the institution's goals are focused more on "bottom-line" economics than on moral responsibility and patient welfare. Conflict is inevitable when nurses, whose primary loyalty is to the welfare of patients, are employed by institutions that eliminate important programs, employ poorly-qualified staff or inadequate numbers of staff, and are otherwise ill-equipped to meet the needs of patients.

CASE PRESENTATION

When Economy Replaces Excellence

Community Hospital is a large metropolitan hospital that boasted the reputation of maintaining excellent nursing care services for many years. As a result of fierce competition and increasing financial strain, the hospital Board of Trustees decided to affiliate with a large hospital corporation. Television and radio advertisements describing the hospital corporation as having state-of-the-art equipment and services were far from reality. Immediately after the official affiliation was finalized, the hospital began dismissing nurses, cutting back supplies, eliminating unprofitable patient care services, and increasing patient charges. It was soon clear to nurses that patients would no longer receive the excellent nursing care that had been the hallmark of that hospital for many years. Nurses who remained on staff were faced with a changing environment that was no longer patient-centered, did not encourage autonomous nursing practice, and fostered ethical and practical dilemmas related to the "bottom-line" orientation. Many felt trapped because of a shrinking job market and years of investment in the hospital retirement program. They also felt powerless to change impersonal policies that were created by faceless bureaucrats hundreds of miles away.

Think About It

How Do Nurses Respond to Bottom-Line Economics?

- What kinds of dilemmas are likely to occur in this situation?
- Recognizing that a nurse's primary responsibility is to patients, how does

the new hospital arrangement affect the nurse-patient relationship?

- Can nursing practice maintain a patient-centered, ethically sensitive focus in this type of setting? Discuss your thinking.

- What alternative solutions to potential problems faced by nurses in this situation can you suggest?

Determine the Nature of the Problem

It is important that we are able to determine the nature of the problem. Is this a problem of moral uncertainty, moral distress, moral dilemma, or moral outrage? Is this a problem of a practical or ethical nature? Ethical considerations should carry more weight than matters of self-interest, though, clearly, we owe some consideration to our own needs. For example, with changing patient demographics and increasing hospital bed vacancies, we face being asked to "float" to unfamiliar settings. This practice redistributes the workload and offers the promise of improved nursing care. However, we frequently object to the prospect of being asked to float. Some nurses complain, "I've never worked there; I would be unsafe to practice in that setting!" They are tempted to refuse to float to unfamiliar settings. These nurses are faced with a moral dilemma. Recall that the nurse has obligations to ensure both the welfare of the patient and meet the needs of the institution. In either case—in assigning a nurse to float or in accepting the assignment—one must be guided by the principles of nonmaleficence and beneficence: the actions that the nurse is expected to perform must be relatively certain to do good and do no harm. In that regard, neither the nurse, the patient, nor the institution will benefit from requiring a nurse to perform tasks for which there is no preparation. To do so would be unethical. When faced with situations of this sort, we should look to our codes of ethics for help. Regarding this particular situation, for example, the ICN *Code of Ethics for Nurses* (2000) is very specific about the nurse's duty: "The nurse uses judgment regarding individual competence when accepting and delegating responsibility." Similarly, the ANA *Code of Ethics for Nurses* (2001) states, "As the scope of nursing practice changes, the nurse must exercise judgment in accepting responsibilities, seeking consultation, and assigning activities to others who carry out nursing care." The Canadian Nurses Association *Code of Ethics for Registered Nurses* (1997) also addresses this type of situation: "Nurses practice within their own level of competence. They seek additional information or knowledge; seek the help, and/or supervision and help, of a competent practitioner; and/or request a different work assignment, when aspects of the care required are beyond their level of competence."

Nevertheless, it could also be said that to refuse an assignment is unethical on a number of levels. We must not abandon patients in need of care. If there is no one else available to care for the patients, we are obligated to give care, albeit only the type of care for which we are prepared and competent. For example, nurses temporarily assigned to specialty units can be asked to give basic, supportive nursing care, but should not be asked to perform technical tasks for which they are unprepared. To do so is both ethically wrong and legally risky. In the same regard, we should not

CASE PRESENTATION

Facing a Dilemma in the Newborn Nursery

Maggie is a nurse employed in the newborn nursery of a small hospital. She is working toward completing her bachelor's degree and has an important exam at 4:30 P.M. Though she is scheduled to leave work at 3:00 P.M., by 4:00 P.M. the nurse from the next shift has not yet arrived. There is an LPN who is capable of caring for the newborns, but hospital policy requires the presence of an RN in the unit at all times. The supervisor is unable to give her any assistance. All the babies are quiet; she expects the evening shift RN to arrive soon and feels the LPN can handle the nursery for a short time. Maggie is torn between honoring her duty to patients versus leaving to take her exam.

Think About It

What Should the Nurse Do?

- Is this a practical or an ethical dilemma? What factors make this either a practical or an ethical dilemma?
- Do you think Maggie's duty to stay outweighs her obligation to take the exam?
- What is the harm that could occur if she leaves before the evening shift RN arrives?
- What is the harm that could occur if she stays and misses her exam?

attempt tasks for which we are not prepared: to do so will compromise fidelity. We should not, however, refuse to accept float assignments simply because we fear the unknown, because familiarity is comfortable, or for other self-interested reasons.

The situation in the previous example constitutes a practical dilemma. Moral and nonmoral claims are in conflict. Based upon the principles of beneficence, nonmaleficence, and fidelity, Maggie has a moral obligation to the patients committed to her and to the institution. On the other hand, her obligation to attend class is a matter of self-interest and is not based upon moral principle. There is the potential for harm to the newborns if she leaves the unit inappropriately staffed. An emergency could arise for which the LPN is not prepared. Possibly the evening shift RN will not arrive at all. If Maggie utilizes Kant's moral imperative—one should do only that which could become a rule for all people—a decision to leave the unit unattended by an RN would be untenable. By leaving, she would create a situation that should not become a rule for all nurses in all situations. A rule suggesting that all nurses should leave patients improperly attended would harm many patients in the future and as a result would harm society's faith in the profession of nursing. Based upon a comparison of moral versus practical considerations and the potential harm that could result if Maggie left the unit improperly attended, it seems clear that she should not leave. This is not meant to imply that nurses should always subjugate personal needs to patient or institutional ones. Staying at work later than scheduled as a result of an occasional, unpredictable circumstance is one thing; being required to stay repeatedly is something entirely different.

NURSES' RELATIONSHIPS WITH INSTITUTIONS

We enter the workforce with very different perceptions than our employing institutions. Having learned that autonomy and accountability are valuable components of the nursing role, we believe we owe primary loyalty to patients. We also expect that our beliefs will be honored and that our opinions and knowledge will be respected. Hospitals and other health care institutions, on the other hand, tend to be sharply hierarchical and bureaucratic institutions that expect nurses' and other subordinates' primary loyalty to be toward the institution (Jameton, 1984). In the only country that openly calls the health care delivery system an industry, institutions' motives sometimes seem to be geared more toward profit and control than compassion and care (Kritek, 1994). Moreover, institutions expect nurses' actions to be directed toward attaining the goals of the system: goals that focus strongly upon ensuring the well-being of the institution itself and sustaining patterns of power and control. Difficulties arise when there is conflict between the goals of nurses and patients and those of the institution.

Problems arise, in part, because the institution's demands for loyalty are often inequitable (Jameton, 1984). Though requiring employees to accede to certain requests, institutions rarely reciprocate with similar loyalty to nurses. For example, due to budget constraints, most institutions are fairly rigid about nurses' work hours. We are expected to arrive ready to begin and complete work according to a set schedule. We are sometimes directed to complete more work than can reasonably be done. Nurses, loyal to the institution and to the duty that they feel toward the patients in their care, are often willing to skip meals and breaks and complete work after "clocking out." In essence these practices, though very stressful for nurses, are financially appealing to institutions.

We need to balance professional obligation and the ideal of compassionate service with basic personal commitments. The ANA *Code of Ethics for Nurses* (2001) supports nurses' professional role, which may include working overtime and attending meetings on one's own time and expense in order to improve patient care or to establish and maintain conditions of employment conducive to high-quality nursing care. However, consistently repeated, self-sacrificing, altruistic behavior on the part of nurses is self-defeating, and does not establish conditions of employment conducive to high quality nursing care. It tends to support and perpetuate a flawed system; as long as nurses continue to work selflessly, the system (rather than the patient) benefits. Nurses willing to work free devalue the work of nurses and perpetuate the expectation that this type of one-sided self-sacrifice will continue. Of course, on rare occasion this sort of problem can occur in any institution, but when we repeatedly accept workloads that are unreasonable, we become complicit in continuing the wrongs. Although working extra appears to fulfill both professional obligations and the ideal of compassionate service, it "may only superficially meet obligations to clients and may actually lead to a less desirable state of affairs not only for nursing colleagues and the nursing profession, but ultimately for clients" (Benjamin & Curtis, 1986, p. 137). In the long run, this type of behavior is harmful to both patients and nurses. Jameton says:

> A basic choice is forced on those who work in hospitals by the existence of prevalent and systematic problems in health care. If one fails to resist exploitation, incompetence, and corrupt practices, one becomes responsible for them. If one resists them, one enters into conflict with conventional conceptions of behavior for employees and thereby risks reprisals. One has to choose between complicity and self-sacrifice. . . . (1984, p. 289)

Jameton's term *self-sacrifice* is related to the willingness of some nurses to risk reprisals for resisting exploitation in the health care system. He does not suggest that nurses sacrifice all issues of self-interest in favor of institutional interests.

In some instances, we base the motivation for altruism on misguided beliefs about duty. Some believe that altruism is necessary to fulfill their duty to patients. Though many philosophers consider altruism and sacrifice a virtue, Ayn Rand (1996) suggested that altruism has a dehumanizing effect. Rand believed that those who are altruistic have a nightmare view of existence—believing that people are trapped in a malevolent universe. Using the term *self-sacrifice* in a fashion nearly opposite that of Jameton, Rand viewed a persistent willingness to sacrifice as flowing from poor self-esteem and inappropriate priority-setting. Moreover, she believed that those with poor self-esteem have difficulty valuing others. Because genuine regard is partially a product of sympathy (imagining oneself in the situation of another), one must value oneself in order to value others. Additionally, nurses who repeatedly sacrifice for the good of an institutional system fail to assume the power to change the wrongs that are committed.

CASE PRESENTATION

When Patients Suffer from Lack of Nursing Care

Tim, an RN, works weekends on the skilled nursing unit of a small rural hospital. Recently purchased by a large corporation, the hospital was forced to dismiss nearly one-third of the staff of the skilled nursing unit. Lately, when Tim comes to work, he feels totally overwhelmed. Although he always considered himself efficient, Tim is distressed because he rarely has enough time to complete his work. He knows that many of the patients suffer because of lack of attention. Those who are bedfast are not turned on a regular schedule, they often wait for assistance with eating until their food is cold, and medications are rarely given on time. Suffering from expressive aphasia and hemiplegia secondary to a CVA, Mrs. Wallace was admitted to the skilled nursing unit after two weeks in the intensive care unit.

Mrs. Wallace has been on the skilled nursing unit for three weeks when her daughter, Nina, notices a large reddened area surrounding a small gray ulcer over her mother's coccyx. Concerned, Nina asks Tim what caused this problem. Even though Mrs. Wallace's nursing care plan calls for attention to activity including frequent turning and sitting in a chair twice daily, Tim suspects that this was not consistently done the previous week. He recognizes that the reddened area is the beginning of a large pressure ulcer, a problem that might have been prevented with proper attention to activity and good nutrition. Tim hesitates to tell Nina that the problem is a potentially serious one that might have been prevented by good nursing care measures. He believes she has a right to know but is hesitant to implicate himself or the other nurses, and he is afraid that he will lose his job if he complains.

Think About It

How Do Nurses Make Decisions When Loyalties Conflict?

- What are the ethical principles implicit in this situation?
- What are Tim's conflicting loyalties?
- The staff on the unit is efficient and hard-working—skipping lunch and staying overtime to complete their work. Do you believe the staff is responsible for the apparently poor nursing care that Mrs. Wallace is getting?
- Do you believe Tim should tell Nina the truth about the pressure sore?
- Should Tim risk losing his job by whistle-blowing?
- Is this an ethical or practical dilemma?
- What harm can result from either option?
- What would you do?

The previous case presentation is another example of a practical dilemma. The conflict that Tim is experiencing is between the principle of beneficence (the desire to do good for the patient) and a sense of loyalty to the institution or the other nurses with whom he works. There may also be an element of self-interest—Tim may not want to be implicated in the harm that the patients are experiencing as a result of the staff cutbacks. Tim's primary loyalty is owed to the patients—Mrs. Wallace, other patients suffering from the shortage of staff, and future patients who could be harmed by perpetuation of the problem. There are strong arguments that he should act to correct the situation. He may choose to take any number of actions: he can work through the administrative hierarchy to improve staffing; he can answer Nina's questions honestly; though his job will certainly be jeopardized, he can inform the media of the problems that were created by the drastic staffing shortages. In any case, if Tim fails to act to solve the problem, he will be complicit in its perpetuation and the subsequent harm to patients.

Another example related to institutions' inequitable demands for loyalty is seen in the customary practice of requiring nurses to complete incident reports. In an effort to prevent litigation, institutions discourage nurses from talking to patients about mistakes that have been made. They much prefer that nurses file incident reports. These documents, geared toward institutional goals, are filed and kept for use in the event the hospital needs a legal defense, in firing or disciplining workers, or in reorganizing services to prevent future incidents (Jameton, 1984). Thus, patient-centered goals based upon the principles of autonomy, fidelity, veracity, and respect for persons are subordinated to institutional subgoals of employee control and risk management.

Nurses' loyalty to the institution is an important mode of control. Without loyalty, administrators cannot manage institutions (Jameton, 1984). For this reason supervisors and administrators sometimes react negatively when nurses support and cooperate with each other to make changes. The ensuing perception of nonsupportive supervisors is a contributing factor for job stress and dissatisfaction (Moore, Kuhrik, Kuhrik, & Katz, 1996). In the end, this can be harmful to nurses and patients alike. Jameton says, "Where institutions as a whole fail to serve patients well, this demand for loyalty can interfere with the nurses' expressions of loyalty to nurses and patients" (1984, p. 121).

NURSES' RELATIONSHIPS WITH OTHER NURSES

Nurses work together in close proximity day in and day out. No other profession is so intimately connected with the essence of life. The knowledge gained from the intimate experiences of birth, illness, life, and death are both powerful and mysterious. Nurses are connected to each other and set apart from others: connected by common experience, language, and knowledge, and set apart through professional mystique. Nurses work together closely, identify with each other, and supervise or are supervised by other nurses. The practice of one affects that of others.

Loyalty is a natural product of long-term acquaintance and close working relationships. Some view loyalty among members as a distinguishing characteristic of a profession. Jameton defines loyalty as:

> showing sympathy, care, and reciprocity to those with whom we appropriately identify; working closely with others toward shared goals; keeping promises; making mutual concerns a priority; sacrificing personal interests to the relationship; and giving attention to these over a substantial period of time. It supports showing respect for persons. And it resolves potential conflicts in autonomy by making values and goals that I see as my own more like values and goals of those who work with me. (1984, p. 118)

Promoting faithfulness and commitment, loyalty is very limited and exclusive in its scope. Though normally viewed as admirable, loyalty is seldom regarded as a cardinal virtue because of the potential for fanaticism and blind injustice (Honderich, 1995).

CASE PRESENTATION

Nurses' Loyalty to the Profession

A few years ago, politically-active nurses in a small state lobbied for a bill mandating nurse representation on government bodies charged with considering health-related issues. Positions included membership on committees, task forces, advisory panels, and so forth. There was also a stipulation that required each public hospital to include one nurse on its governing board. As the largest group of health care professionals, nurses believed their knowledge and experience would be a welcome addition. Though there was strong and unified nursing support, the bill was fiercely opposed by both the state hospital association and individual hospitals. When public hearings were held, the politically-active nurses found themselves testifying for the bill in opposition to commanding and articulate nurse administrators. Representing individual hospitals, nurse administrators cited everything from nurses' lack of economic expertise to a gossipy tendency to spill industry secrets as reasons to oppose nurse members on hospital governing boards. The bill failed.

Think About It

Examining Differences in Loyalty

- Can you think of moral justification for the diverse positions of nurses?
- To whom is each group of nurses loyal?
- How would you characterize each group's stance in relation to the professionalization of nursing?
- How would you account for the diverse positions of the nurses?

In practical matters, loyalty is a productive virtue. It enhances unity, strength, and power. Facing bureaucratic, economic, and political forces, our loyalty to each other and to the profession adds strength to our call for improved patient care, public welfare, nursing autonomy, and optimum employment conditions.

While having the potential to strengthen the profession of nursing and improve the welfare of patients, loyalty among nurses can also be harmful. Misguided or fanatical loyalty can lead to a confused sense of obligation. Though our primary obligation is to patients, those of us who are overly loyal to other nurses might act in ways that are harmful to patients' health status. For example, a nurse having blind loyalty to another might cover up a coworker's incompetent practice, illegal drug use, or other actions that have the potential to harm present or future patients. For this reason, we must be careful to maintain objectivity in balancing loyalty to nurses and the profession against the obligation owed to patients.

NURSES' RELATIONSHIPS WITH PHYSICIANS

Nurses' relationships with physicians are an important factor in the quality of patient care. Ideally, the work of nurses and physicians should be complementary and synergistic. Because both professions hold claim to the primary goal of patient health, one would expect a sense of collegiality and collaboration between nurses and physicians. When this type of relationship exists, it is rewarding and productive. When there is conflict between nurses and physicians, the relationship is stressful and damaging to nurses, physicians, and patients alike. Because nurses and physicians work in close proximity, conflict that occurs between them is a strong contributor to the lack of job satisfaction for nurses.

Nurse-physician relationships have generally reflected the prevailing gender roles in society. These roles were well defined for centuries. The traditional nurse was expected to obey the physician, much as the wife was expected to obey her husband. Physicians demanded obedience, and nurses hesitated to disagree with physicians, even if there was good reason to do so. Unfortunately, these "time-worn attitudes" linger in both professions (Benjamin & Curtis, 1986, p. 86).

Given the bureaucratic nature of most health care institutions, particularly hospitals, the relationship between physicians and nurses is complex and peculiar. Generally, nurses are employees of the institutions, while physicians are independent practitioners who have the privilege of institutional practice. Physicians, who are not employees of the institutions, have no formal chain-of-command relationship with the nurses who care for their patients. Curtin and Flaherty (1982) write, "This tradition of self-employed 'guest practitioners' in health care institutions having so much power over the large groups of 'full-time employees' of the institutions defies explanation, but it is a fact of life in health care" (p. 144). Though they issue orders to nurses directly, physicians are not employed by, subordinate to, or even responsible to the institutional administration. These dual lines of authority are confusing, and have the potential to severely limit the autonomous decision-making role of the nurse (Benjamin & Curtis, 1986, p. 82). Because most nurses are employees with either expressed or implied contracts with institutions, they have an obligation to perform the tasks required by the institutions. One of the major tasks that most institutions require of nurses is the implementation of physicians' orders. When nurses question or disagree with physicians, they may feel distressed, believing they are being disloyal to both the physician and the institution.

Another contributor to conflict in the nurse-physician relationship is the rapid advent of advanced practice nursing. Having an expanded knowledge base and a scope of practice that includes many functions that were once the sole domain of physicians, advanced practice nursing can contribute to the tensions that exist between nurses and physicians. The outmoded tradition of the nurse who obeys the physician is in direct conflict with the autonomous nurse who thinks independently, makes nursing diagnoses, and implements independent nursing actions (Benjamin & Curtis, 1986).

What actions should be taken by the nurse who questions or disagrees with an order or action of a physician? The nurse must remember that the primary obligation is owed the patient, not the physician. Nurses are autonomous practitioners. They have the knowledge and experience, and the legal and ethical responsibility, to make independent judgments even when carrying out physicians' orders. If medical care constitutes incompetent, unethical, or illegal practice, the nurse is clearly obligated to disobey orders (American Nurses Association, 2001). When deciding what course to take in situations in which nurses disagree with physicians' orders, Benjamin and Curtis (1986) suggest that nurses apply the test of the **spectrum of urgency.** At one end of this spectrum are problems that are minor and may be solved at a leisurely pace. At the other end are urgent problems that require quick solutions and immediate actions. The low-urgency end of the spectrum includes situations in which there is little risk of serious harm, or there is significant time available to examine all aspects of the situation. The high-urgency end of the spectrum consists of emergencies in which life-saving actions must be carried out at once. Nurses may have time to discuss and negotiate satisfactory solutions to problems at the low-urgency end of the spectrum, but problems at the high-urgency end of the spectrum require quick, sometimes drastic action.

CASE PRESENTATION

Making a Decision in an Urgent Situation

Marta is night shift charge nurse in the emergency department. She has advanced certification and twenty-five years of experience. Marta works well with the other members of the emergency room staff, and is comfortable and efficient in situations of extreme urgency. The emergency department is usually staffed by board-certified emergency physicians. Because one of the regular physicians recently moved to another state, there has been a series of physicians with various degrees of preparation and ability moonlighting in the department, particularly on night shift. During an unusually busy shift, an ambulance arrives with a middle-aged man having severe chest pain and dyspnea. His condition quickly deteriorates, and after a few minutes he experiences cardiac and respiratory arrest. The physician on duty, Dr. Andrews, is a family practice physician moonlighting after his regular shift at a local community health center. Marta perceives Dr. Andrews as nervous and hesitant. During the first phase of the "code," Dr. Andrews seems uncertain of every detail. As the nurse in charge, Marta begins instituting a seldom-used protocol that was developed for use in the event that the nurses are faced with a cardiac arrest when no physician is present. All the nurses are trained in intubation techniques, but hospital policy prohibits them from performing that particular procedure. Marta suggests to Dr. Andrews that he intubate the patient. After several clumsy attempts, Dr. Andrews angrily orders Marta to call an anesthesiologist at home to come and intubate the patient. Marta realizes that the patient's chances of survival are best if he is intubated quickly. She asks the unit clerk to call the anesthesiologist. Over his angry objections, Marta removes the laryngoscope and endotracheal tube from Dr. Andrews's trembling hands and proceeds to intubate the patient quickly and successfully. The patient responds to resuscitation attempts and is discharged five days later.

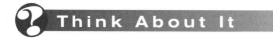

Think About It

Was Marta's Decision Correct?

- What is your immediate response to the situation in which Marta finds herself?
- Where would you place this situation on the "spectrum of urgency"?
- What are the arguments in favor of Marta's actions?
- What are the arguments in favor of Marta's following Dr. Andrews's orders?
- Do you consider Marta's actions to be based upon ethical principle?
- Did Marta place herself at risk of reprisal or legal action?
- What would you have done?

Nurses are charged with making thoughtful, fair, and knowledgeable decisions in relation to questioning physicians' orders, while also being careful to consider the overall harm that can result from any given action. Recognizing that the physician's goal, like that of the nurse, is the welfare of the patient, we must be mature and objective when questioning orders. Nurses have an ethical obligation to protect the patient from medical incompetence. Nevertheless, we must be careful in this regard, keeping in mind the overall harm that can result from the practice of constantly and inappropriately questioning insignificant aspects of physicians' orders.

NURSES' RELATIONSHIPS WITH SUBORDINATES

While maintaining an awareness of the primary obligation owed to patients, nurses must be sensitive to those who work beside them. Each person is a moral agent and must be recognized as worthy of dignity and respect. As the coordinator of patient care, the professional nurse is accountable for the quality of nursing care rendered to patients. This accountability includes supervision, delegation of nursing care functions, and disciplining of other health care providers. The inherent practical, moral, and legal implications of these functions are facets of the role of professional nurse that must be undertaken with sensitivity and respect.

The structure of health care delivery in some institutional settings makes the professional nurse responsible for delegating a number of nursing functions to subordinate staff members. The nurse has a moral obligation to ensure that each patient receives excellent nursing care, to respect the value of each individual, and to make sure the situation is conducive to high-quality nursing care (ANA, 2001). Following is an excerpt from the ANA *Code of Ethics for Nurses* regarding the nurse and delegation of nursing activities:

Since the nurse is accountable for the quality of nursing care given to patients, nurses are accountable for the assignment of nursing responsibilities to other nurses and the delegation of nursing care activities to other health care workers. The nurse must make reasonable efforts to assess individual competency when assigning selected components of nursing care to other health care workers. This assessment involves evaluating the knowledge, skills, and expertise of the individual to whom the care is assigned, the complexity of the assigned tasks, and the health status of the patients. The nurse is also responsible for monitoring the activities of these individuals and evaluating the quality of the care provided. (ANA, 2001)

As the coordinator of patient care, the nurse is accountable for all nursing care that patients receive, whether from the nurse or subordinates.

In addition to delegation, the supervisory role of professional nurses occasionally includes disciplining of subordinates. Disciplining is a difficult task that must be done with insight, respect, compassion, and logic. The nurse must be keenly aware of the effect of disciplinary action upon others and must focus on the intended goal. The traditional methods of discipline, such as punishment and chastisement, are damaging to the spirit and counterproductive in practice.

Nurse managers' method of disciplining may set the tone for the entire nursing unit. Discussing poor leadership, Dilley says, "Nurse managers from hell can be easily identified. They use coercion—as in, 'do as I say or you'll find yourself on the night shift.' They belittle their employees in front of patients or other staff. They communicate by memo rather than face-to-face. They change policies without input from others. They are rude and thoughtless" (2000, p. 9).

A good nurse manager may also set the tone of the unit through the style of discipline. Quoting the great teacher, Maria Montessori, Leah Curtin (1996) writes, "'Our aim is to discipline for activity, for work, for good; not for immobility, not for passivity, not for obedience'" (p. 51). Curtin suggests that the most meaningful method is self-discipline, which corrects the problem, strengthens the character of the worker, and improves performance. She defines self-discipline as a process by which the rules are internalized and become a part of the individual's personality. This process is possible only if the person knows the rules, understands their purpose, and agrees that they deserve compliance. To achieve this result, the nurse must model the expected standard daily and have few rules—all of which are applied consistently, change infrequently, and apply to all personnel equally. The nurse has a moral obligation, to both patients and personnel, to uphold rules that protect the health or safety of patients, other employees, the institution, and oneself as leader (Curtin, 1996, p. 51).

DISCRIMINATION AND HARASSMENT

Claims of discrimination or harassment in the workplace are becoming more frequent. In fact, millions of Americans have experienced employment discrimination. Swart, Wendt, and Slonaker (1996) report that 27 percent of workers believe they have experienced discrimination on the job. Discrimination is ethically prohibited. Because this prohibition entails treating others fairly and equitably, the ethical principle of justice is a key point when discussing issues of discrimination. In their 1991 position statement on human rights, the ANA wrote, "Actions that are termed 'unjust' are of three basic types: first, discrimination or arbitrarily unequal treatment in legislating, administering, or enforcing rules; second, exploitation, taking advantage of another person to gain unfairly; and third, making false or derogatory statements about people or their work that aren't fair" (p. 1). Discrimination is also legally prohibited. The Bill of Rights of the United States Constitution, the Civil Rights Act of 1964, the Americans with Disabilities Act of 1990 (ADA), and the Civil Rights Act of 1991 provide legal protection against discrimination in the workplace.

Racial Discrimination

The Civil Rights Act of 1964 made it unlawful for an employer to fail or refuse to hire or to discharge any individual, or to otherwise discriminate against any individual, because of the person's race, color, religion, sex, or national origin. Unlawful acts include discrimination in terms of compensation or payment, conditions of employment, or privileges of employment. Considered one of America's strongest civil rights laws, the Civil Rights Act of 1964 primarily protects the rights of African-Americans and other minorities. Attempting to correct a long tradition of racial discrimination, this act ensures that minorities receive fair and equal treatment from government, other persons, and private groups, including schools and employers. Enforced by the Equal Employment Opportunity Commission (EEOC), the act also specifically forbids discrimination by any program that receives money from the federal government.

The Civil Rights Act of 1964 enjoins employers to provide equal employment opportunities to individuals from the initial recruitment or application process through termination of employment. When considering claims of discriminatory practices, the legal system looks at two discriminatory outcomes: disparate treatment and disparate impact. *Disparate treatment* occurs when an individual is treated differently by a superior or by organizational policy. For example, if a supervisor passes over all Hispanic nurses who apply for promotion, regardless of their qualifications or abilities, disparate treatment exists. *Disparate impact* occurs when employers consistently apply policies that appear to be fair to all employees but actually adversely affect one group. For example, in January 2000, 346 men received a $5 million settlement in a disparate impact claim. The men were denied medical and dental insurance coverage for their children because of a former requirement that children of employees and pensioners live with them full time (EEOC, 2001). Denial of coverage for these men was considered disparate impact, because certain social and ethnic groups are less likely to have intact families living together in one home.

Because stereotypes are slow to change, it can be very difficult for nonmajority group members to enter and succeed in any occupational group. Though the landmark civil rights legislation was passed decades ago, there is some indication that discrimination continues to exist in the health care system. Swart, Wendt, and Slonaker (1996) studied a group of nurses who had filed discrimination claims. Among nurses reporting discrimination, 47 percent based their claims on race discrimination.

Another source of race discrimination may be a lack of recruitment and retention of minority nursing students. According to Dowell (1996), student, faculty, and administrative populations in many schools of nursing still reflect uniformity and homogeneity. Citing several studies, Dowell identifies barriers to recruitment of minority groups, including the following: lack of full scholarships, scarcity of minority groups in certain geographic areas, lack of effective minority recruitment strategies, a negative attitude from administrators, and a lack of minority role models.

Both the ICN *Code of Ethics for Nurses* (2000) and the ANA *Code of Ethics for Nurses* (2001) identify racial discrimination as an ethical issue. Racism is prohibited by both. The American Nurses Association is active in identifying and eradicating racism in the profession. According to their position statement on discrimination and racism in health care, "ANA abhors the recent rise in racism and discriminatory behavior in this country. . . ." and " . . . is committed to addressing the need for racial and ethnic diversity among nurses" (1998).

Discrimination Against Persons with Disabilities

The Americans with Disabilities Act of 1990 (ADA) was signed into law on July 26, 1990. Seen by some as the most significant piece of legislation since the Civil Rights Act of 1964, this act provides comprehensive protection to Americans with disabilities. Challenged to combine the legal concepts of disability and equality, the aim of Congress in drafting this legislation was to ensure equality for the disabled without creating "undue" hardships on employers (Guido, 1997). The ADA considers one to have a covered *disability* if there is record of physical or mental disability that causes an impairment substantially limiting one or more of the major life enjoyments of the person, and if the person actually has such an impairment. *Major life enjoyments* include such activities as the average person can perform with little or no difficulty, such as caring for oneself, performing manual tasks, walking, seeing, hearing, speaking, learning, and working. A *physical impairment* includes any physiologic disorder or condition, cosmetic disfigurement, or anatomical loss affecting any body system. A *mental impairment* includes any mental or psychological disorder, such as mental retardation, organic brain syndrome, emotional or mental illness, and learning disabilities. Mental or psychological conditions that result from such conditions as diabetes, cancer, AIDS, alcoholism, and drug abuse qualify under this definition (Guido, 1997).

Related to the Civil Rights Act of 1964, the ADA has several provisions. The act ensures that people with disabilities are not excluded from job opportunities or adversely affected in other aspects of employment unless they are unqualified or unable to perform the job. This protection extends to application, salary, promotion, discharge, transfer, and all other aspects of work. The ADA prohibits the practice of requiring medical examinations before employment except for drug testing, which may be performed. Medical examinations may be done only after a job offer has been extended. Employers may question individuals about their educational qualifications, experience, and their ability to perform the job safely with or without accommodation. To avoid the suggestion of discrimination, the prospective employer may not ask questions about disabilities, past medical problems, or previous workers' compensation claims. Upon request from disabled employees, employers must make necessary physical accommodations to the workplace, such as wheelchair accessibility, telephone systems for the hearing impaired, and so forth, but may be exempted from hiring persons with disabilities if the necessary accommodations cause *undue hardship* because they are extremely expensive or difficult to implement. The employer must have investigated the required accommodations and offer data proving the hardship. Undue hardship is based on cost, numbers of employees, and type of business (Guido, 1997).

The ADA does not require employers to hire individuals with disabilities. It demands, however, that employers base employment decisions solely upon job qualifications and ability, without regard to physical or mental disabilities. It also protects employers from financial ruin in the case of undue hardship related to making workplace accommodations for disabled persons.

Sexual Harassment and Discrimination

Sexual harassment is a widespread problem. A 1998 survey found that 42 percent of all women and 15 percent of all men experienced some form of sexual harassment (ANA, 2001). Sexual discrimination and harassment is not new in nursing. In the nineteenth century certain occupations were redefined as feminine. Nursing and teaching, for example, became accepted as feminine lines of work, and women in these occupational groups were seen and treated as "ladies." Florence Nightingale struggled with this identity: "In effect, she violated the gender norms of the day and threatened male power. Very much aware of her threat to the men, she continually emphasized that she was doing only what a proper lady should do—extending the role by accepting what society said women were especially qualified to do" (Bullough, 1990, p. 6). While allowing women to function as nurses, this attitude sustained the social order. Defined today as sexual harassment, there was an effort to sustain male power by treating women as sexual objects and inferiors.

Sexual harassment is defined as unwelcomed sexual advances, requests for sexual favors, and other verbal, non-verbal, or physical conduct of a sexual nature (EEOC, 1990). According to Friedman (1992), "sexual harassment refers to conduct, typically experienced as offensive in nature, in which unwanted sexual advances are made in the context of a relationship of unequal power or authority" (p. 9). Recognizing sexual harassment as a significant problem, federal and state courts have struggled with the issue for the past several decades. In October of 1991, the problem was brought to the attention of the public with the Senate confirmation hearings of Supreme Court nominee Clarence Thomas. A direct result of these hearings, the Civil Rights Act of 1991 was signed into law on November 21, 1991. This act defines sexual harassment and identifies two categories of the offense—quid pro quo sexual harassment, and hostile work environment sexual harassment.

When submission to or rejection of the sexual conduct of an individual is used as a basis for employment decisions, *quid pro quo sexual harassment* is said to occur. There are four requirements to prove quid pro quo sexual harassment. The employee must show first that there was unwelcome harassment in the form of sexual advances or requests for sexual favors; second, that the harassment was based on sex; and third, that submission to the unwelcome sexual advances was required for receiving job benefits or that refusal to submit to the advances resulted in job detriment. Fourth, the individual who claims to be a victim of sexual harassment must be a member of a group that is lower on the chain of command than the person making the unwelcome advances. In quid pro quo harassment suits, employers are liable for the conduct of supervisory personnel (Guido, 1997).

Hostile work environment sexual harassment occurs when the employee is subjected to sexual innuendos, remarks, and physical acts that are so offensive as to create an abusive work environment. The two factors that must be shown in claims of hostile work environment are that the harassment unreasonably interfered with work, and that the harassment would affect a reasonable person's work. The employer is only liable in such an instance when it can be shown that there was knowledge of the harassment. In hostile work environment sexual harassment cases, it is not necessary that the conduct be directed toward the individual who files the complaint, merely that the employee's psychological well-being was affected because the conduct was observed or known. This can occur, for example, with the unwanted posting of pornographic pictures or cartoons, sexually explicit comments or jokes, or sexual propositions. It is not necessary to prove that terms of employment are attached to this type of sexual harassment (Guido, 1997).

Although 90 percent of sexual harassment claims are filed by women (Wolfe, 1996), men can also be the object of real or perceived sexual harassment or discrimination. Kelly, Shoemaker, and Steele (1996) discuss the problem of underrepresentation of men in schools of nursing. Male student nurses in the study reported that they experienced a fear of being perceived as unmanly, felt isolated, and were excluded from activities and discussions. In addition to the same type of sexual discrimination experienced by women, there are potential areas for sexual discrimination targeted specifically against men. These might involve such behaviors as stereotyping all male nurses as being gay, or as assigning an inequitable portion of tough patients to men because of perceived physical stamina or strength.

Sexual harassment entails emotional costs such as anger, humiliation, and fear, and direct costs such as counseling and lawyer's fees. To avoid these costs, nurses must be sensitive in recognizing and protecting themselves and their colleagues from sexual harassment. Madison and Minichiello report on a study of nurses that identifies cues for recognizing harassment as follows:

- Invasion of space: someone corners you or enters your personal space.

- Confirmation: another person or colleague recognizes and confirms your suspicions of harassment.

- Lack of respect: past or present behavior of the harasser is perceived to be disrespectful.

- Deliberate nature of behavior: harassment is intentional, planned, orchestrated.

- Perceived power of control: circumstances put the harasser out of the control of the harassed organizationally, hierarchically, and physically.

- Overly friendly behavior: behavior is considered too friendly, or falsely friendly.

- Sexualized work place innuendos, explicit jokes, or pictures are common. (2000, p. 407)

Prevention of sexual harassment in the workplace is difficult. Sexual harassment is difficult to identify, difficult to prove, and many nurses are afraid to report incidents, fearing reprisal. Monarch (2000) suggests some guidelines for sexual harassment policies. A good policy should meet the following criteria: provide a clear description of prohibited conduct; assure employees who file complaints that they will be protected from retaliation; assure confidentiality to the greatest extent possible; identify reporting and investigative procedures that are free of chain-of-command entanglements; guarantee prompt investigations; assure immediate and appropriate action when sexual harassment is found to have occurred; pledge thorough investigation; identify sanctions; and offer counseling to the person complaining of sexual harassment.

SUMMARY

In the professional realm, nurses are faced with the dichotomy of striving to meet their primary obligation to patients while dealing with problems among providers and within the institutional system. Nurses must be prepared to examine personal beliefs, prioritize obligations, and devise morally sound solutions to problems. Solutions must reflect an overall respect for persons and recognize the moral agency of individuals. Nurses are guided in this endeavor by personal values and beliefs and by professional codes of ethics.

CHAPTER HIGHLIGHTS

- As a moral agent, each person has the duty to pursue solutions to moral problems.
- Solutions to practical and ethical problems in the professional realm must be sensitive to personal values and beliefs.
- Nurses must be able to identify and prioritize conflicting obligations.
- It is important for nurses to determine the nature of conflicts in the professional realm.
- Problem resolution requires thoughtful consideration and weighing of alternative solutions.
- In solving problems, nurses must recognize that each person is an autonomous being, worthy of respect.
- Nurses must seek solutions to moral problems related to conflicting role expectations in the institutional setting.
- Nurses must seek solutions to moral and practical problems related to relationships among nurses, physicians, and subordinates.
- Discrimination is prohibited by the ethical principle of justice, because it entails claims related to fair and equitable treatment of persons.

DISCUSSION QUESTIONS AND ACTIVITIES

1. Explore the U.S. Equal Employee Opportunity website at: http://www.eeoc.gov. html. Identify three recent court cases involving discrimination or harassment. Report the court decisions to the class.

2. Explore the ANA website at http://nursingworld.org.htm. Read two position statements on discrimination or harassment. How do these position statements fit with your experience in the health care system?

3. Describe potential problems in the professional realm that fall into each of the following categories:

   - Conflicts of obligation
   - Conflicts of principle
   - Practical dilemmas
   - Conflicts of loyalty

4. Discuss with your classmates situations that could reasonably occur in the work setting that would constitute an appeal to conscience.

5. Review the ANA Code for Nurses with Interpretive Statements. List each statement that applies to problems related to nurses' relationships with other professionals. Discuss the practical application of each of these statements.

6. Interview nurses who have been in practice one year or less. Ask them to compare their expectations of the work environment with the reality that they faced upon graduation.

7. Discuss the conflict that results as shrinking institutional budgets require cutbacks in nursing staff.

8. List the positive and negative aspects of loyalty. Do you feel loyalty is a virtue?

9. Describe the ideal professional relationships that can occur between nurses and physicians.

10. Role-play a situation in which a nurse is sensitive and respectful in disciplining a subordinate-focusing on the goal of improving performance rather than punishing.

11. Discuss racial discrimination, discrimination against persons with disabilities, and sexual harassment in terms of ethical principles and legal mandate.

REFERENCES

American Nurses Association (2001). *Code of ethics for nurses*. Washington, DC: Author.

American Nurses Association (2001). *Position statements: Sexual harassment*. Washington, DC: Author. Retrieved January 25, 2001 from the World Wide Web: http://www.nursingworld.org

American Nurses Association (1998). *Position statements: Discrimination and racism in health care*. Washington, DC: Author. Retrieved January 25, 2001 from the World Wide Web: http://www.nursingworld.org

Americans with Disabilities Act of 1990, Pub. L. No. 101–336, § 2, 104 Stat. 328 (1991).

Benjamin, M., & Curtis, J. (1986). *Ethics in nursing* (2nd ed.). New York: Oxford University Press.

Bullough, V. (1990). Nightingale, nursing and harassment. *Image: Journal of Nursing Scholarship*, *22*, 4–7.

Canadian Nurses Association (1997). *Code of ethics for registered nurses*. Author.

Childress, J. (1978). Appeals to conscience. *Ethics, 89*, 316–321.

Civil Rights Act of 1964, 41 U.S.C.A. § 2000e *et seq.*

Civil Rights Act of 1991, P.L. 102-166, 105 Stat. 1071 (1991).

Curtin, L. (1996). Ethics, discipline and discharge. *Nursing Management, 27*(3), 51–52.

Curtin, L., & Flaherty, M. J. (1982). *Nursing ethics: Theories and pragmatics.* Bowie, MD: Brady.

Dilley, K. B. (2000). Out from under their thumbs. *American Journal of Nursing 100*(5), 9.

Dowell, M. (1996). Issues in recruitment and retention of minority nursing students. *Journal of Nursing Education, 35*(7), 293–297.

EEOC (2001). Web page. Retrieved January 25, 2001 from the World Wide Web: http://www.eeoc.gov.html

EEOC (1990). *Policy guidance on current issues of sexual harassment.* Washington DC: Author. Retrieved January 25, 2001 from the World Wide Web: http://www.eeoc.gov/docs/current issues.html

Friedman, J. (1992). *Sexual harassment.* Deerfield, FL: Health Communications.

Gadow, S. (1980). Existential advocacy: Philosophical foundation of nursing. In S. F. Spicker and S. Gadow, eds., *Nursing: Images and ideals, opening dialogue with the humanities* (pp. 90–91). New York: Springer.

Guido, G. (1997). *Legal issues in nursing* (2nd ed.). Norwalk, CT: Appleton & Lange.

Honderich, T., ed. (1995). *The Oxford companion to philosophy.* New York: Oxford University Press.

International Council of Nurses (2000). *The ICN code of ethics for nurses.* International Council of Nurses, Geneva Switzerland. Retrieved January 23, 2001 from the World Wide Web: http://icn.ch/index.html/

Jameton, A. (1984). *Nursing practice: The ethical issues.* Englewood Cliffs, NJ: Prentice-Hall.

Kelly, N., Shoemaker, M., & Steele, T. (1996). The experience of being a male student nurse. *Journal of Nursing Education, 35*(4), 170–174.

Kritek, P. B. (1994). *Negotiating at an uneven table: A practical approach to working with difference and diversity.* San Francisco: Jossey-Bass.

Madison, J., & Minichiello, V. (2000). Recognizing and labeling sex-based and sexual harassment in the health care workplace. *Journal of Nursing Scholarship, 32*(4), 405–410.

Monarch, K. (2000). Protect yourself from sexual harassment. *American Journal of Nursing, 100*(5), p. 75.

Moore, S., Kuhrik, M., Kuhrik, N., & Katz, B. (1996). Coping with downsizing: Stress, self-esteem and social intimacy. *Nursing Management, 27*(3), 28–30.

Rand, A. (1996). The ethics of emergencies. In J. Feinberg, ed., *Reason and responsibility: Readings in some basic problems of philosophy* (9th ed., pp. 541–545). Belmont, CA: Wadsworth.

Swart, J., Wendt, A., & Slonaker, W. (1996). Employment discrimination experiences of registered nurses. *JONA, 26*, 37–43.

Wolfe, S. (1996). If you're sexually harassed. *RN 5*(2), 61–64.

CHAPTER 10

Practice Issues Related to Technology

There is an appointed time for everything, and a time for every affair under the heavens.

(Ecclesiastes 3:1)

OBJECTIVES

After completing this chapter, the reader should be able to:

1. Discuss the impact of technology on nursing and health care.
2. Apply beneficence and nonmaleficence to decisions about technology.
3. Discuss issues and dilemmas related to current technology and to life-sustaining interventions.
4. Relate the concept of medical futility to health care decisions.
5. Relate economics to decisions regarding health technology.
6. Discuss considerations in decisions about cardiopulmonary resuscitation and artificial sources of nutrition for patients.
7. Describe legal issues associated with health care technology.
8. Discuss issues and dilemmas associated with technologies affecting reproduction, genetics, and organ transplantation.
9. Describe nursing considerations for patient care in the midst of technology.

INTRODUCTION

Nursing care is inextricably intertwined with ever-expanding advances of scientific knowledge and technology. Few would deny the benefits of medical advances, often referred to in terms such as *wonders* or *miracles*. However, the many benefits brought to the health care arena by technology are often accompanied by serious dilemmas for both practitioners and patients. Technology brings to the fore many questions related to issues of living and dying, and the changing definitions of both that are brought on by scientific advances. Dilemmas include availability of technologies, what patient situations warrant the use of available technologies, and who decides when to initiate and when to withdraw particular interventions. Additionally, nurses must be concerned about the amount of nursing energy and attention that technology requires. As much as we say that nursing focuses on holistic caring for the patient, nurses are faced with increasing demands to focus attention to technology rather than on their patients.

This chapter focuses on common issues related to technology encountered in today's health care settings. Issues of technology, patient self-determination, and economics are intertwined. Nurses who are directly involved in dilemmas, as well as those who are more on the periphery, must be aware of considerations regarding the effect of technology on patient care. These considerations include values, attitudes, communication, and attention to the humanistic caring role. The term *technology* includes the vast range of scientific advances that affect health and health care. Changing technologies bring with them the challenge of dealing with new issues, and nurses need to be prepared to face this challenge.

BENEFITS AND CHALLENGES OF TECHNOLOGY

Scientific advances in the past one hundred years have been phenomenal. They include medications, surgical techniques, machines and equipment, diagnostic procedures, specialized treatments, expanded understanding of the causes of and progression of disease, gene diagnosis and therapy, and greater insight into what is required for people to stay healthy. New interventions have saved lives, improved quality of life, alleviated suffering, and significantly decreased the incidence of some diseases. Before the advent of many modern health-related technologies, people experienced illness and death as an inevitable part of the cycle of their lives. Although death was not necessarily welcomed, it was expected as the natural outcome when the body could no longer ward off the effects of certain diseases or injuries. If someone was born with, or developed, a deformity, it may have been seen as a curse, but was also considered part of who the person was. Life began when the infant started breathing, and life ended when the heart and breathing stopped.

Current technology makes it possible to restart arrested hearts, use machines to breathe for people, correct deformities, assist the body in dealing with disease through use of medications and other interventions, eliminate diseased parts through surgery, and even to replace malfunctioning or diseased vital organs. The ability to prolong life, or at least to extend the functioning of the physical being, has prompted the necessity of dealing with some very important issues. One dilemma relates to questions of quality of life, and whether physical existence is synonymous with living. Another issue relates to whether the availability of certain technologies means they should always be used. Many issues relate to decisions about how and for whom technologies will be used.

Quality of Life

The ability to keep people alive and physically functioning through use of technology has led to much reflection and discussion about what constitutes life and living. Some people believe that biological life must be preserved, regardless of the effect on the person whose body is being kept alive. A frequently-asked question is whether a person is truly alive in situations where there is merely physiological functioning, without awareness of oneself or others. Many suggest that living implies a quality that goes beyond physical existence. **Quality of life,** a subjective appraisal of factors that make life worth living and contribute to a positive experience of living, means different things to different people. It is difficult to find a clear and concise definition of quality of life, because of the multidisciplinary usage and variable cultural understanding of the concept. Farquhar (1995) points out that definitions of quality of life derive from both lay and "expert" sources and range from global understandings of the concept, such as satisfaction with life, to focused definitions used for research, for example, health or functional ability. Ideas incorporated in understandings of the concept include fulfillment, satisfaction/dissatisfaction, conditions of life, happiness/unhappiness, experiences of life, and factors such as comfort, functional status, socioeconomic status, independence, and conditions in one's environment.

Farquhar (1995) suggests that deciding what weight to give different dimensions of the concept presents problems in defining quality of life. For instance, when evaluating personal quality of life, which does a person rank as more important, happiness, or functional status, such as the ability to get around and care for oneself? Nurses need to understand patient perspectives of what constitutes quality in their lives in order to incorporate these factors into goal setting and care planning.

Quality of life is a personal perspective that is determined by each individual. Recognizing this, we should not judge the quality of another's life based on our own values. If judgments are made about a person's worth and quality of life based on factors such as contributions to society, age, mental capacity, or ability to function, discrimination against those who are judged to have a lesser quality of life may easily follow. Perceptions of quality of life often change with age and life experiences. For example, persons with debilitating health concerns may rate the quality of their lives quite positively, although others might feel that they could never live with such limitations. When patients and families are confronted with technological options, nurses need to help them clarify their perceptions regarding quality of life, and discuss not only how life might be extended, but also how quality of life may be affected by various options.

Principles of Beneficence and Nonmaleficence

When dealing with issues of technology, the principles of **beneficence** and **nonmaleficence** may be in conflict. A particular technology, which may be implemented with the intention of *doing good* (beneficence), may result in much suffering for the patient. Inducing such suffering is counter to the maxim of *do no harm* (nonmaleficence). In some circumstances this is accepted as part of the treatment process, such as pain associated with surgery or side effects of chemotherapy. We are willing to endure the discomfort because there is an expectation of recovery, that we will ultimately be or feel more healthy. In circumstances in which there is little or no expectation of recovery or improved functioning, the essential question is whether the harm imposed by technology outweighs the good intended by its use. Suffering associated with technology may include physical, spiritual, and emotional elements for both patient and family. Making decisions regarding use of technology may cause pain, and there is suffering in living with unknown results of these ongoing decisions. Relief of suffering, a goal of healing from its earliest days, needs to be addressed in all patient encounters.

CURRENT TECHNOLOGY: ISSUES AND DILEMMAS

Current technologies related to organ and tissue transplantation, genetic engineering, reproduction, and sustaining life have profound potential for affecting our lives and health in positive ways. Their use also presents dilemmas for patients, families, professionals, and society. Nurses generally do not make the decisions regarding implementing or withdrawing particular technologies (except perhaps in situations like initiating cardiopulmonary recuscitation following specific protocols), yet we are involved as the caregivers of those receiving interventions and in many levels of patient care that involve technology. One of nursing's primary responsibilities is to help patients and families deal with the purposes, benefits, and limitations of the specific technologies. This section focuses primarily on the issue of withdrawing or withholding treatment as a prime example of a dilemma related to technology. Other issues related to technology are discussed briefly, and the reader is encouraged to further explore particular areas as the need or interest arises.

Treating Patients: When to Intervene and to What End

One of the most controversial bioethical topics of recent years centers around withholding or withdrawing life-sustaining treatments when they are deemed to have poor outcomes or offer no benefit. Decisions about withholding or withdrawing medical treatment are generally made by physicians in consultation with patients and family members. Approaches to dealing with these decisions reflect varying attitudes and concerns and may be confusing for all involved. A brief look at history sheds light on current attitudes regarding dealing with contemporary medical treatment. Questions related to the ethical limitations of medical care date back to the time of Hippocrates, when physicians were taught that the goal of medicine was to relieve suffering and reduce the effects of disease by lending support to natural processes. Medicine was not intended for situations in which the body was overpowered by disease, since interventions might merely prolong the suffering. The accepted ethical stance recognized the limitations of medicine, and withheld treatments that held little potential for healing (Jecker, 1995).

The scientific era that began emerging in the seventeenth century fostered a change in this ethical stance. Rather than revering and working with natural processes, con quering and dominating nature became the goal of science. In the nineteenth century, as medicine began to align more with science and biologic causes for diseases were discovered, the goal of medicine became the conquest of disease by exercising power over nature. Jecker notes that ethical problems involving aggressive medical treatments where there is little likelihood of success or poor quality of expected outcomes "are the outgrowth of a scientific tradition whose mission is to control and dominate, whose proving ground is nature, and whose means is an unfailing faith in the scientific method" (1995, p. 144). Within this narrow focus of curing disease, ethical issues of personal quality of life and dimensions of suffering are often unrecognized and neglected. With their attention to healing and caring, nurses play an important role in calling attention to concerns that go beyond the narrow focus of curing.

Issues of Life, Death, and Dying

Ethical dilemmas faced in health care settings often relate to issues of and attitudes toward living and dying. Important questions that are deliberated by those involved include "When does life begin?," "When does life end?," "How can we be sure that someone has died?," and "Who decides?" Technology has stretched the boundaries and clouded the waters surrounding life's beginning and ending. Perspectives vary from the belief that life begins at conception to the view that it begins when an infant can survive outside the womb. Technology makes this discussion even more complex and raises questions such as "What happens when conception cannot occur 'naturally' and artificial processes are employed either in vivo or in vitro?" and "Is the laboratory embryo a life?"

Today, many low birth weight infants and those with certain birth defects, who would not have survived in prior eras, survive with the support of machines, medications, and surgical procedures. In the process, however, some babies are kept alive only to die after months of expensive treatment. Others survive to face chronic health problems, with their associated financial, emotional, and physical strains on families and the health care system. There is no definitive way to predict which infants will have problems as they grow and develop. Dilemmas arise regarding how much effort to invest in "saving" a few infants who have a high probability of living only a short time or with significant health problems.

Ask Yourself

When Does Life Begin?

- What are your beliefs about when life begins? What shaped these beliefs?
- Consider that you are a member of a special task force called together by your hospital to establish guidelines for allocating dwindling funds for support of low birth weight infants in the neonatal intensive care unit. What criteria would you use to determine which of the infants who cannot survive without technology at birth receive such interventions?
- If an infant will die without technology and the technology is withdrawn, do you consider that a natural or unnatural end of life? Why?

In our society, death has become an unnatural event, frequently associated with hospitals and other institutions, surrounded by tubes, machinery, and heroic efforts. Determining when life ends has become a critical issue related to use of technology, prompting the involvement of courts in decision making. The general attitude, especially among health care providers, is that death is the enemy to be overcome or kept at bay for as long as possible, regardless of the age or health condition of the person. Thus death is often viewed as a failure on the part of the health provider. It is understandable, therefore, that many health care providers have difficulty dealing with death as a possible outcome for patients, thus finding it a difficult topic to discuss. Another reason that the topic of death may be avoided is that discussing death requires us to face issues of meaning in life and anxieties and fears regarding our own mortality. However, lack of discussion of death as a possible outcome may lead families and patients to have unreasonable expectations and false hopes of what the system can offer. Demands for inappropriate interventions, or accusations that not enough was done, may arise from such situations. Patients and families need support in recognizing and honoring their responses, beliefs, and fears regarding death. By facing our own issues about death, we are better able to facilitate this process with patients.

In many cultures, death is viewed as part of our life cycle which comes in its own time. Health care focused on curing is provided when there is reasonable hope of benefit, but people recognize when it is time for care to mean letting go and facilitating the transition through the dying process. In such cultures, dying often occurs at home, surrounded by family and friends.

Ask Yourself

What Are Your Views of Death and Dying?

What many people fear most regarding death is suffering and dying alone.

- How does technology contribute to this concern or attitude?

- What has your experience been related to death, what has shaped your attitudes regarding death, and what are your fears related to death?

- How can nurses minimize or deal with the effects of technology on patients in the dying process?

- How can nurses support patients and families in recognizing and honoring their own responses and beliefs regarding death?

- If machines and medication are keeping a body functioning, even if the person is apparently unaware, is that person still alive? Discuss your response.

- Do you think that brain wave activity in the midst of severe deterioration of major systems constitutes living? Discuss your response.

Personal attitudes prompt different expectations and scenarios when we are faced with decisions about heroic efforts and life-sustaining technologies. We must be aware of our own attitudes concerning living and dying, as well as the beliefs and expectations of patients, families, and other health care providers. Such awareness alerts us to situations in which there are differing attitudes among the parties involved, and provides an opportunity for opening lines of communication before a serious dilemma arises. Consider, for example, the patient who tells the nurse that he feels that his body is just giving up in spite of all the medications and treatments he is receiving, and he would like to go home to die peacefully, yet the physician is considering another surgery that is helpful about 30 percent of the time. In such a situation it would be important for the nurse to explore this area further with the patient, and either communicate his wishes to the physician or facilitate the patient's talking with the physician about his wishes.

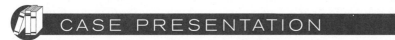

CASE PRESENTATION

A Child with Leukemia

Lucia, a twelve-year-old child with leukemia, has relapsed in spite of routine chemotherapeutic interventions. This child has suffered the side effects of the treatment, including nausea, hair loss, and frequent hospitalizations with infections, and is deteriorating physically. She says she feels as if she is being tortured with all the needles, spinal taps, and bone marrow samples; that she has no friends; and that this kind of life is not worth living. A bone marrow transplant (the only hope for a cure at this point) would mean subjecting her to intensive chemotherapy, total body irradiation, and weeks in isolation following the transplant. The family is told that there is a 40 percent chance that the transplant will be effective. The procedure is very expensive, and the family has already had to obtain a second mortgage for their home because their insurance has not covered many of the expenses to date.

Think About It

Factors Influencing Choices Regarding Medical Technology

- What factors do you think need to be considered in making the decision about having the bone marrow transplant?
- How do percentages of risk and benefit affect your decision making?
- In this situation, do you think a 40 percent chance of success is enough to go ahead with the transplant? What if it were 60 percent? What about 20 percent?

- How can you help patients and families use statistical information in deliberating their decisions? What other factors would you help them to consider?
- Who should be involved in making this decision?

We must remember that dying is more than a medical occurrence; it is a spiritual process touching the individual, family, and community. Although medical interventions can assist and support those in the dying process, current technologies can prolong suffering by prolonging the dying process, and separate people from their families by actual physical barriers and institutionalization. Relieving suffering and supporting a dignified death are important elements of the nursing role. Addressing patient needs may require nurses to make decisions to go against institutional policy regarding such things as visitors and visiting hours, in order to ensure that the patient is not alone, or to risk confrontations with physicians over pain management or other aspects of care.

Medical Futility

Ethical and legal arguments for initiating or discontinuing life-sustaining treatments are based primarily on the relative benefits and burdens for the patient. "Although many health care professionals feel reluctant to discontinue life-sustaining treatments, most philosophical and legal commentators find no important ethical or legal distinction between not instituting a treatment and discontinuing treatment already initiated" (Rushton, 1994, p. 517). Withholding or removing life-sustaining treatments in situations in which the burden or harm has been determined to outweigh the benefits is, in essence, allowing the person to die as a result of the natural progression of the illness process. This is different from **euthanasia**, which is causing the painless death of a person in order to end or prevent suffering. Curtin (1996) suggests that it is not reasonable to say that removal of artificial interventions cause death; rather, it is the condition (such as disease or accident), in response to which artificial interventions were initiated, that causes death.

In deliberations regarding withholding, initiating, or withdrawing life-sustaining interventions, **medical futility** related to the patient's situation has been discussed as a major factor. Medical futility refers to situations in which interventions are judged to have no medical benefit, or in which the chance for success is low. Futility is often discussed in relation to cardiopulmonary resuscitation (CPR), but it relates as well to interventions that preserve patients in persistent vegetative states or dependent on the technology of tertiary care settings. One difficulty associated with medical futility is that there is no set definition of the concept, only suggested parameters that vary greatly in guiding health care providers. Lo (1995) suggests that there are strict definitions of futility that would justify unilateral decisions by physicians to withhold or withdraw interventions, and *loose*, value-laden definitions of the concept that do not justify such unilateral decisions. Strict definitions of futility include interventions that have no pathophysiologic rationale, have already failed in the patient, will not achieve the goal of care, and situations where maximal treatment is failing. Determination of futility in these situations "is based on objective data and judgments within the expertise of the physician. Physicians have no ethical duty to provide interventions that are futile in such strict senses; indeed, they generally have an ethical obligation not to provide them even if they are requested" (Lo, 1995, pp. 74–75).

Loose definitions of futility include situations that prompt variable interpretations and thus are more confusing—for example, situations in which the likelihood of success is very small; no worthwhile goals of care can be achieved; patient quality of life is unacceptable; and prospective benefit is not worth the resources required. In these situations, the meaning of futility must consider perceptions of the patient and family and judgments of the health care team. In the absence of clear external guidelines, these less-clear situations require more skillful nursing care, as persons draw on their own understandings and resources shaped by personal beliefs and cultural values.

Ask Yourself

What Constitutes Medical Futility?

- What do you think about these definitions of futility? Where would you envision potential problems or dilemmas based on these definitions?

- Would you consider an expensive treatment that works 20 percent of the time to be futile? What if it only works 5 percent of the time? Explain.

- Should medical futility be an issue when treatments are not expensive? Explain.

- Do you think a decision about futile treatment should be different with children and younger adults than with the elderly? Discuss your response.

- How would you see a patient's inability to pay for treatment affecting decisions about futility?

Because personal values come into play, health care providers, patients, and families may have differing views of what is a benefit or burden. Because of the difficulty in defining and developing clear guidelines for medical futility, recent literature focuses less on the concept of futility, and more on the process of working with the patient and family to explain fully the medical circumstances, and negotiate care that is in the best interest of the patient. For example, a patient or family may find hope and be willing to consider a treatment that has a 5 percent likelihood of success, while the health care providers see this as a futile effort. When considering quality of life, the perspective of the patient and family is essential in any determination of futility. Deciding when it is not worth continuing life-sustaining treatment is another circumstance in which the views of the parties involved may differ. Consider, for example, a seventy-two-year-old quadriplegic patient on a ventilator at home who has been deteriorating and having frequent infections. She had to be resuscitated when recently hospitalized for severe respiratory infection. The physician discussed the situation with the patient and the family and suggested a **do not resuscitate (DNR) order,** which is a written directive placed in the patient's medical chart indicating that cardiopulmonary resuscitation is to be avoided. (See further discussion of DNR orders later in this chapter.) Even though the patient and most family members indicated agreement, the daughter who is the caregiver said she wants every effort made to keep her mother alive, saying that God will take her mother when He is ready. In another situation, health care providers might view continuing treatments that prolong a patient's life a few more days to be causing unnecessary suffering, while for the patient and family this is important "saying goodbye" time.

CASE PRESENTATION

Mr. Mason and His Son

Mr. Mason is a seventy-eight-year-old retired, widowed ironworker. He has been estranged from his adult son, an only child, for many years. He was recently diagnosed with advanced lung cancer. He recognized that he needed to make some plans for his immediate future, so he contacted his son and allowed him power of attorney. Mr. Mason is admitted to your unit in severe pain. He is somewhat confused, and you are unable to elicit information from him about his wishes regarding life-sustaining measures. You carefully begin discussing this difficult subject with his son, as it is your hospital's policy that everyone admitted to your oncology unit be informed about advance directives. Following are three possible twists this case could take, each of which is based on a real-life situation.

Ending 1. Mr. Mason's son begins to sob uncontrollably, saying, "I was never a very good son. I left home when I was barely nineteen and didn't even write or call for many years. I am just getting to know my dad, and now this happens. I want as much time with him as possible. He told me a few days ago that he was ready to die and didn't want to be kept alive on machines. But it is so unfair to me. I want him alive and more time with him. Please, do everything you can to keep him alive. I need some more time with him. I need for him to forgive me."

Ending 2. Mr. Mason's son seems impatient, continually looking at his watch as you talk to him. Finally, seeming exasperated, he says, "Look, he's going to die anyway, right? Two things: first, I'm a busy man, and the quicker we get this over with the better. Second, I have an appointment in twenty minutes with a real estate agent, and later with Dad's stockbroker. I'd really like to start arranging to sell his house and cash in some of his stocks. My son starts college in two months, and we could use the money. I suppose you think this is cruel, but realistically, would Dad rather we spend the money he worked so hard for on keeping him alive, when he's bound to die anyway, or on his grandson's education? It's pretty clear to me. I say, just let Dad go, that would be the best for everyone concerned."

Ending 3. The son quickly acknowledges that he understands the question. Without hesitation he says, "Do all you can to keep him alive. The tyrant was mean to me all of my life. I hate him. I want him to suffer as long as possible."

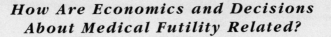

Think About It

Family Reactions to Medically Futile Situations

- What is your response to the son's statement in each of these scenarios? Include both your thinking response and your feeling response.
- How would your feelings lead you to advise one option over another?
- How do you think the nurse should react to each response?
- What values and dilemmas are evident in each scenario?
- Identify your personal and professional values related to each scenario.
- Who should make the decision? Do you feel conflicting loyalties?
- How would you respond to the son's decision?

Economics and Medical Futility. The cost of health care, particularly in relation to technology, has brought economic factors into discussions of futility. Some suggest that the principle of justice indicates that if a particular intervention is judged to be of limited or no benefit for one person, it should be discontinued so it is available for another patient who can make better use of the scarce resource. Lantos (1994) notes that political and economic developments in medicine in recent years, particularly prospective payment, have prompted physicians and hospitals to look more closely at futile treatments. Under prospective payment systems, physicians and institutions lose money if patients are maintained on particular treatments beyond a predetermined length of time. Lantos argues that the development of prospective payment systems delegated the responsibility to limit excessive treatments to physicians as a kind of social mandate. He further suggests that it is ethical and justifiable for physicians to limit access to treatments that are expensive while offering limited benefits, and that, given limited health care resources, such decisions are socially responsible. Such an argument is consistent with utilitarian ethics, a perspective often used by government agencies when deciding about distribution of goods and services.

Ask Yourself

How Are Economics and Decisions About Medical Futility Related?

- Under what circumstances do you feel physicians or institutions should be able to limit a patient's access to expensive treatments?
- How do you think economics affects decisions about medical futility?
- How might patient care be affected by these decisions?
- What are potential legal ramifications of such decisions?

Do Not Resuscitate Orders

Cardiopulmonary resuscitation (CPR) is an area in which nurses have an active role in initiating or withholding life-sustaining treatment. Considering whether to initiate CPR with a patient requires attention to professional, ethical, legal, and institutional considerations. Principles utilized to justify decisions regarding resuscitation include autonomy, self-determination, nonmaleficence, and respect for persons.

The general practice regarding CPR is that it must be initiated unless: (1) it would clearly be futile to do so, or (2) the practitioner has specific instructions not to do so. The legal definition of do not recuscitate (DNR) is not to initiate CPR in the event of a cardiac or pulmonary arrest. As noted previously, DNR orders are written directives placed in a patient's medical record indicating that the use of cardiopulmonary resuscitation is to be avoided. DNR orders should be documented immediately in a patient's health care record, noting the reason the order was written, who gave consent and who was involved in the discussion, whether the patient was competent to give consent or who was authorized to do so, and the time frame for the DNR order (Thibault-Prevost, Jensen, & Hodgins, 2000). In situations of the strict definitions of medical futility noted above, Lo (1995) suggests that decisions to withhold or stop CPR are appropriately made by physicians and that, in such situations, resuscitation need not be offered as an option for patients. Some suggest that nurses are as well qualified as physicians to write DNR orders. Because nurses are the professionals who are in close and continuous contact with patients, they are perhaps better able to help patients and families articulate their views regarding end-of-life care and concerns (Martin & Redland, 1988; American Nurses' Association, 1992a; Thibault-Prevost, Jensen, & Hodgins, 2000). DNR decisions require open communication among the patient or surrogate, the family, and the health care team. This communication needs to include explicit discussion of the efficacy and desirability of CPR, balanced with the potential harm and suffering it may cause the patient. People often overestimate the effectiveness of CPR, and do not understand that CPR is not always medically indicated. Many people derive their concept of CPR from what they see in the media. In their study of how CPR is portrayed on television, Diem, Lantos, and Tulsky (1996) discovered that rates of survival after CPR in television dramas were much higher than the most optimistic survival rates in the medical literature. In order to make informed decisions regarding CPR, patients and families need to understand their clinical condition and prognosis. People rarely appreciate that CPR is a harsh and traumatic procedure, and that patients with multiple, severe, chronic health problems who receive CPR rarely survive to discharge (Quill, 2000; Moss, 2001).

Tomlinson and Brody (1988) note that the relevance of considering the patient's or family's values in justifying DNR orders may vary, depending on the rationale given for the decision. In situations in which there would be no medical benefits, patient autonomy and consent are considered less relevant. However, when rationale for the decision is based on the patient's quality of life, either after or before CPR, determination of whether the benefit of continued life outweighs the risk of harmful consequences, such as debility or suffering, must flow from the values of the patient or patient's surrogate. Competent patients have the right to refuse CPR and may request DNR orders after they have been informed of the risks and benefits involved. Good communication is the most critical key factor in assuring that any DNR decision is acceptable to all parties involved.

CASE PRESENTATION

Mistaken Resuscitation

Jacob has had a chronic lung condition for the past ten of his thirty-two years. The condition causes some restrictions on his life, but he has kept up with a regular job and is very involved in his church. He is currently hospitalized with a severe respiratory infection. Although his condition did not seem to be that serious, when he was admitted he made sure that there was a DNR order in his chart, noting that he has a firm religious conviction that the Creator, and not the doctor, is to decide when it is time for him to die. Because of a staff shortage, Lashanda, a registered nurse who usually works on another unit, has been assigned to Jacob's unit. Although she has been working on the other side of the unit, she is presently covering the whole unit while other staff are at lunch. As she answers a call light from Jacob's roommate, she notices that Jacob is not breathing and has no pulse. Since she is unfamiliar with Jacob's DNR request, she immediately calls a "code" and initiates CPR, figuring that there would be no question that this would be the appropriate action for someone this age. Although Jacob is successfully resuscitated with no serious sequelae, he is intensely angry, saying that it was an interference in the Creator's plan.

Think About It

Decisions Regarding Resuscitation

- What do you think about Jacob's request for a DNR order? What ethical principles are involved in his choice?
- What do you think about Lashanda's response in the situation? Do you think she acted appropriately under the circumstances?
- How do you think you might respond in a similar situation? What principles would guide your actions?
- Describe potential legal ramifications in this situation.
- What guidelines would your state's laws regarding DNR status offer to LaShandra? Would they support her actions?

DNR orders apply only to resuscitation. The fact that CPR might be considered futile does not necessarily imply that other life-sustaining interventions are futile or that other treatments will not be used. Health care providers often fail to make this distinction, thus causing confusion for patients as well. Many institutions require more specific instructions regarding what is and is not to be done for a patient. These interventions might include treatment of physiological abnormalities like fever or cardiac arrhythmias, nutrition, or use of mechanical ventilation and CPR. Plans for and parameters of DNR orders need to be discussed with all members of the health care team so that the goal of care is clear. The presence of DNR orders requires nurses to become even more focused on providing supportive and comfort interventions, and to ensure that there is no reduction in the level of care for the patient and family. A DNR order means only that, in the event of cardiac or respiratory arrest, there are to be no attempts to resuscitate. Presuming no arrest occurs, the patient may recover from the problem necessitating hospitalization and return home.

At a more philosophical level, Scofield suggests that decisions to not resuscitate ask us "individually and collectively, to arrive at a consensus on how to integrate death and decisions about it into the legitimating values of our moral universe. Deciding what kind of life we want involves deciding what kind of death we can face" (1995, p. 184). He notes that death, which was once considered fate, is now often a matter of a choice that we do not want to have to make. This is the dilemma that faces those involved in DNR decisions.

Nursing Considerations Related to DNR Orders.   Although it is generally considered the domain of the physician to write a DNR order, nurses need to be aware of parameters surrounding such orders. Nurses need to know which patients under their care have DNR orders, and these orders need to be documented clearly in a patient's chart, and perhaps at the bedside, and reviewed periodically as the patient's condition changes. If a patient or appropriate surrogate indicates to the nurse the desire not to be resuscitated and there is no order in the chart, the nurse should document the request in the patient's chart and bring this to the immediate attention of the physician. The nurse may wish to explore the request with the patient or surrogate, and may need to facilitate discussion of the issue between patient and physician. Orders should specify which interventions are to be withheld, and considerations regarding circumstances in which they are to be withheld. All persons involved in the care of the patient need to know about the orders. Since attitudes affect one's approach to others, nurses need to reflect on their own attitudes toward decisions regarding withholding of interventions, both in general and in particular patient situations.

Artificial Sources of Nutrition

Maintaining nutrition is a natural life-sustaining measure and a common part of the nursing role. Once a person has difficulty with functions associated with nutrition, such as chewing or swallowing, or is not conscious enough to participate in these activities, decisions about artificial sources of nutrition must be made. Ethical dilemmas arise concerning whether to classify such interventions as feeding or as medical treatments, as ordinary or extraordinary measures. ANA's (1992b) policy on *Forgoing Nutrition and Hydration* stresses the importance of determining whether food and fluid are more beneficial or harmful to a patient, noting that artificially-provided nutrition and hydration may not be ethically justified.

Utilizing artificial sources of nutrition may present dilemmas in situations involving persons in persistent vegetative states or end-stage dying processes for whom this intervention is maintaining physical life. We know that withholding food will eventually lead to starvation and death and, under most circumstances, is not considered an ethical action. However, it is considered appropriate to withhold or discontinue life-sustaining medical interventions when they are not benefiting the patient or are contrary to the patient's wishes. There are fewer complexities surrounding decisions to withhold artificial sources of nutrition than there are regarding decisions to withdraw medical interventions.

As with any such decision, we must consider the wishes of the patient or surrogate. Quality of life is an important factor, and if interventions contribute to, more than relieve, a patient's suffering, the principle of nonmaleficence may sway one toward a decision of not implementing or of discontinuing such therapies. Evidence suggests that tube feeding does not improve outcomes, and has substantial risks in some patients, particularly those with dementia or multisystem illness (Finucane, Christmas, & Travis, 1999; McCann, 1999; Moss, 2001). Curtin reflects that if a person is willing and able to eat and drink, even when death is imminent and the patient is suffering, attempts to quicken death by withholding ordinary nourishment is morally repugnant. However, "in situations in which death is inevitable and the conditions of living intolerable (involve extensive technological isolation from human touch, futile pain and pointless extensions of dying), highly sophisticated means of feeding are not in a patient's best interests and may be withheld or withdrawn" (1996, p. 82). Once artificial measures have been implemented, it is psychologically more difficult to decide on their removal. Curtin suggests that, unless a rational adult refuses them, such measures should be continued as long as sentient life is a reasonable expectation, but that they may be terminated when there is a reliable prediction of permanent unconsciousness. With any technological intervention we must consider whether its use is prolonging living or prolonging dying. When competent patients refuse food or fluid, respect for persons directs nurses to honor this refusal. Nurses need to help family and other caretakers understand that people who are dying often have a decline in appetite, and that the care of keeping the person comfortable does not need to include efforts to maintain nutrition. Involved parties may view the use of such interventions from different perspectives.

Legal Issues Related to Technology

As noted in Chapter 7, what is considered an ethical decision by some may not be upheld as a legal action. In the area of health care technology, the courts have intervened in some decisions related to withholding or withdrawing life-sustaining treatments when there has been disagreement among the involved parties. Legal precedents regarding issues such as what constitutes clear evidence of a person's wishes related to these treatments and what is considered standard practice have been set in the process. Examples of two such cases are presented here. When one looks at dilemmas faced by families, health care providers, institutions, and the legal system in situations such as these, the importance of having advance directives becomes evident. **Advance directives** are instructions indicating one's wishes regarding health care interventions or designating someone to act as a surrogate in making such decisions in the event that one loses decision making capacity. These directives are discussed in Chapter 11.

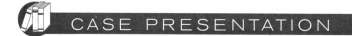

CASE PRESENTATION

Karen Quinlan

The well known case of Karen Quinlan (Devettere, 1995; Pence, 1995) is a story of a twenty-one-year-old woman who, in 1975, was found to have suffered cardiopulmonary arrest at home alone after having been drinking at a local bar. After the ambulance crew restored heartbeat through CPR, she was admitted to the local hospital and placed on a ventilator. Within a few days she was transferred to a larger hospital where she was kept alive with the assistance of a respirator and feeding tube. Over months she lost weight, developed contractures, and was given no hope of regaining awareness. After much deliberation, the family asked that the respirator be discontinued, but the hospital indicated that it could not grant the request unless the father was named as her guardian. When the father asked the court to appoint him guardian with authority to make decisions to discontinue extraordinary interventions, the court appointed him guardian of her property, but not of her person, and appointed a **guardian *ad litem*** to represent Karen. The guardian ad litem felt responsible for preserving Karen's life, and opposed removing the respirator. The physician's lawyer argued that removing a respirator from a living person was not standard medical procedure, and the judge sided with this view. When the family appealed the ruling to the New Jersey Supreme Court, the decision of the lower court was reversed and the father was appointed as her guardian. When the father requested that the respirator be removed, the physicians initiated a process of weaning her from it, resulting in her being able to breathe without the machine. Totally unconscious with severe contractures, she was transferred to a nursing home, where she died ten years later.

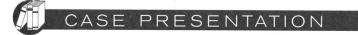

CASE PRESENTATION

Nancy Cruzan

In another well known case, Nancy Cruzan (Angell, 1990; Annas, 1990; Pence, 1995) was found unconscious and not breathing after her car went into a ditch in the winter of 1983. Although emergency personnel restored her breathing, she never regained consciousness. After a year of being sustained through the use of a gastrostomy tube for artificial nutrition, it was determined that she was in a persistent vegetative state. When her parents, acting as her guardians, asked that the artificial feeding be discontinued because she had indicated previously that she would not want to be kept alive in this condition, the physicians and hospital refused. When the case went to court, the evidence supporting discontinuing the feeding was based primarily on a statement she had made to a roommate that she would not want to live if she were a vegetable. The judge ruled that the medical nutrition could be removed, but that decision was appealed to the Missouri State Supreme Court by a guardian *ad litem*. The Missouri court reversed the previous decision, claiming that there was no clear and convincing evidence that this would be her wish, that she was not terminally ill or suffering, and that there was no reason to act contrary to the state's interest in preserving life, regardless of how minimal that life had become. An appeal to the United States Supreme Court upheld the decision that medical nutrition could not be withdrawn because of the lack of clear and convincing evidence. In 1990, almost eight years after her accident, Nancy's parents appealed again to the local court with the evidence of three of her friends who stated that she had told them that she would not want to live in a vegetative state. At that time, the physician agreed that it was no longer in her best interests to be medically nourished, and the judge agreed that there was now clear and convincing evidence indicating that it was in her best interests to terminate artificial nutrition.

Think About It

When the Courts Intervene

- As you reflect on these two cases, which position do you support, that of the family or that of the guardian ad litem?
- Which court decisions do you think are more valid? Defend your position.
- Describe ethical dilemmas and principles involved in these situations.
- If one of your family members was in a similar situation, how do you think you would respond? Would you expect solidarity or disagreement with this position from other members of your family?
- Consider that you are a nurse caring for Karen or Nancy at various stages in her situation. How would you respond to the various parties involved as decisions about her care are being discussed?
- What do you think about the role of the legal system in decisions regarding use of technology?

Palliative Care

Two primary obligations that we have to people who are dying are comfort and company (Moss, 2001). When life-sustaining interventions are no longer of benefit or are not desired by the patient, the focus of care becomes palliative, that is, directed toward comfort and support. **Palliative care** is comprehensive, interdisciplinary, and total care, focusing primarily on comfort and support of patients and families who face illness which is chronic or not responsive to curative treatment (Critchley et. al., 1999; Billings, 2000; Moss, 2001). Palliative care focuses on the best quality of life for patient and family through meticulous control of pain and other symptoms, a personalized plan to optimize quality of life as defined by patient and family, and spiritual and psychosocial care. Palliative care requires delivery of coordinated and continuous services in home, hospice, skilled nursing facilities, or hospital, and includes support in bereavement. Members of the palliative care team include nurses, physicians, spiritual support persons, pharmacist, social services, mental health services, and pain services.

The backbone of palliative care is good nursing care that continues to support the dignity and self-respect of patient and family. In addition to providing care to the patient and the family, nurses often coordinate palliative care teams. When families are in disagreement about when it is time to stop other interventions and focus on palliative care, the nurse's ability to communicate effectively with and facilitate communication among those involved is crucial. Families often need time to see what we see regarding the patient's condition and expected outcomes of various interventions. We have to be willing to take as much time as necessary and as often as needed to explain and negotiate care decisions. Robin Shirley (personal communication, January 18, 2001) shares the following process that she uses in her role of palliative care nurse.

Palliative Care Conference

- Have a holistic view of the patient, including present health status, prognosis, significant relationships, living situation, family dynamics, decision-making capacity, advance directives or surrogate, and spiritual support.

- If the patient does not have decision-making capacity and there is no surrogate, seek to have a surrogate named.

- Prior to scheduling the conference, inform the surrogate that the purpose of the meeting is to determine the best way to provide quality end-of-life care to the patient and family, and stress the need for all family and significant persons, including spiritual support persons, to participate. The conference is set at a time when most people can be there. Primary nurse, physician, and other involved health care team members are included.

- In opening the meeting, the palliative care nurse describes the process that will be followed in order to allow everyone an opportunity to speak and ask questions, and to arrive at a consensus regarding what is truly best for the patient.

- The meeting is opened by introducing everyone present and their role or relationship with the patient. In order to prevent disorder that can occur with the high emotions of the circumstances, those present are then asked one by one to name things that the patient enjoyed in life. This process also helps the physician and other care providers to step back from the clinical picture and see the patient as a person with individual values and meaning. Next, the physician is asked to discuss current status and prognosis, allowing an opportunity for family to ask any questions. The primary nurse is then asked to discuss daily care and interactions with the patient, and to respond to any questions. Through this process the family is often able to acknowledge that their loved one will not return to the state they once enjoyed, which leads to the beginning of acceptance and consideration of what is truly best for the patient at this time.

- Everyone in turn is then asked what they know or believe to be the desires of their loved one regarding end-of-life care. This includes the values of the patient, and what family members consider to be in the best interest. This process often prompts tears and reminiscing. Spiritual support persons may comment about the patient's spiritual values and considerations, or intervene as needed to support those participating.

- Throughout this process the palliative care nurse periodically re-states what the general consensus of the group seems to be. This helps to clarify what is being said, and provides those not in agreement an opportunity to bring up concerns or issues. The meeting generally concludes with consensus regarding what is best for their loved one and discussion regarding comfort measures desired by the family and which the care providers feel will best suit the patient. (In some situations more than one meeting may be needed before consensus is reached.)

- All involved frequently join around the patient's bedside following the meeting for prayer and reminiscing. The family usually has open visitation, and are involved as much as they wish in care for the patient.

- Documentation of the process, participants, content, and outcomes is completed in the patient's record and ongoing follow-up is initiated.

Examples of Potential Dilemmas with Other Technology

In addition to life-sustaining interventions, advances in technology affect nursing and health care in other arenas as well. Examples of a few such technologies are briefly presented here. Nurses who work with patients whose care involves such technologies need to be aware of potential ethical issues associated with their use, as well as the benefits of such interventions. The intention here is to alert the student to some of the questions and dilemmas that may be associated with these technologies. The student is encouraged to explore these areas further, reflecting on personal values related to each technology.

Reproductive Technology.   Because the inability to conceive and bear children can be a very distressing experience for a couple, any technology that can facilitate the process may well be viewed as a life-affirming gift. Such technologies include artificial insemination by donor, in vitro fertilization, and surrogate embryo transfer. While scientists develop and refine these technologies to benefit people, ethicists and others raise questions related to moral implications of their use. Some questions focus on the potential for changing society's concept of family and parenthood. For example, in the case of surrogacy, is the mother of the baby the woman whose ovum is joined with her husband's sperm, or the woman who donates her body for the baby's development and birth? We must consider whether the use of such technologies might relegate childbearing into little more than the production of a product. Other ethical questions arise regarding who has custody of frozen embryos, and whether these embryos have rights. A related consideration is the potential that women may become more exploited than liberated by the use of these technologies. Because these interventions are expensive, questions arise regarding who should pay for them, and for whom they should be made available. For example, Roberts (2000) notes that these technologies are more available to white women than to women of color. Ethical considerations regarding these technologies, she asserts, must include an emphasis on social justice and attention to societal attitudes about who should or should not have children, and what kind of children should be born.

Genetic Diagnosis, Engineering, and Screening.   Advances in molecular biology, new reproductive technologies, and the Human Genome Project have prompted rapid breakthroughs in genetic research. This research has advanced our knowledge of the use of genetic interventions as possible remedies for diseases caused by genetic disorders. The possibilities of these interventions, however, raise ethical as well as legal and social justice questions (Frankel & Chapman, 2000). **Genetic diagnosis,** which is usually done within an in vitro fertilization program, involves a process of biopsy of embryos to determine the presence of genetic flaws and gender prior to implantation. At present, such diagnosis is aimed at couples who have a high risk of conceiving a child with a serious genetic disorder, with the intent that only embryos that are free of genetic flaws would be implanted. **Genetic engineering** is the ability to alter organisms genetically for a variety of purposes, such as developing more disease-resistant fruits and vegetables, or eventually being able to alter embryos genetically so that the fetus and baby will be healthier. Through **genetic screening** it is possible to determine if persons are predisposed to certain diseases, and whether couples have the possibility of giving birth to a genetically impaired infant. The implications of having such technologies available include the potential for correcting some genetic defects in embryo, eliminating some very serious genetic diseases, and producing food that is more nourishing and resilient. Frankel and Chapman (2000) make a distinction between the therapeutic use of these interventions, and the possibility that these interventions may be used to modify human characteristics beyond those that are needed to sustain or restore health. The possibility of their use to enhance certain human characteristics has significant social implications. For example, such interventions could offer control over the genetic inheritance, including the biological properties and personality traits of our children. They suggest that the ability to discard "undesirable" traits and improve those that are "desirable" may lead to a form of **eugenics,** meaning "good birth." The eugenics movement of the early twentieth century sought to promote traits that proponents felt were desirable for society, while weeding out what they considered undesirable. In the United States and elsewhere around the world, eugenics led to efforts to discourage procreation among people deemed to be "socially inferior" through compulsory sterilization of many people, particularly those who were poor, in prison, or in mental institutions. Another concern that these authors raise is that these technologies may lead to the imposition of a skewed or harmful definition of what is normal regarding human traits, and what is considered abnormal or undesirable. Because individuals and societies tend to impose their values and standards on others, this could lead to serious transcultural implications.

Concerns related to these technologies are as varied as their potential benefits, particularly the recognition that relaxing criteria related to a person's value or rights in one arena may lead to abuses or exploitation in other circumstances. Ethicists often speak of these concerns in terms of a *slippery slope* where, for example, one decision based on relaxing criteria supporting the value of human life makes it easy to slide into acceptance of lower standards as ethical guides. For example, one concern is that genetic engineering might produce organisms that could be harmful to humans; another is that employers or insurers might use information gained from genetic screening to exclude people with particular traits from certain jobs or from being insured. Might genetic screening and diagnosis lead to abuses, such as forbidding people with certain traits to have children, insurers refusing to cover epenses if insured mothers give birth to genetically-impaired infants, or prohibiting the birth of babies with particular genetic features deemed undesirable by those in power in a society? These areas include other broad societal implications, such as who pays for the procedures, who determines guidelines for their use, and to whom they are made available.

Organ and Tissue Procurement and Transplantation.
Organ transplantation is no longer considered as extraordinary or uncommon a health care event as it was in the not too distant past. As techniques become more refined, the possibility of a transplant becomes a hope for more and more people afflicted with the failure of a vital organ. Because the demand for organs is great and the supply limited, dilemmas related to allocation of scarce resources emerge. Questions arise regarding eligibility of recipients for organ transplant. Should these determinations be made based on a potential recipient's expectation of survival posttransplant, or ability to pay for the procedure, or power and prestige, or some combination of these and other factors? Transplantation may involve organs from dead or living human donors, animals, or artificial appliances, and there are dilemmas associated with each. This discussion focuses on human donor issues.

Because transplantation requires well-nourished organs, procurement must occur as soon after death as possible. Thus, having criteria for determining when death occurs is imperative. Irreversible cessation of cardiopulmonary functioning is one such criterion. However, until CPR has been attempted, how is one to know if the cessation is irreversible? If CPR is initiated, organs to be donated may be damaged, raising an issue of how to deal with a person's desire to be an organ donor with a consideration for CPR. Questions regarding when and how intensively to initiate CPR become important issues regarding organ donation. If a person has been maintained on life support technology, brain death is the most likely criteria to be used, which leads to issues regarding what constitutes brain death. Some suggest that current criteria for brain death which indicate that all functions of the entire brain must cease are more stringent than necessary, and that irreversible cessation of higher brain functions would be sufficient criteria. Such a change in brain death criteria would open the possibility of harvesting organs from people in persistent vegetative states or in permanent comas, and with this would come questions about the ethics of doing so.

The scarcity of available organs and the long waiting lists of potential recipients raise the possibility that people may be declared dead prematurely. This scarcity of organs also affects organ procurement from living human beings. With living donors, issues related to voluntary informed consent and the buying and selling of organs are of concern. There are places in the world where organs are taken from poor people or prisoners, without their knowledge or against their will, and sold to procurement centers in more affluent countries. Desperate straits have prompted some individuals to sell an organ to raise money for personal or family needs, raising a question about whether there can be true voluntary informed consent under such circumstances.

In cases of sudden accidental death, family members may be asked to consider donation of viable organs. Consider whether there can be true voluntary consent when the family is in the midst of crisis and shock. With the urgency for a decision due to time factors for harvesting organs, coercion could be a factor. In some settings nurses are asked to approach patients or families about considering organ donation. In such situations nurses need to be clear about their own feelings regarding organ procurement and transplantation, and they must remember that attention to family needs takes precedence over the time constraints of organ harvesting.

NURSING PRACTICE IN THE MIDST OF TECHNOLOGY

Nursing practice continues to evolve with expanding knowledge and scientific advances in many arenas. As technology has been developed and refined, related nursing responsibilities have expanded. In the midst of these changes, the essence of nursing remains the human focus of caring for patients and families—being attentive to the needs of persons whose lives are affected by the technology. Integrating caring and technology and juggling the demands of each present challenges for nurses in any area of practice. As new technologies become available, they will bring with them associated issues of concern. Regardless of the technology, important considerations for nursing relate to attitudes and values, communication, and maintaining the human focus of care.

Attitudes and Values

The importance of self-awareness related to values, beliefs, and reactions is especially significant when dealing with issues related to technology. The process of being more attentive to personal perspectives regarding such issues as quality of life, living, dying, medical futility, and allocation of scarce resources may be facilitated by pondering questions such as those posed throughout this chapter. Such awareness enables the nurse to differentiate personal values from those of patients and others involved in the situation. Principles of self-determination and autonomy counsel the nurse to understand that individuals may judge benefits of an intervention from varying perspectives. Recognizing where personal values may be different enables nurses to be more attentive to fostering good communication, encouraging others to make their own decisions, avoiding judgment about the rightness or wrongness of the decision based on personal values, and accepting those decisions even if they are different from what the nurse would do.

As the various examples presented in this chapter suggest, many dilemmas that emerge surrounding technology relate to differing values among the parties involved. Facilitating discussion of values among patients and families may help them to clarify their own perspectives. Nurses also need to be alert to situations in which there may be differences in values among the patient, family, and physician. Encouraging timely communication may avert a major dilemma, or facilitate more effective resolution of the concern. Nurses who cannot reconcile their values with a particular situation need to take the necessary steps to remove themselves from that situation so as to not compromise patient care or personal integrity. In so doing, it is essential to avoid abandoning the patient by ensuring that there are others who will provide the needed care for the patient.

The Importance of Communication: Who Decides?

As has been noted, there are many factors involved in making decisions about withholding or withdrawing life-sustaining treatments and utilizing other technologies. Nurses need to determine who is involved in making the decision, and how the nurse fits into the scenario. Utilizing the decision-making process described in Chapter 6 may assist in this process. Nurses need to be aware of institutional policies and protocols regarding various technologies. Such policies should include approaches to reaching decisions about particular patients; ways of dealing with conflicts that may arise; protection of patient rights; description of roles of those involved in the decision-making process; and directions for documenting the decision in the patient's chart. In most situations, the patient or the patient's surrogate has the ultimate authority to decide which interventions to use or withhold.

Because nurses are in close and continual contact with patients, they are often perceived as more available and more approachable than physicians. Patients or family members may discuss their concerns about interventions more readily with the nurse, seeking information or advice. It is important to know what they have been told by the physician, determine the patient's and family's level of understanding about the situation, and whether they have the necessary information to make an informed decision. If information is needed in such areas as risks, discomforts, side effects, potential benefits, likelihood of success, treatment alternatives, or estimated costs, advocating for the patient in this regard is an expected nursing response. Nurses are in a key position to utilize conversations with patients and families to discover areas of confusion and to elicit information about the patient's wishes regarding interventions.

Sometimes people just need to talk out their concerns and sort through sometimes conflicting messages coming from the head and the heart. Providing a listening presence can help people vent emotions, speak their fears, and clarify their concerns. At times the concern may be such that the nurse must advocate for the patient by facilitating communication with the physician, support people such as family or pastor, or other appropriate persons, such as a patient representative or member of the ethics committee. Collaboration among all involved is important to ensure an informed choice. Effective communication can be facilitated by providing an environment that is not rushed; using terms and language that are understood by the other person; allowing time for and encouraging questions; practicing attentive listening; and offering a caring presence.

Caring: The Human Focus

In the context of expanding scientific and technological knowledge, nurses have the responsibility for helping patients and families benefit from what technology offers, while always remembering the human focus of care. Davis (1991) suggests that when medical treatment is deemed futile, nursing care in its fullest meaning is most essential. This is evident especially in nursing's role in palliative care. However alert, and in whatever stage of living and dying, an individual has a life story that continues to unfold, a story that continues to intertwine with lives of others. In the midst of the technology, nurses can encourage family and loved ones to talk with, touch, and be in touch with the patient. In this way nurses acknowledge the primary importance of relationships, even in a health care setting filled with machines, noises, and other evidences of advanced technology.

Attention to the human focus includes helping patients and families become more comfortable with the sometimes formidable array of machines and equipment, and make sense of the large amounts of clinical data that are generated. Incorporating family members in caring for the patient provides time for connecting and observing the patient in both good and bad moments, and engenders a more realistic view of the patient's condition. Rather than engendering anxiety and mistrust by shutting the family out of the patient's life and experiences at critical moments, nurses should encourage them to share directly in the patient's journey. This provides families more experiences upon which to base hard decisions.

The nursing role of providing care and comfort is paramount in any health care setting, and has many facets. It may take the shape of explaining, as often as necessary, the purpose and problems related to interventions. Caring requires that the nurse see the experience from another's point of view, so that questions, fears, concerns, and frustrations may be addressed appropriately. Providing care and comfort also requires that the nurse support and encourage behaviors that enable patients and families to choose in accordance with their own beliefs and values. Being proficient in technical skills with the intent of doing what is best for the patient is part of human care, as is the ability to be with and wait with persons as they struggle through difficult situations.

SUMMARY

Many of the major ethical dilemmas encountered by nurses and other health care providers today are associated with advances in scientific knowledge and technology. In order to recognize and to deal with such dilemmas, nurses need to clarify their own values, and to appreciate differences in values among the various people involved in making patient care decisions. The potential of technology has raised very deep questions about life and death that must be addressed on individual, professional, and societal levels. Issues of quality of life, relief of suffering, and futility of interventions are some facets of these questions. Decisions about when to intervene and reasonable goals of interventions are made more difficult because of varying perceptions of the value of such interventions, nondefinitive outcomes, and issues related to availability of interventions. Principles of beneficence, nonmaleficence, justice, and autonomy provide the basis for arguments on different sides of issues related to technology. Nurses must take into account their responsibilities to patients and the profession, as well as personal integrity, when dealing with ethical dilemmas engendered by technology. Nurses must remember that, in the midst of the technology with its associated dilemmas, there are persons who need the human focus of care that is basic to nursing practice.

CHAPTER HIGHLIGHTS

- The use of technology in health care has prompted the need to address important ethical questions regarding life, death, and allocation of resources.
- Utilization of health care technology may give rise to conflicts between the principles of beneficence and nonmaleficence.
- Appropriate utilization of health care technologies requires that health care providers, patients, and families understand the purposes, benefits, and limitations of specific technologies.
- Attitudes and beliefs concerning life and death affect how health care providers, patients, families, and the legal system approach issues related to health care technology. Ethical dilemmas may arise when there are differing opinions related to the use of technology among the parties involved.
- Determination of medical futility is an important consideration in decisions to withhold or withdraw life-sustaining interventions. Ethical decisions regarding these measures require consideration of whether they are prolonging living, or prolonging dying.
- Economics may factor into decisions related to medical futility, availability of technology, and accessibility to many interventions.
- Withholding or withdrawing life-sustaining treatments in situations in which the burden or harm has been determined to outweigh the benefits constitutes allowing a person to die, and is not euthanasia. Dilemmas may arise regarding whether to classify the use of specific interventions as ordinary or extraordinary measures. The courts have sometimes been involved in making this determination.
- Patient self-determination and distributive justice must be considered in decisions regarding technology. Vigilance is required to ensure that people are not harmed, exploited, controlled, discriminated against, or excluded from care by the use of health care technologies.
- Nurses are in a key position to help patients and families articulate their preferences regarding technological interventions, and to facilitate communication with other health team members in this regard. This role requires familiarity with

patient and family decisions and institutional policies regarding life sustaining interventions, and awareness that when medical care is deemed futile, nursing care in its fullest meaning is most essential.

DISCUSSION QUESTIONS AND ACTIVITIES

1. Develop advance directives for yourself, considering interventions you would choose and parameters regarding these choices. Discuss and compare your directives with classmates.

2. Discuss your beliefs regarding determinants of the beginning and end of life.

3. Describe quality of life as it relates to health care decisions.

4. Discuss potential *slippery slope* elements related to reproductive and genetic technologies, and organ procurement and transplantation.

5. Plan and engage in a debate in your class focused on economic and justice issues related to health care technologies.

6. Observe several patients who are receiving technological interventions, and note how the technology is affecting them and their families; issues surrounding its use; the focus of nursing care; and your reaction to the situation. Describe strengths of the nursing care you observe, and aspects that you might do differently if you were providing care. Talk to nurses and patients regarding the impact of technology on their health and care.

7. Discuss your view about nurses writing DNR orders.

8. How would you handle a situation where you feel the physician's decision regarding life-sustaining interventions is inappropriate for your patient?

9. Choose one of the topics discussed in this chapter and explore the web sites of the ANA, the CNA, and the ICN regarding policies or positions statements on this issue. You may include information from other disciplines as well. Compare and contrast positions of the various organizations. Discuss your views about this issue, and how they compare with the positions of the professional organizations.

ANA—http://www.nursingworld.org

CNA—http://www.cna-nurses.ca

ICN—http://www.icn.ch

10. Role-play a palliative care conference with students in the class, using a real or hypothetical patient case situation.

REFERENCES

American Nurses' Association (1992a, April 2). Position statement: Nursing care and do-not-resuscitate decisions. Author. Retrieved January 7, 2001, from the World Wide Web: http://www.nursingworld.org/readroom/positio/ethics/etdnr.htm

American Nurses' Association (1992b, April 2). Position statement: Forgoing nutrition and hydration. Author. Retrieved January 7, 2001, from the World Wide Web: http://www.nursingworld.org/readroom/position/ethicsetnutr.htm

Angell, M. (1990). Prisoners of technology: The case of Nancy Cruzan. *New England Journal of Medicine, 322*, 1226–1228.

Annas, G. J. (1990). Nancy Cruzan and the right to die. *New England Journal of Medicine, 323*, 670–672.

Billings, J. A. (2000). Palliative care: Recent advances. *British Medical Journal 321*, 555–558.

Critchley, P., Jadad, A. R., Taniguchi, A., Woods, A., Stevens, R., Reyno, L., & Whelan, T. J. (1999). Are some palliative care delivery systems more effective and efficient than others? A systematic review of comparative studies. *Journal of Palliative Care, 15*(4), 40–47.

Curtin, L. (1996). *Nursing: Into the 21st century.* Springhouse, PA: Springhouse.

Davis, A. J. (1991). Ethical issues in nursing research: My own experience. *Western Journal of Nursing Research, 13*, 414–415.

Devettere, R. J. (1995). *Practical decision making in health care ethics: Cases and concepts.* Washington, DC: Georgetown University Press.

Diem, S. J., Lantos, J. D., & Tulsky, J. A. (1996). Cardiopulmonary resuscitation on television. *New England Journal of Medicine, 334*(24), 1579–1582.

Farquhar, M. (1995). Definitions of quality of life: A taxonomy. *Journal of Advanced Nursing, 22*, 502–508.

Finucane, T. E., Christmas, C., & Travis, K. (1999). Tube feeding in patients with advanced dementia. *Journal of the American Medical Association, 282*(14), 1365–70.

Frankel, M. S., & Chapman, A. R. (2000). *Human inheritable genetic modifications: Assessing scientific, ethical, religious, and policy issues.* Washington, DC: The American Association for the Advancement of Science.

Jecker, N. S. (1995). Knowing when to stop: The limits of medicine. In J. H. Howell & W. F. Sale, eds., *Life choices: A Hastings Center introduction to bioethics* (pp. 139–148). Washington, DC: Georgetown University Press.

Lantos, J. D. (1994). Futility assessments and the doctor-patient relationship. *JAGS, 42*, 868–870.

Lo, B. (1995). *Resolving ethical dilemmas: A guide for clinicians.* Baltimore: Williams & Wilkins.

McCann, R. (1999). Lack of evidence about tube feeding: Food for thought. *Journal of the American Medical Association, 282*(14), 1381.

Martin, D. A., & Redland, A. R. (1988). Legal and ethical issues in resuscitation and withholding of treatment. *Critical Care Nurse, 10*, 1–8.

Moss, A. H. (2001). What's new? Progress in palliative care, CPR, and advance directives. Seminar at Raleigh General Hospital, Beckley, WV. January 18, 2001.

Pence, G. E. (1995). *Classic cases in medical ethics.* New York: McGraw-Hill.

Quill, T. E. (2000). Initiating end-of-life discussions about seriously ill patients: Addressing the "elephant in the room." *Journal of the American Medical Association, 284*(19), 2502–2507.

Roberts, D. (2000). Race, gender, justice, and reproductive health policy. Presentation at *New century, new challenges: Intensive bioethics course XXVI,* Kennedy Institute of Ethics, Georgetown University, Washington, DC, June 9, 2000.

Rushton, C. H. (1994). Guidelines on forgoing life-sustaining medical treatment. *Pediatric Nursing, 20*, 517–521.

Scofield, G. R. (1995). Is consent useful when resuscitation isn't? In J. H. Howell & W. F. Sale, eds., *Life choices: A Hastings Center introduction to bioethics* (pp. 172–187). Washington, DC: Georgetown University Press.

Thibault-Provost, J., Jensen, L. A., & Hodgins, M. (2000). Critical care nurses' perceptions of DNR orders. *Journal of Nursing Scholarship, 32*(3), 259–265.

Tomlinson, T., & Brody, H. (1988). Ethics and communication in do-not-resuscitate orders. *New England Journal of Medicine, 318*, 43–46.

SUGGESTED READINGS

Devettere, R. J. (1995). *Practical decision making in health care ethics: Cases and concepts.* Washington, DC: Georgetown University Press.

Howell, J. H., & Sale, W. F., eds. (1995). *Life choices: A Hastings Center introduction to bioethics.* Washington, DC: Georgetown University Press.

Jonsen, A. R., Veach, R. M., & Walters, L., eds. (1998). *Source book in bioethics: A documentary history.* Washington, DC: Georgetown University Press.

Pence, G. E. (1995). *Classic cases in medical ethics.* New York: McGraw-Hill.

CHAPTER 11

Practice Issues Related to Patient Self-Determination

The task set before us is to find the golden mean between moral autonomy and the cooperative action necessary to contemporary life.

(Curtin, 1982)

OBJECTIVES

After completing this chapter, the reader should be able to:

1. Discuss autonomy and paternalism as they relate to patient self-determination.
2. Describe factors that may threaten autonomy in health care settings and situations in which autonomy may be limited.
3. Examine the interaction of justice and autonomy.
4. Discuss informed consent as it relates to patient self-determination.
5. Examine legal and ethical elements of informed consent.
6. Describe the nursing role and responsibilities related to informed consent.
7. Discuss the place of advance directives in health care decisions.
8. Discuss patient autonomy related to choices for life and health.
9. Describe the nursing role and responsibilities related to patient lifestyle and health choices.
10. Discuss the nursing role regarding complementary therapies.
11. Describe confidentiality in relation to health care choices.

INTRODUCTION

The role of the patient and that of the healer, and the implied responsibilities of each, have varied throughout history and in different cultures. In some cultures, decisions regarding "what is best" for the patient are deferred to the healer, who is presumed to know what will bring about healing. Indeed, until recent years, the physician was often viewed in this light. Such paternalism has been challenged in recent years, and greater emphasis has been placed on the role and rights of patients in making health care decisions. This chapter focuses on practice issues related to patient self-determination. Discussion of these issues includes both ethical and legal components, and is intertwined with issues of technology and economics.

AUTONOMY AND PATERNALISM

Self-determination derives from the principle of autonomy. **Autonomy,** which is discussed in detail in Chapter 3, denotes having the freedom to make choices about issues that affect our life and to make decisions about personal goals. Autonomy, which means self-governing, implies respect for persons, the ability to determine personal goals and decide on a plan of action, and the freedom to act on the choices made. The value placed on the primacy of the individual implicit in autonomy is primarily an Anglo concept, and may not be fully accepted in other cultures. Sherwin (1992) suggests that the notion of autonomy is more than a sense of an isolated self, and must include an appreciation for the self in relation to others, recognizing that choices are made in the context of community. Implications of this view for health care include viewing patients as members of a social world, in which health care decisions affect others and are made in conjunction with trusted persons.

Factors that may threaten autonomy in health care settings include: a prevailing paternalistic attitude that promotes the dependent role of the patient; assumptions that a patient's values and thought processes are the same as those of the health care provider; failure to appreciate a difference in knowledge level regarding health matters; and a focus on technology rather than caring. Persisting paternalistic attitudes have contributed to increased numbers of patients and families struggling with health care providers over control of health care decisions. **Paternalism** "derives from the privileges associated with the patriarchal family, where fathers are granted the right and responsibility to use their supposedly superior knowledge and judgment to make decisions on behalf of other family members" (Sherwin, 1992, p. 138). Paternalism (or parentalism, as discussed in Chapter 3) implies well-intended actions of benevolent decision making, leadership, protection, and discipline. In the health care arena paternalism manifests in the making of decisions on behalf of patients without their full consent or knowledge. Although the principle of beneficence suggests that decisions are focused on the patient's well-being, the power inherent in such a hierarchical arrangement can be abused, and decisions made may reflect the interests of the health care provider more than those of the patient. Consider, for example, many elderly patients in nursing homes who are routinely sedated "for their own protection" because of "agitation and confusion." It is worth pondering whether medication used in this way is for the benefit of the patient, or to make life easier for the staff.

CASE PRESENTATION

Determining What Is Best for the Patient

Mr. Zumma, a former butcher who is eighty-four years old, has had evidence of memory loss and periodic confusion for about eighteen months. He has been functional at home, able to do personal care, household chores, and shopping, and has been on no medication. One night he came into the bedroom with two straight razors and told his wife to stay still so he could slit her throat. She was able to escape by exiting through a nearby door and running to a neighbor's house. Reluctant to call the police because "he is not a criminal," she called her son, who came and calmed his father down. At the advice of another family member, Mrs. Zumma contacted a geriatric psychiatrist, who immediately hospitalized Mr. Zumma and started him on Haldol. When he got worse, the physician increased the dose of the medication. Although he was walking and talking when he was admitted, after one day in the hospital the patient became incontinent, could not walk, was drooling, and had to be restrained. The decline in his condition throughout the week in the hospital concerned Mrs. Zumma, and she approached the psychiatrist about taking him on a previously planned vacation. The psychiatrist indicated that this would be impossible, and that the patient would need to go to a nursing home. With persistence, however, Mrs. Zumma was able to convince the psychiatrist to discontinue the medications, after which Mr. Zumma's condition improved and he walked out of the hospital and did well on the vacation trip. Although he still gets confused, he remains functional at home without medication, where his wife makes sure that all sharp or dangerous objects are kept hidden.

Think About It

When Interventions Do More Harm than Good

- How did paternalism factor into the case of Mr. Zumma?
- What ethical issues are evident in this case?
- If you were the nurse caring for Mr. Zumma, and his wife approached you with her concerns about his condition, how would you respond?
- Describe patient and family values that you believe influenced decisions about Mr. Zumma's care.

Inherent in the authoritarian medical model is the "belief that neither patients nor health care professionals other than physicians possess the appropriate skills and capacities to exercise decision-making power. In particular, patients (and their guardians) are thought to be too uneducated, too emotionally distraught, or too stupid to make adequate decisions in the face of illness" (Sherwin, 1992, p. 145). What this attitude does not address, however, is that decisions about health require more than scientific expertise. Such decisions must take into account factors such as the patient's values, culture, spiritual and other beliefs; evaluation of risks, benefits, and economic considerations; and effects on lifestyle and role. For this to occur, patients must be engaged in the decision-making process as autonomous agents in relationship with others who may need to be part of the process.

How Far Does Autonomy Go?

Although the principle of autonomy has become a key consideration in health care ethics, it does have limits. Practitioners are not obligated to honor requests from patients or families for interventions that, in the best judgment of the practitioner, are outside accepted standards of care or that are contrary to the practitioner's own ethical views. Autonomy may also be limited by availability of resources and economic circumstances.

In discussions of patient self-determination, the principle of justice needs to be considered along with that of autonomy. **Justice** implies fair, equitable, and appropriate treatment in light of what is due or owed to persons, recognizing that giving to some may deny receipt to others who might otherwise have received these things. In determining who deserves what portion of finite health care resources, autonomy and justice may conflict where needs or demands for health care by autonomous patients outweigh available resources. The rights of family members and of society must be considered in relation to the needs of individuals. Hardwig (1995) suggests that the medical and nonmedical impact of treatment decisions on both the patient and the family needs to be considered. He reflects that patient autonomy implies the responsible use of freedom, which means considering the needs of family and society as well as our own desires. He raises the question of whether it is legitimate to ask families to make sacrifices of major resources to meet the needs of one member. The limited availability and expense of many medical interventions bring such questions to the fore. Since people can be maintained on very expensive treatments for prolonged periods of time, justice requires us to ask not only who deserves an intervention, but also who is expected to pay for it. Although the moral relevance of considering the interests of the family is generally not addressed in current ethical theory, dilemmas faced by patients, families, and practitioners include these issues, and it is well worth pondering their implications.

Ask Yourself

Should There Be Limits to Patient Autonomy?

- Can you think of health care situations in which the interests of the family should take precedence over those of the patient? Upon what criteria do you base this decision?

- How would you describe nursing's role regarding patient autonomy?

- How have you experienced paternalism in nursing?

- How do you feel about the suggestion that the physician is most qualified to make health care decisions? What have you experienced in this regard?

INFORMED CONSENT

Informed consent provides legal protection of a patient's right to personal autonomy. The concept of informed consent is one that has come to mean that patients are given the opportunity to autonomously choose a course of action in regard to plans for health care. The choice includes the right to refuse interventions or recommendations about care, and to choose from available therapeutic alternatives. This is usually discussed in relation to surgery and complex medical procedures, but also includes consent to more common interventions that may have undesirable side effects, such as immunizations and contraceptives. Exceptions to informed consent include emergencies in which there is no time to disclose the information, and waivers by patients who do not want to know their prognosis or risks of treatment.

The emergence of informed consent as we know it has been affected by several factors. One factor has been the institutionalization of health care in hospitals, with their associated technologies and life-prolonging techniques over which people have little control and limited understanding. When health providers visited in the home, informed consent was not as necessary, because people had more control and better understanding of traditional remedies (Devettere, 1995). The courts, however, have exerted the most significant influence on shaping the doctrine of informed consent.

The history of the concept dates back to at least three landmark legal cases. In *Slater v. Baker & Stapleton* (1767), a decision was made that prohibited "unauthorized touching." This decision held that a person has a right to know what is to be done to his or her body. It did not require any participation in the decision-making process. In the 1905 case of *Mobe v. Williams* (Husted & Husted, 1995, p. 61) and the case of *Schloendorff v. The Society of New York Hospital* (1914), separate rulings established the patient's right to know what was to be done, and also the right to give or withhold consent. These decisions did not address the patient's right to be informed about risks of treatment or nontreatment or about the existence of alternative therapies. In the case of *Salgo v. Leland Stanford, Jr.* (1957), the California Supreme Court ruled in favor of a patient who had not been informed of the risks of aortography and subsequently became paralyzed. This ruling established a patient's right to be advised of the risks involved in any proposed treatment (Husted & Husted, 1995).

Ethical and Legal Elements of Informed Consent

We must remember that, although the informed consent doctrine has foundations in law, it is essentially an ethical imperative. "Ethically valid consent is a process of shared decision-making based upon mutual respect and participation, not a ritual to be equated with reciting the contents of a form that details the risks of particular treatments" (President's Commission, 1983, p. 2). The two major legal elements of informed consent that are inherent in the ethical imperative are *information* and *consent*.

Information. The information component of informed consent includes both disclosure and understanding of the essential information. Figure 11–1 lists the information that must be included in an informed consent. People need access to sufficient information to help them understand their health concerns and make decisions regarding treatment. The information provided need not be "textbook" detail, but does need

Figure 11–1 **Content of Informed Consent**

> • The nature of the health concern and prognosis if nothing is done.
> • Description of all treatment options, even those that the health care provider does not favor or cannot provide.
> • The benefits, risks, and consequences of the various treatment alternatives, including nonintervention.

to offer enough explanation for the person to have a clear picture of the situation, what is being offered, the alternatives and their risks, benefits, and consequences. Determining the adequacy of information disclosed in an informed consent is based on one or more standards: (1) *the professional practice standard*—the disclosure is consistent with the standards of the profession; (2) the *reasonable person standard*—the disclosure is what a reasonable person in similar circumstances would need in order to make an informed decision; and (3) the *subjective standard*—the disclosure is what the particular person wants or needs to know. Informed consent implies that the person has received the information and understands what is provided. Verification of understanding can be accomplished through discussion, in which patients have an opportunity to ask questions and are asked to describe their understanding of the nature of the intervention, alternatives, risks, and benefits.

Consent. Consent to something implies the freedom to accept or reject it. This means that consent to health care interventions must be voluntary, without coercion, force, or manipulation from health care providers or family. Force entails making someone do something against his or her will. Coercion and manipulation may be overt or subtle, and may include threats, rewards, deception, or inducing excessive fear. The voluntary nature of consent does not prohibit health care providers from making recommendations or attempting to persuade patients to accept their suggestions. However, we must be alert to situations in which persuasion takes on qualities of coercion or manipulation.

CASE PRESENTATION

Language and Informed Consent

Mohano is a sixty-seven-year-old deaf man who was admitted to the hospital with atrial fibrillation. The nurse notes that he is alert, apparently oriented, and able to follow simple directions that she acts out, although he does look apprehensive as she cares for him. Mohano's social history indicates that he was brought into the hospital by a community worker who looks in on him because he is deaf and illiterate and has no family in the area. She had indicated that he came to the area as a migrant worker a number of years ago, along with a brother who died the previous year. She had also noted that two of his five siblings were also deaf, and they had developed a type of sign language that was understood only by family members. At the interdisciplinary care conference, the medical resident who is in charge of his case voices frustration because of the need to get the patient's permission to do a stress test and to talk to him about medications and risk for stroke. He suggests that they should just get the patient to make an X on the form so they can go ahead with the treatment protocol because it is in the patient's best interest to do so. The social worker suggests that they get an interpreter for the deaf to come in and try to talk to him through sign language, although she is not sure he will understand.

Think About It

Obtaining Informed Consent When There Is No Common Language

- What ethical dilemmas are evident in this case?
- What do you think about Mohano's decision-making capacity?
- Do you think it is possible to obtain an informed consent from Mohano? Support your position with discussion of elements of informed consent and decision making capacity.
- In a situation such as this, it is evident that the patient has a language, although it is not understood by the health care providers, and that he has been able to care for himself with some assistance. How would these factors enter into determination of his decision-making capacity?
- How does the inability of the health care provider to communicate with a patient affect determination of the patient's decision-making capacity?
- What are the implications of denying Mohano important services because of lack of common language and subsequent inability to ensure informed consent?

Nursing Role and Responsibilities: Informed Consent

While the practice of documenting informed consent for a procedure usually ends with the signing of a consent form, the process is much more complex. Following the rules laid out previously, informed consent must include explicit verification that the patient is aware of all options, the possible outcomes of each option, and the likely outcome with nontreatment. The patient must also recognize the implications that each option will have upon his or her lifestyle. The nurse must be sensitive to the fact that the very act of asking a patient to sign a form giving permission for a particular treatment may constitute a form of coercion. It is the nurse's responsibility as advocate for the patient to ensure that all criteria for autonomous decision making are met. If the nurse believes that the patient does not understand the implications of any part of the process, including nontreatment and alternative options, or that the patient is unable to deliberate and to reason on the various choices, it is the responsibility of the nurse to intervene. Legally the nurse must act if it becomes apparent that the patient is not informed. Actions may include notifying the physician and requesting further information for the patient, or stopping the process until it is ensured that the decision can be made autonomously. Although the mechanics of the process usually require the nurse to obtain the patient's signature on a consent form, the primary concern of the nurse is to ensure that all criteria for autonomous decision making are met.

Witnessing a patient's signature on a consent form implies accountability on the part of the nurse. Sullivan (1998) notes that the nurse's signature attests that the patient is giving consent willingly, is competent in that moment to give consent, and that the patient's signature is authentic. She cautions nurses who are not present when the treatment is explained to the patient to verify the patient's understanding of the procedure, inquire if there are any questions that need to be discussed with the physician, and to not let a patient sign a consent form if there is any indication of coercion. She also stresses the importance of nurses documenting their communication with the patient and with the physician regarding any questions, concerns, or teaching related to the informed consent. Any special circumstances, such as the patient's inability to read or write, or the use of an interpreter if the patient speaks a different language, should also be documented.

Nurses in advanced practice roles are accountable for providing information and obtaining informed consent for interventions that they initiate under their scope of practice. The question of the nurse's right to inform a patient of the risks inherent in a certain procedure or alternative courses of action in other settings is not as clear. In 1977 Jolene Tuma, a nursing instructor, in the course of initiating chemotherapy, answered an elderly patient's questions about cancer treatment alternatives. The patient indicated that she did not want to question the physician because he was not open to considering other therapies. Tuma was also asked to describe the therapies to the patient's son, who was upset by this. Although the patient decided to continue chemotherapy, she died two weeks later. After the patient's death, the son told the physician of Tuma's action. The physician subsequently brought charges against Ms. Tuma for disrupting the physician-patient relationship. She was fired from her job and lost her nursing license as a result. Ms. Tuma pursued an appeal of the decision. In 1979 the Idaho Supreme Court ruled that she could not lose her license for "unprofessional behavior" because there was no statutory description of this offense. The court did not address, however, the nurse's right to inform the patient (Becker, 1986; Benjamin & Curtis, 1986; Husted & Husted, 1995).

Unfortunately, this leaves the nurse in a sort of limbo in regard to ensuring informed consent. Although the nurse is legally required to act on behalf of the patient to guarantee true informed consent, there is no clear course of action when a nurse believes that the patient has not been informed or does not understand the information, and the physician is uncooperative in remedying the situation. Institutional and legal constraints may impede the nurse from following the ethically correct course of action.

Ask Yourself

What Is the Nurse's Responsibility Regarding Informed Consent?

- In the case described above, do you feel that Jolene Tuma's actions were appropriate? Support your position.
- What ethical issues are apparent in situations such as this?
- How does the nurse-patient relationship factor into such a situation?

ADVANCE DIRECTIVES

Given the dilemmas that can arise regarding the use of technology, we must encourage and assist people to make their wishes known concerning the use of such interventions. For those who are mentally alert and capable of making decisions, informed consent is needed prior to initiating any life-sustaining interventions. To ensure that our wishes regarding treatment are followed in the event that we have lost decision-making capacity, advance directives are needed. **Advance directives** are instructions that indicate health care interventions to initiate or withhold, or that designate someone who will act as a surrogate in making such decisions in the event that we lose decision-making capacity. Such directives can be considered as a kind of informed consent for future interventions. Advance directives support people in making decisions on their own behalf, and help to ensure that patients have the kind of end-of-life care they want. In order to help patients be as clear as possible about their choices, the various life-sustaining measures that may be considered in end-of-life care should be discussed openly and clearly. Patients should be encouraged to express verbally, or in writing, their wishes about tube feedings, breathing machines, cardiopulmonary resuscitation, and dialysis. Consideration of interventions should include how long they might want to stay on an intervention if it is initiated and their condition continues to decline or is not improving. In addition to enabling people to have choices in their dying process, the presence of clearly understood advance directives can alleviate stress on family and clinicians when dealing with end-of-life concerns.

Perhaps the most important factor in decision making regarding end-of-life care is clear and open communication between the patient or the surrogate and health care providers. We need to do more than merely seek to know which potential life-sustaining technology a person does or does not want. We need to see and get to know the person who is making these decisions. Eliciting a clear statement of personal values is basic to this process. What does the person value in life? What constitutes quality of life for the person? What are his or her personal beliefs and concerns about dying? We must recognize the influence of cultural, societal, spiritual, and family norms and perspectives on personal values. For example, in some cultures, speaking of death and dying is believed to bring bad luck. Family wishes may influence personal choices, and in some cultures the patient may defer decisions about end-of-life care to the family. When discussing different interventions, we need to ensure that patients understand what the procedure is and what it involves. They also need to appreciate that risks risks and benefits of life-sustaining interventions vary with age, health condition, and circumstances that prompt the consideration of the intervention. For example, the literature shows no evidence that tube feedings prolong life or improve quality of life for patients with dementia or multisystem illness (Finucane, Christmas, & Travis, 1999; McCann, 1999; Moss, 2001). We need to understand why the patient or family wants a particular intervention, and what it is that they think it will do for them.

Advance directives include living wills and durable powers of attorney. **Living wills** are legal documents giving directions to health care providers related to withholding or withdrawing life support if certain conditions exist. Statutes regulating living wills vary from state to state, so nurses must be familiar with their own state laws. Living wills guide decisions by indicating a person's desires regarding life-sustaining interventions; however, they also raise issues of concern. Directives in living wills may be vague, and can address only the interventions a person does not want. In some states, only persons who are terminally ill or whose death is imminent are allowed to make living wills. Particularly in emergency situations, there may be a concern that a document that has been developed when a person was in good health may not reflect the patient's current desires.

Durable power of attorney allows a competent person to designate another as a surrogate or proxy to act on her or his behalf in making health care decisions in the event of the loss of decision-making capacity. Although there is no particular legal form required, the designation must be in writing and must be signed and dated by the person making the designation and two witnesses other than the designated surrogate. The designating person may revoke the designation at any time by changing the person named as surrogate, or by destroying the document. The authority of the surrogate does not become effective until it has been determined that the person has lost decision-making capacity. The authority of the surrogate is effective only for the duration of the loss of decision-making capacity. For example, in the case of a person who has a temporary loss of consciousness, the surrogate's authority to make decisions would end once the person regained consciousness and the ability to make decisions for self.

The presence of a living will or durable power of attorney and surrogate designation should be documented in a patient's health record. Nurses should routinely ask patients whether they have such documents and be able to discuss the importance of such directives with patients and families. The American Nurses Association (ANA) *Position Statement on Nursing and the Patient Self-Determination Act* recommends including the following questions in nursing admission assessments:

> Do you have basic information about advance care directives, including living wills and durable power of attorney? Do you wish to indicate an advance care directive? If you have already prepared an advance care directive, can you provide it now? Have you discussed

your end-of-life choices with your family and/or designated surrogate and health care workers? (ANA, 1991)

It is well known that patients may indicate concerns to nurses that they have not discussed with their physicians. Issues related to advance directives may be one such concern.

Decision-Making Capacity

Informed consent requires that the patient or surrogate have the ability to make a reasonable decision regarding health care concerns. A surrogate or health care proxy is someone who makes medical decisions on the patient's behalf if the patient is incapable of doing so. Conscious adults are presumed to have decision-making capacity, unless there is evidence to the contrary. **Decision-making capacity** is a medical determination relating only to the issue at hand, as people may have the ability to make decisions about some areas and not others. For example, a person may be able to make decisions about health, while unable to make reasonable decisions about household matters. Persons may have decision-making capacity at some times and not others, and in each specific situation, there must be a determination that they have, or do not have, the capacity. The fact that a person makes a decision that seems unreasonable to the health care provider does not necessarily mean a lack of decision-making capacity; it may merely reflect a difference in values. If the decision seems unreasonable, however, it is wise to explore the patient's capacity regarding decision making.

Elements of Decision-Making Capacity. When evaluating a patient or surrogate for decision-making capacity, several elements must be present. These are listed in Figure 11-2. First, the patient must be able to understand all relevant information, including the nature of the health care problem, the prognosis, treatment options and recommendations, and the risks, benefits, and consequences of each. Second, the patient must be able to communicate this understanding and her or his choices. Third, the patient must possess a set of values and goals that enable evaluation regarding whether this health care decision will be of benefit in terms of personal goals. Fourth, the patient must have the ability to reason and to deliberate about available choices, which includes the ability to grasp notions such as risk and percentage, cause and effect, and chance and probability. Although it is not unreasonable to see some indecision, or

Figure 11-2 **Elements of Decision-Making Capacity**

The patient must:
- have the ability to understand all information.
- have the ability to communicate understanding and choices.
- have personal values and goals that guide the decision.
- have the ability to reason and deliberate.

even a change of mind once a choice has been made, a great deal of vacillation between choices suggests the need to re-evaluate decision-making capacity. Nurses are in a key position to observe patients and families for the presence of these elements of decision-making capacity. As patient advocates, nurses need to assess, document, and communicate to appropriate members of the health care team any concerns in this regard.

Physicians usually have legal authority and responsibility to determine decision-making capacity. In at least one state, however, an advanced practice nurse or a psychologist can also legally certify incapacity (WVNEC, 2000). Determining incapacity is best done in consultation with family or others who have the patient's best interest in mind. We must make a distinction between decision-making capacity and competence. Decisions about **competence,** which is the ability to make meaningful life decisions, require a legal action. Legally, persons are considered competent unless there is a ruling by a judge that they cannot make meaningful life decisions. Legal declarations of incompetence generally stay in effect for the remainder of the person's life, and include a court-appointed guardian to be the surrogate decision maker for the person.

When a patient lacks decision-making capacity, someone else must be identified as a surrogate to make decisions for the patient. In the case of children, the surrogate is usually a parent or legal guardian. With adults, the surrogate may be a spouse, parent, adult children, other relatives, or other person named as surrogate in the patient's advance directives. In situations in where a patient has no advance directives, or has not named a surrogate to make decisions in the event of incapacity, health care providers should work with family and others to identify a surrogate. The legal process for choosing a surrogate varies from state to state and you need to be familiar with the process in your state. The person chosen as surrogate should be someone willing to serve in this role and who can make health care decisions in accordance with the patient's wishes, or that are consistent with the patient's best interest if these wishes are not known or cannot be reasonably discerned. The surrogate should demonstrate care and concern for, and have regular contact with the patient. In addition, the surrogate should be willing and able to participate fully in the decision-making process, and engage in face-to-face contact and communication with caregivers. Close family members such as parents, adult children, adult siblings, and adult grandchildren are often considered first if the patient has not designated a surrogate. However, close friends or neighbors may at times be better qualified to make these decisions. The decisions made by the surrogate should reflect the patient's values, including cultural and spiritual perspective, to the extent that these are reasonably known.

Patient Self-Determination Act.   The **Patient Self-Determination Act,** which went into effect December 1991, is a federal law requiring institutions such as hospitals, nursing homes, health maintenance organizations, and home care agencies receiving Medicare or Medicaid funds to provide written information to adult patients regarding their rights to make health care decisions. Such decisions include the right to refuse treatments, and to write advance directives for guiding decisions should they become incapacitated. The ANA notes that nurses have a responsibility to facilitate informed decision making with patients, particularly regarding end-of-life care, and that nurses have a critical role in implementing the Patient Self-Determination Act (PSDA) within all health care settings.

> The formation of advance directives is an important decision, and will inevitably involve nurses who are the most omnipresent professionals in health care facilities. It is imperative that the decision making that will fall to patients and their families as they make choices about end-of-life care be facilitated by nurses. (ANA, 1991)

In spite of the PSDA, only a small percentage of patients have advance directives, and many clinicians are not aware of the wishes of the seriously ill patients for whom they care (Haynor, 1998; LoBuono, 2000). Paternalistic attitudes of some clinicians may result in their disregarding advance directives because of their belief that they know what is best for the patient in the current circumstances. Developing advance directives must be part of the ongoing process of communication between patients or their surrogates and clinicians (Canadian Nurses Association, 1998; Haynor, 1998; Forbes, Bern-Klug, & Gessert, 2000; Schlenk, 1997). Open discussion of end-of-life decisions should occur routinely within primary-care settings, before the physical and emotional stress of serious illness or hospitalization.

Nursing Role and Responsibilities: Advance Directives

What is the nursing role and responsibility regarding advance directives? Whatever the work setting, nurses have a key role and responsibility in ensuring that patients have an opportunity to complete advance directives, and in interpreting and following through with patient's wishes as expressed through these directives. As nurses, we need to know our state's statutes that guide and govern advance directives. We also need to be aware of the policies and procedures regarding advance directives where we work. Tilden (2000) urges us to complete our own advance directives. Doing so helps us to reflect on our own values, beliefs, and concerns associated with end-of-life issues, to learn more about the specific forms and processes involved, and ultimately to have more empathy with patients going through this process. Information concerning advance directives is often provided to patients on admission to a facility by a clerical worker. Because there may be limited explanation of this information to patients or opportunity for questions, we need to explore patient and family understanding of the information received. We can use this as an opening to stress the importance of having such directives, and to advocate for patients who may need assistance in developing advance directives. This is also a beginning opportunity for us to help patients explore personal values, their understanding of themselves in the context of their current situation, and significant cultural or other issues that may influence decision making. As nurses, we need to be familiar with our patients' directives for care, and ensure that care is consistent with the patient's wishes as expressed in the advance directives. Nursing's advocacy role in this regard includes informing other health team members of the presence and content of advance directives, alerting appropriate team members to changes in patient wishes or to evidence of changes in the patient's decision-making capacity, and intervening on behalf of the patient when wishes expressed in advance directives are not being followed. As nurses, we have an important role in increasing public awareness about advance directives through patient and community education, through research, and through education of nurses and other health care providers.

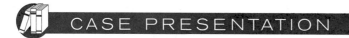

CASE PRESENTATION

The Absence of Advance Directives

Ninety-year-old Mr. Moshe did not have advance directives when he was admitted to the hospital with Alzheimer's disease and renal failure. Although he was coherent at times and could converse with caregivers, the doctor determined Mr. Moshe did not have decision-making capacity and named his daughter Zelda, with whom he had been residing, as his surrogate. The nursing staff questioned this choice because of their concerns about the quality of care Mr. Moshe had been receiving from Zelda and her husband Josh. As Mr. Moshe's health began to deteriorate rapidly, the nurses inquired about his DNR status. Josh replied he wanted Moshe kept alive, and that this was what Mr. Moshe wanted also. Zelda concurred with this. Although Zelda's four siblings called frequently inquiring about their father, Zelda would not inform them about their father's condition nor allow them access to him. Because of this conflict and their concerns regarding the motives for his DNR status, the nurses notified the physician about the family issues and requested an ethics committee consultation to determine the best interests of the patient. The nurses also noted that the physician had not signed the surrogate form as required by their state law, so legally there was no surrogate. The ethics committee representative convened a family meeting that included all five siblings, the physician, the primary nurse, and a member of the pastoral care team. After explaining that the purpose of the meeting was to discuss the type of care that would be in the best interests of their father, not to resolve family issues, the physician was asked to discuss Mr. Moshe's current health status and prognosis. Each of the children were given the opportunity to ask questions of the physician and primary nurse. Then each family member was asked to voice what their father valued in life, and what they believed to be his wishes regarding end-of-life care. Even though some of the siblings had not spoken to each other for nearly ten years, they each stated the same thing, that their father had told them he would never want to be on life support. Zelda, who was asked to speak last, agreed, much to the dismay of her husband, that her father would not want to be placed on life support. The siblings also requested that they be allowed to visit their father and to call and check on him. When they were informed that there currently was no legal surrogate for their father, they all agreed to have Zelda continue in that role, providing she allow them access to him. They stated that even though they were upset with her, they believed she loved him and provided good care for him. To close the meeting all family members were invited to go join together at their father's bedside where they shared prayer and family stories. Mr. Moshe died that night.

Think About It

Considering the Patient's Best Interests

- Because Mr. Moshe was coherent at times, do you think the physician should have asked him what he would want regarding life support?
- What do you think of the physician's choice of a surrogate for Mr. Moshe? What factors do you think he considered in appointing Zelda as surrogate? Are there factors you think he should have considered he may not have?
- As the nurse caring for Mr. Moshe, what would be your concerns regarding his situation? How do you think you would have responded in this situation?
- How did the process of the family meeting address the communication that is needed for making end-of-life decisions?

CHOICES CONCERNING LIFE AND HEALTH

Although discussion of patient autonomy frequently centers around issues of informed consent and end-of-life decisions, issues related to self-determination can arise in any area of nursing practice. In every area of practice nurses must deal with the effects of lifestyle choices on patients' health and healing. Many people who come into our care are suffering from ill effects of such things as overeating; tobacco, drug, or alcohol use; sexual activity; or work-related stress. Our job is to deal with the present health concern while encouraging change toward healthier living. However, patients are often not willing to follow the treatment plan and make the changes needed for healthier living. Dealing with patients whose health problems are clearly related to lifestyle choices, yet who are not willing to change their behaviors, may present dilemmas for nurses. Although nurses may acknowledged that the autonomous person has the right to choose healthy or unhealthy behaviors, it may be difficult to be as caring toward those who are perceived to have brought problems on themselves.

This is another area where the principle of justice may temper the bounds of autonomy. In situations where resources are limited, questions arise regarding whether it is ethical to put resources into treatments for people whose health problems are brought on by unhealthy life choices. This is countered by the question of whether it is ethical to refuse treatment or provide a lesser level of care to someone because the provider does not agree with the lifestyle choices.

Choices Regarding Recommended Treatment

What are nurses to do when patients are well informed and apparently able to follow plans of care, yet do not? Certainly one hears of physicians who refuse to continue to

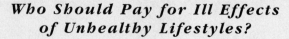

Ask Yourself

Who Should Pay for Ill Effects of Unhealthy Lifestyles?

It is interesting that in the time of Hippocrates physicians were taught that they should not treat persons whose bodies were overmastered by their disease because it was an inappropriate use of medical resources.

- How do you feel about this?
- Would this same stance be considered ethical today?
- To what extent do personal lifestyle choices impinge on the rights of others if significant health care resources are needed to pay for the ill effects of these choices?

Autonomy implies that persons have the right to make choices about things that affect their lives, whether these choices have a positive or negative effect, unless these choices impinge on the rights of others.

- Is it just to expect society to pay for the health care services required for treating the effects of unhealthy behaviors?
- How would you go about allocating health care resources in relation to unhealthy lifestyle choices?

care for patients who do not comply with instructions-smoking cessation, for example. In a climate of limited resources this is a question worthy of contemplation. The first tenet of ANA's revised *Code of Ethics for Nurses* (2001) remains consistent with the 1985 *Code for Nurses*, stating that nurses in all professional relationships practice "with compassion and respect for the inherent dignity, worth, and uniqueness of every individual, unrestricted by considerations of social or economic status, personal attributes, or the nature of health problems" (p. 4). Further, the nurse must not be affected by the patients' individual differences in background, customs, attitudes, and beliefs. Health care practices are an integral part of patients' backgrounds, customs, and beliefs. Therefore, it is clear that refusal to participate in a plan of care, regardless of the outcome, is the prerogative of the patient, and must not affect the caring attitude of the nurse. Unhealthy life practices are part of the whole person, and should be taken into consideration when revising plans of care.

CASE PRESENTATION

A Challenging Patient

Rochelle, a thirty-six-year-old woman who is a known cocaine addict, presented to the emergency room (ER) with severe left leg pain and swelling. The triage nurse reviewed her chart and presenting problem, noting that she had been seen two days prior for chest pain and left leg pain. Assuming these complaints were evaluated then, the nurse sent her to the "fast track" area to be seen by the Nurse Practitioner (NP). The NP noted that her chart was flagged regarding her cocaine addiction and that the physician who had seen her at the previous visit, after doing an EKG, CBC, electrolytes (which were normal), and a urine drug screen (which was positive for cocaine), discharged her with diagnoses of chest pain and illicit drug use. The NP's assessment revealed no shortness of breath, cough, or chest pain; severe swelling and skin tightness of the left leg, with exquisite tenderness and positive Homan's sign, were suggestive of deep vein thrombosis. When the NP went to the ER physician saying that the patient needed to be evaluated by him, she was told to keep the patient over there and do the work-up because he had a patient with a similar problem in the ER.

When the ultrasound confirmed extensive deep vein thrombosis, the NP told the patient the situation and that she needed to be hospitalized. The patient immediately said that she could not stay because she had no one to watch her nine-year-old-daughter, and she began to put on her shoes to leave. The NP told her that she could choose to leave but that the reason she (the NP) wanted her to stay was that this was a very serious problem from which she could die. Rochelle's response was to start crying, saying that she thought she would go home anyway because she had nothing to live for since her husband had died, so she would go home to die. When the NP called Rochelle's primary physician to alert him to the situation, he responded that he would come in to see her only if Rochelle agreed to stay; otherwise, it would be a waste of his time. After considerable effort, the NP contacted Rochelle's mother, who reluctantly agreed to keep her granddaughter when the NP explained the situation, and Rochelle agreed to stay.

Think About It

Dealing with Patients Who Make Apparently Unhealthy Choices

- What issues of patient self-determination are evident in this case?
- How do you see lifestyle choices affecting Rochelle's care? What ethical issues must be considered here?
- Take an honest look at how you think you might react to Rochelle, knowing that she frequently shows up in the ER and is a cocaine addict?
- As the nurse in this situation, how would you deal with the patient's saying she could not stay? What do you think of the way the NP handled it?
- Evaluate ethical issues involved in the responses of the various health care practitioners in this case.
- Interestingly, Rochelle was indigent, African-American, and without health insurance, and the woman in the ER with similar complaints was middle-class, Caucasian, and had health insurance. Discuss the implications of these factors in this case.

Ultimately, choices about health care practices belong to patients. If allowed to choose, patients should not be labeled in a negative way for choices with which nurses do not agree. It is not appropriate for professionals who express the belief that all competent patients have the right to autonomous choice, to then make value judgments about the choices made, and subsequently label patients as noncompliant. In fact, it is worth pondering whether the term *noncompliant* even belongs in nursing vocabulary. The notion of compliance relates to a paternalistic view that health care providers know what is best for patients and that, providing patients follow these directions, they will get well. Nurses should speak more appropriately in terms of motivation to follow a mutually agreed upon plan of care that incorporates patient and family values and beliefs. We must remember that patients have a right to refuse interventions, and they have a right to seek therapies other than those offered by conventional Western medicine.

Complementary Therapies. Many people utilize therapies that may be termed complementary, alternative, or unconventional in regard to Western allopathic medicine (Eisenberg, Kessler, Foster, Norlock, Calkins, & Delbanco, 1993; Eisenberg, et al., 1998). Examples of **complementary therapies** include acupuncture, herbal and nutritional interventions, healing touch, massage, and guided imagery. Most people tend to use such therapies along with conventional modalities, but some will choose to use them in lieu of what is offered by medical practitioners. Most people do not inform their medical practitioner that they are using these therapies.

Several issues regarding the use of complementary therapies need to be considered. First, people have a right to use modalities other than conventional medicine to address their health care needs. Second, nurses and other health care practitioners need to develop at least a talking knowledge, and better yet a working knowledge, of such therapies in order to be better able to discuss their use with patients,. Many therapies work as an adjunct to medical interventions, some may interact in unhealthy ways, and the efficacy of many modalities is not yet known. Nurses need not be practitioners of other modalities in order to discuss them with patients any more than they need to be able to do surgery in order to discuss it. Nurses should create an atmosphere that encourages nonjudgmental discussion of all modalities being considered or employed, with a goal of using whatever is beneficial for the particular patient. Transcultural considerations (which are discussed in Chapter 18) may influence a person's choice of treatment modalities. Third, complementary modalities should not be discounted merely because they are not understood within the Western medical framework; however, it is also important to counsel patients to explore the validity of claims made about a particular therapy. Fourth, as research continues and expands in the area of complementary therapies, the question of whether informed consent will need to at least acknowledge these therapies as treatment options must be addressed. Fifth, nurses who are skilled in complementary therapies need to be clear about what is within their scope of practice according to their state's nurse practice act. The ethical stance with complementary therapies, as with other interventions, requires offering an explanation of the intervention and receiving permission from the patient or family prior to initiating the therapy. Because these therapies can affect conventional interventions, practitioners should apprise other health team members of their use and dcument both treatments and their effects.

Controversial Choices

The value of patient self-determination is cited to support two decisions that have been the focus of much controversy in this country for many years: abortion and active euthanasia. Both of these choices are surrounded by ethical and religious opinion and debate. Abortion in particular is an example of an issue in which legal answers have been sought for ethical dilemmas. The potential for transmission of HIV infections within health care settings raises controversial issues regarding testing and disclosure. This discussion presents some of the arguments on both sides of these issues.

Nurses need to be very clear about their own values regarding each of these issues, and find a balance between personal values and professional obligations to patients and families. Nurses must sort out their own beliefs about what is right and wrong, so that they can differentiate between tasks and roles that are consistent with their ethical stance and those that are not, and make responsible practice decisions accordingly. Davis & Aroskar (1991) suggest that in the process of reasoning through dilemmas such as those involved with these issues, the least that can be expected is that the nurse not abandon the patient. "The most that can be hoped is that each nurse regard the rights of others as precious, as she would want her own regarded, and that within this complex context she view her obligations to self, to the patient, to nursing, and to her place of employment" (p. 136).

Abortion. The abortion debate sparks passionate, emotion-laden arguments in political, social, legal, religious, and moral arenas. Issues of self-determination arise regarding the mother's right to control her body and her life (right to choose) in contrast to rights of the unborn fetus to a chance at life (right to life). Those in the right-to-life camp believe that abortion constitutes murder of an unborn person, suggesting that it is a legal as well as an ethical matter. This has raised questions about the role of government in dealing with this ethical concern. Those who hold to the right to choose maintain that the right to privacy regarding health care decisions includes a woman's reproductive choices, implying that governmental regulation is an infringement on this privacy.

Values in relation to life are fundamental considerations in regard to abortion. Such values include beliefs about when life begins, considerations regarding quality of life for children who are unwanted, and concerns about the mother's life and health. Some believe that life starts at conception, while others hold that life begins only when a fetus is viable outside the womb. Discussions regarding viability continue to change as technology enables the survival of babies of lower and lower birth weights, and results in saving some imperiled newborns of the same gestational age as some aborted fetuses.

Opponents of abortion hold the position that because a fetus possesses humanity, it must be accorded all human rights, including the right to life. Proponents of abortion argue that, based on autonomy, a woman has a right to her own body, and that no woman should be forced to bear a child that she does not want. Because abortion is a situation in which two lives are involved, dilemmas arise regarding who has rights, and whose rights take precedence.

> Some take the position that pregnant women, no matter what the circumstances of conception, have obligations toward the life and well-being of the fetus that overshadow any discussion of the woman's rights. . . . So we have a moral argument, where the stakes are high, in which some people support abortion on demand based on the woman's autonomy. At the same time we have people who oppose abortion perhaps except to save the life of the mother or not at all, based on the sanctity of life principle and the personhood of the fetus. To think in a simple way about this ethical dilemma, on the one hand the fetus is viewed as an object or thing while on the other, the woman is viewed as an object or thing. (Davis & Aroskar, 1991, pp. 130–131)

From either perspective, the consideration of abortion presents a dilemma for those involved.

There is no agreement about the morality of abortion in our society. It is a complex issue with many facets to consider. Although debate generally focuses on areas related to rights of the woman or the fetus, Mahowald (1995) suggests that it is also important to consider the morality of circumstances that provide fertile ground for abortion. She notes that immoral conditions that sometimes occasion abortion include: poverty, lack of social and medical supports for pregnancy and parenthood, stereotypic views of sex roles and biological parenthood, and a eugenic mentality that welcomes only "premium babies," those babies that meet the parents' desired specifications (p. 107). She stresses the need for society to direct more effort into rectifying these conditions.

A Broader Look at Reproductive Rights.   Roberts (2000) addresses ethical concerns related to reproductive rights that extend beyond abortion to such areas as contraceptive choices, decisions about cesarian sections, and reproductive-assisting technologies. She discusses particularly how race and gender affect the ethics of policies and practices in these areas. She reflects that the early birth control movement in the United States became tied to the **eugenics** movement that advocated policies encouraging so called "genetically superior" people to have children, while discouraging so-called "genetically inferior" people from having children, even through forced sterilization. She points to the historical example of the first public birth control clinics in the United States that were established in the South and directed toward poor black women. Another example is a class action law suit in Alabama that uncovered that hundreds of thousands of women in the United States, the majority of whom were black, were being coercively sterilized through government welfare programs that conditioned health care and benefits on sterilization. This lawsuit prompted the 1970's federal regulation requiring informed consent and a waiting period before sterilization.

A more contemporary example is found in the area of welfare reform, where some states deny benefits to women on welfare for children they have while they are receiving welfare. Roberts suggests that while the abortion debate relates to compulsory motherhood, where women's value is linked to their ability to reproduce, contraceptive policies often devalue poor women and women of color as mothers in that such policies are aimed at preventing these women from having children. She cautions that various societal norms can lead to reproductive regulation of women, and that we need to expand the meaning of reproductive freedom to include the right to have a child—the right to decide to be a mother. She notes there are as many policies that have sought to deter women from having children as there are those that have sought to force women to have children.

Roberts raises some very important questions regarding the dangers of eugenics in population control, such as deciding that some people are unfit to have children because of their biology or socioeconomic status, and suggesting that reproduction is the cause for social problems. A very important ethical issue that she points out is the racial disparity in reproductive policies and practices. Technologies that help women to have children are more available to white women, contrasted with policies and practices that are aimed at deterring women from having children being targeted toward poor women, particularly women of color. Such policies raise questions about who is valued in society, and how we use reproductive technologies to encourage the birth of certain "valued" children versus those perceived to be of less value. Reproductive policies that flow from such attitudes, she asserts, affect not just individuals, but group status and social structure. Dealing with issues regarding the ethics of reproduction then requires social justice and addressing power relationships in the broader society.

Active Euthanasia. As noted in Chapter 10, technology has caused death to become an unnatural event in the lives of many people. Lo (1995) noted that active euthanasia was illegal in all states, and assisted suicide was explicitly prohibited in two-thirds of states. However, public dissatisfaction with end-of-life care prompted efforts to legalize these acts. The Supreme Court ruled in 1997 that state laws prohibiting assisted suicide are not unconstitutional. Because of the concern that health care providers will not adhere to personal wishes regarding end-of-life issues, fears about prolonged suffering resulting from prolongation of dying, and the lack of control that each of these engenders, many people consider the possibility of active euthanasia or assisted suicide. **Active voluntary euthanasia** is an act in which the physician both provides the means of death and administers it, such as a lethal dose of medication. With **assisted suicide** the patients receive the means of death from someone, such as a physician, but activate the process themselves. Justification offered by proponents of these acts include respect for the person's autonomy in choosing to end his or her life if it is deemed intolerable due to conditions of a lingering terminal illness, and compassion exhibited in relief of the patient's suffering. Opponents argue from a stance of the sanctity of life, saying that any such act violates the prohibition against killing human beings. They hold that suffering can almost always be relieved, and they voice concerns about potential abuses, such as involuntary euthanasia to contain health care costs, if such acts were permitted (Lo, 1995).

It is particularly important to consider the reason for a patient's request for assisted suicide or euthanasia. When the patient indicates that life has become intolerable, we must determine why this is so. Often, inadequate pain management and depression are factors that enter into this perception, which, when treated appropriately, can change the patient's perspective. This may not always be the case, however, and nurses need to be able to support patients and families as they struggle with questions regarding whether natural death is always the best and most loving choice (Hooks & Daly, 2000). Attending to the nature and cause of a person's suffering and providing comfort care throughout the dying process are important components of the nursing role that may influence choices regarding active voluntary euthanasia or assisted suicide.

Issues Related to HIV/AIDS. We know that human immunodeficiency virus and acquired immunodeficiency syndrome (HIV/AIDS) is a major worldwide health concern, and that the virus is generally contracted through sexual contact. Although most cases of HIV/AIDS have resulted from a choice to have unprotected sexual relations, we must remember that not all HIV/AIDS results from lifestyle choices. The ANA *Code for Nurses* directs nurses to care for patients regardless of their values or lifestyle; thus, nurses need to be aware of potential judgmental attitudes toward persons with HIV/AIDS, and be alert to how these attitudes may affect the quality of their care.

Because of the risk of exposure to HIV in health care settings, questions arise regarding issues of autonomy and confidentiality in relation to HIV testing and status. One issue relates to whether patients can be required to submit to HIV testing in situations of potential or actual percutaneous exposure of health care workers to their blood. In order to protect persons from potential discrimination, confidentiality of HIV testing and status is generally assured by law; thus, it is generally illegal to perform HIV testing without a person's written consent. "Ethically speaking, HIV testing over the patient's objections violates the patient's autonomy and privacy as well as the spirit of informed consent . . . consent for HIV testing is important because stigma and discrimination may occur if other people know that the patient is seropositive" (Lo, 1995, p. 332).

Because of concerns about potential stigma in work or home settings related to having a documented HIV test, regardless of its result, patients may refuse a test even if they are sure it will be negative. In order to ensure confidentiality and to encourage patient agreement to testing in the event of exposure of a health care worker to a patient's blood, Lo (1995) suggests an approach of anonymous testing of the patient. Such an approach would necessitate paying for the test by a source other than the patient's insurer (such as an employee health fund), recording the results in a location other than the patient's medical record (such as a special occupational health file), and labeling the blood sample with a code rather than the patient's name. In this way the health care worker could know if he or she is at risk, while protecting the patient from potential stigma resulting from the test.

Another issue that has become a public concern relates to potential exposure of patients to the blood of a seropositive health care worker. Questions arise whether HIV testing among health care workers, or at least those involved in certain invasive procedures, should be mandatory; whether seropositive health care workers should have restrictions on their practice; and whether the HIV status of health care workers should be made known to patients. Some argue that if it becomes mandatory for health care workers to be tested, then it should be mandatory for all patients as well. Principles of autonomy, confidentiality, and nonmaleficence become part of this discussion. Health care workers, as well as patients, have a right to autonomy and confidentiality regarding health matters, particularly where discrimination could result from disclosure. At the same time, nonmaleficence directs them to do no harm to patients, and the doctrine of informed consent requires advising patients of potential risks related to interventions being considered. Economic factors enter into the discussion as well. At the present time, presuming health care workers follow universal infection control precautions, the risk of a patient contracting HIV from a seropositive health care worker is low, in contrast to the high cost of mandatory testing. Requiring such testing could well divert money from other, more effective areas of health promotion and protection.

Current issues related to HIV/AIDS may become less of a concern as technology advances toward more effective prevention and treatment of the disease. However, ethical concerns surrounding these issues apply to other health problems of similar nature. Nurses and other health care workers must be aware of any factors in their own health that might put their patients at risk, and take necessary precautions to protect patients from harm. It is also essential that nurses follow universal precautions aimed at protecting themselves and others from harm. If behaviors on the part of health care workers are observed that might put patients at risk, the imperatives of beneficence and nonmaleficence direct nurses to do what is necessary to protect the patient. Actions may include approaching the person involved, reporting the situation to appropriate persons within the agency, and working with groups to institute changes to prevent similar situations from occurring.

Although cases of HIV/AIDS must be reported, as with other infectious diseases, caregivers cannot disclose a person's HIV status without consent. The legal and ethical right to confidentiality regarding HIV/AIDS raises an ethical issue related to protection of others when the infected individual continues behaviors that may expose others to the infection. In some circumstances, physicians are allowed limited disclosure without consent, such as to the patient's spouse. In such situations the imperative of confidentiality must be weighed against the duty to warn others in order to protect them from potential harm. At the present time there are no clear directives in this area for health care providers.

Confidentiality

The imperative of **confidentiality** in health care, which is discussed in Chapter 3, can be traced at least as far back as the Hippocratic vow not to reveal secrets. In order to care for people with health concerns, nurses must be privy to very personal, and sometimes secret, information. Without assurance of confidentiality, many people would not disclose information that is important in diagnosis and treatment of, and caring for, health concerns. This is especially true in situations where there is stigma attached to, or other risks for social repercussions from, the information disclosed. Nurses need to remember that a patient's trust is sacred, and any breach of confidentiality, no matter how small it might seem to the nurse, is a violation of this trust. As with so many other areas, there are situations where other factors override confidentiality. In circumstances such as court cases, the law might require disclosure. In situations where secrets entrusted to the nurse suggest potential harm for the patient or others, the duty to warn may take precedence over confidentiality. For example, if a patient tells a nurse about suicide plans that the nurse believes are genuine, and the patient is not willing to be hospitalized, protection of the patient may require the nurse to initiate the process of involuntary hospitalization.

SUMMARY

This chapter discussed considerations for nursing practice related to patient self-determination. The concept of self-determination derives from the principle of autonomy, and denotes the right and freedom to make choices about issues that affect one's life. Principles of justice, beneficence, and nonmaleficence may temper the bounds of autonomy in some circumstances. The doctrine of informed consent is both a legal and ethical imperative for protecting a person's right to self-determination in health care decisions. Informed consent implies the right to accept or reject recommended treatment plans. As patient advocates, we need to be alert for situations in which patient autonomy may be limited, or in which there is a lack of sufficient information for the patient or family to make informed decisions. Nurses have a particular responsibility for facilitating informed decision making regarding patient choices for end-of-life care. Nursing's professional code directs nurses to provide services with respect for the rights and dignity of the patient regardless of a person's background or the nature of the health concern. If professional responsibilities expected of a nurse in a patient care situation are inconsistent with the nurse's ethical stance, integrity and accountability, she should remove herself from that situation after ensuring that there are others to assume care for the patient. A nurse's attention to the many-faceted issues surrounding patient self-determination may be the factor that ensures the patient's involvement in important health care decisions.

CHAPTER HIGHLIGHTS

- Self-determination derives from the principle of autonomy, and implies having freedom to make choices about issues affecting one's life, an ability to make decisions about personal goals, and an appreciation for self in relation to others.

- Autonomy may be threatened by factors such as paternalism; presumptions that a patient's values, knowledge level, and ways of dealing with issues are consistent with those of health care providers; and greater attention to technology than caring. In some situations, principles such as justice or nonmaleficence may temper the bounds of autonomy.

- Decisions about health care require attention to patient values, culture, and beliefs; effects of lifestyle and role; others who are affected by a patient's choices; and evaluation of risks, benefits, and economic considerations.

- Practitioners are not required to honor requests for interventions that are outside accepted standards of care or contrary to the practitioner's ethical views.

- Informed consent provides legal and ethical protection of a patient's right to personal autonomy regarding plans for health care, including the right to refuse interventions and to choose from available alternatives. Information necessary in an informed consent includes: the nature of the concern and prognosis if nothing is done; description of treatment options; and benefits, risks, and consequences of treatment options or nonintervention.

- Decision-making capacity, which is a medical determination and essential for informed consent, includes evidence of the ability to understand information, to communicate understanding and choices, to evaluate decisions in relation to personal values and goals, and to reason and to deliberate. Conscious adults are presumed to have decision-making capacity, unless there is evidence to the contrary.

- Nursing responsibility regarding informed consent includes verifying that the patient is aware of options and the implications of each, and advocating for patients to ensure that criteria for autonomous decision making are met in situations where the physician has not attended to these criteria. Nurses in advanced practice must obtain informed consent for interventions that they initiate within their scope of practice.

- Advance directives, which include living wills and durable powers of attorney, provide instructions regarding health care interventions in the event that one loses decision-making capacity. The Patient Self-Determination Act provides legal support for ensuring that patients are informed of their rights regarding health care decisions.

- In dealing with patient lifestyle choices, nurses must remember the instructions in the ANA *Code for Nurses* to provide services with respect for human dignity and to avoid value judgments related to differences in background, customs, attitudes, and beliefs.

- Nurses need to be aware of their own values and beliefs regarding various lifestyle and health care choices, and know how these affect their care with patients.

- Nurses must recognize the patient's right to use complementary therapies, become more knowledgeable about other modalities, and create an atmosphere encouraging of nonjudgmental discussion of such interventions.

- Ethical codes direct nurses to maintain confidentiality regarding patient health status and choices, except in special circumstances in which the "secrets" revealed suggest potential harm for the patient or another.

DISCUSSION QUESTIONS AND ACTIVITIES

1. Discuss your understanding of patient self-determination, including its ethical and legal basis, and nursing practice considerations.

2. Describe dilemmas that nurses may face related to patient self-determination and suggest approaches for dealing with such dilemmas.

3. Explore how practicing nurses in your institution perceive their role regarding

informed consent. What dilemmas related to consent have they encountered and how did they deal with these issues?

4. Analyze your own values regarding abortion and active voluntary euthanasia. How would you respond to a patient under your care who was deliberating such a choice?

5. Explore your state's statutes regarding advance directives, HIV testing and disclosure, euthanasia, assisted suicide, and abortion. What are the implications of these regulations for nursing practice in your state?

6. What are your views on mandatory HIV testing for health care professionals? What about limiting the practice of seropositive health care workers? Review current literature to determine recommendations by professional organizations concerning these issues.

7. Determine how your institution meets requirements of the Patient Self-Determination Act. Discuss the adequacy of the process and nursing's involvement.

8. What is the process for obtaining support and guidance for dealing with ethical concerns and dilemmas in your institution? If there is an ethics committee, how are referrals made? Who is on the committee, and how are members chosen? Talk with a member of an ethics committee, and discuss how they see their role and the effectiveness of the committee.

9. Select a case situation in which there are ethical concerns that warrant referral to the ethics committee. With classmates, role-play the ethics committee discussion, decisions, and actions regarding the case. Explain why you take position that you do, and how you feel about the outcome.

10. Choose one of the issues discussed in this chapter and explore the web sites of the ANA, the CNA, and the ICN regarding policies or positions statements on this issue. Compare and contrast positions of the various organizations. Discuss your views about this issue and how they compare with the positions of the professional organizations.

> ANA—http://www.nursingworld.org
>
> CNA—http://www.cna-nurses.ca
>
> ICN—http://www.icn.ch

REFERENCES

American Nurses Association. (1985). *Code for nurses with interpretive statements*. Washington, DC: Author.

American Nurses Association. (1991). *Position statement on nursing and the Patient Self-Determination Act*. Kansas City, MO: Author.

American Nurses Association. (2001). *Code of ethics for nurses*. Kansas City, MO: Author.

Becker, P. H. (1986). Advocacy in nursing: Perils and possibilities. *Holistic Nursing Practice, 1*(1), 54–63.

Benjamin, M. & Curtis, J. (1986). *Ethics in nursing* (2nd ed.). New York: Oxford University Press.

Canadian Nurses Association (1998, May). Advance directives: the nurse's role. *Ethics in Practice.* Retrieved January 9, 2001 from the World Wide Web: http://www.cna-nurses.ca/pages/ethics_sec . . .cs%20in%20practice/advance_directives.htm

Curtin, L. (1982). Autonomy, accountability, and nursing practice. *Topics in Clinical Nursing, 4,* 7–14.

Davis, A. J. & Aroskar, M. A. (1991). *Ethical dilemmas and nursing practice* (3rd ed.). Norwalk, CT: Appleton & Lange.

Devettere, R. J. (1995). *Practical decision making in health care ethics: Cases and concepts.* Washington, DC: Georgetown University Press.

Eisenberg, D. M., Kessler, R. C., Foster, C., Norlock, F. E., Calkins, D. R., & Delbanco, T. L. (1993). Unconventional medicine in the United States. *New England Journal of Medicine, 328,* 246–252.

Eisenberg, D. M., Rogers, B. D., Ettner, S., Appel, S., Wilkey, S., Van Rompay, M., & Kessler, R. C. (1998). Trends in alternative medicine in the United States, 1990–1997. *Journal of the American Medical Association, 280*(18), 1569–1575.

Finucane, T. E., Christmas, C., & Travis, K. (1999). Tube feeding in patients with advanced dementia. *Journal of the American Medical Association, 282*(14), 1265–1370.

Forbes, S., Bern-Klug, M., & Gessert, C. (2000). End-of-life decision making for nursing home residents with dementia. *Journal of Nursing Scholarship, 32*(3), 251–258.

Hardwig, J. (1995). What about the family? In J. H. Howell & W. F. Sale, eds., *Life choices: A Hastings Center introduction to bioethics* (pp. 53–67). Washington, DC: Georgetown University Press.

Haynor, P. M. (1998). Meeting the challenge of advance directives. *American Journal of Nursing, 98*(3), 26–32.

Hooks, F. J., & Daly, B. J. (2000). Hastening death. *American Journal of Nursing, 100*(5), 56–63.

Husted, G., & Husted, J. (1995). *Ethical decision making in nursing* (2nd ed.). St. Louis, MO: Mosby.

Lo, B. (1995). *Resolving ethical dilemmas: A guide for clinicians.* Baltimore: Williams & Wilkins.

LoBuono, C. (2000). A detailed examination of advance directives. *Patient Care for the Nurse Practitioner, 3*(11), 31–32, 35–36, 39–42, 47–48, 51.

McCann, R. (1999). Lack of evidence about tube feeding: Food for thought. *Journal of the American Medical Association, 282*(14), 1381.

Mahowald, M. B. (1995). Is there life after Roe v. Wade? In J. H. Howell & W. F. Sale, eds., *Life choices: A Hastings Center introduction to bioethics* (pp. 96–110). Washington, DC: Georgetown University Press.

Moss, A. H. (2001). What's new? Progress in palliative care, CPR, and advance directives. Seminar at Raleigh General Hospital, Beckley, WV. January 18, 2001.

President's Commission for the Study of Ethical Problems in Medicine and Biomedical and Behavioral Research. (1983). *Making health care decisions,* pp. 1–6, Washington, DC: U.S. Government Printing Office.

Roberts, D. (2000). Race, gender, justice, and reproductive health policy. Presentation at *New century, new challenges: Intensive bioethics course XXVI.* Kennedy Institute of Ethics, Georgetown University, Washington, DC, June 9, 2000.

Salgo v. Leland Stanford Jr. (1957). 317 P. 2d 170 (Cal. Dis. Ct. App; 1951).

Schlenk, J. S. (1997). Advance directives: Role of nurse practitioners. *Journal of the American Academy of Nurse Practitioners, 9*(7), 317–321.

Schloendorff v. The Society of New York Hospital (1914) 211 NY125, 105 N.E. 92 (1914).

Sherwin, W. (1992). Paternalism. In *No longer patient: Feminist ethics and health care* (pp. 137–157). Philadelphia: Temple University Press.

Slater v. Baker & Stapleton. (1767). High Court of Justice, King's Bench Division. English Reports, vol. 95, pp. 860–863.

Sullivan, G. H. (1998). Getting informed consent. *RN* (April), 59–62.

Tilden, V. P. (2000). Advance directives. *American Journal of Nursing, 100*(12), 49, 50.

West Virginia Network of Ethics Committees (WVNEC) Newsletter, 9(3). Morgantown, WV: Center for Health Ethics and Law (www.wvethics.org).

CHAPTER 12

Scholarship Issues

My experience tells me that people instinctively trust those whose personality is founded upon correct principles.

(Covey, 1992, p. 18)

OBJECTIVES

After completing this chapter, the reader should be able to:

1. Describe scholarship issues encountered by nurses in academic and clinical settings.
2. Discuss principles basic to academic honesty and the ethical treatment of research data.
3. Describe principles and nursing standards undergirding the protection of human rights in research.
4. Explain why informed consent is mandated for research involving human subjects, and describe the elements required for this consent.
5. Discuss the nursing role regarding protection of human rights in research.
6. Describe principles guiding personal response to dilemmas regarding nursing scholarship.

INTRODUCTION

Scholarship issues face students, teachers, researchers, and clinicians from the moment a person enters a nursing program and throughout that person's professional career. This chapter discusses principles that undergird ethical behavior in academic matters, in conducting research, and in the treatment of data both during the research process and in presentations or publication. Respect for all persons, including ourselves, is basic to ethical behavior regarding scholarship. Personal values affect how we approach situations that present ethical dilemmas. It is essential that nurses be knowledgeable about principles guiding ethical conduct, whether dealing with academic assignments, research data, or research with human subjects.

ACADEMIC HONESTY

Integrity in upholding the principles of veracity and fidelity is expected of nurses in any setting and is at the core of academic honesty. Veracity refers to truth telling, which is an essential ingredient for trust among humans. Husted and Husted (1995) suggest that true interaction and communication cannot occur where there is no trust. These authors describe fidelity as promise keeping, suggesting that it is the form that truth takes in an agreement between persons such as nurse-patient, researcher-participant, or student-teacher. Integrity implies respect for self and others, and a personal commitment to principled behavior over time in our personal and professional lives. When integrity is present, there is no need for monitoring a person's behavior; rather, there is an implicit trust that we represent ourselves in a truthful way. Honesty and integrity are key considerations in both academic and clinical situations. Personal values such as honesty serve as the basis for professional integrity.

Students at all levels face many stresses in regard to academic performance, and nursing students are no exception. Pressures may come from many areas, such as family expectations, personal goals of being accepted into graduate school, needing a certain grade to receive tuition reimbursement, or self-expectations that say "I always get good grades." When pressures become intense, values such as honesty and integrity may become challenged.

Issues of academic honesty include plagiarism, cheating, and forgery. **Plagiarism** is taking another's ideas or work and presenting them as our own. Examples include submitting written, oral, or visual materials-such as a paper, report, speech, or thesis-that have been knowingly copied or obtained, in whole or in part, from another's work without appropriate acknowledgment. **Cheating** refers to dishonesty and deception regarding examinations, projects, or papers. Examples include receiving help from or giving help to another student during an exam, allowing another to copy our work, or doing work for another student that is to be submitted by that student. **Forgery** includes fraud or intentional misrepresentation, for example, altering or causing a grade to be altered in an academic record or presenting false data on admission records (West Virginia University, 1999–2001).

Implicit in academic honesty is a trust that work submitted by a student, whether papers, projects, or exams, is indeed the work of that student. When material from

Ask Yourself

What Are Your Perspectives on Academic Honesty?

- One of your closest friends is in a different section of the same course, and his section meets two days after yours. You know he has been very stressed because of his mother's illness and that he needs good grades to keep his scholarship. You have just taken the mid-term exam, and he asks you to give him an idea of the topics covered so he can focus his studying. What would you do? How do you feel in this situation? What principles would guide your decisions?

- During an exam you notice two students passing what appears to be notes between them. You are fairly sure that the instructor has not seen this. How do you feel in response to this? What would you do, and why?

- You are struggling with an assignment that is due in just a few days. A classmate says she has a paper that her cousin did for this same course three years ago that she is using as a guide, changing the text so that it seems like her writing. She offers to let you see her cousin's paper to do the same. What do you think about her plan? How would you respond? What would guide your decision?

other sources are included in papers, students must utilize appropriate referencing so as to avoid plagiarizing. One university catalog suggests that academic dishonesty indicates an "inability to meet and face issues . . . creating an atmosphere of mistrust, disrespect, and insecurity" (West Virginia University, 1999–2001, p. 48). The breach of trust and potential consequences within a student-teacher relationship that academic dishonesty engenders are self-evident. Litigation is another potential consequence in severe situations. Because of the value of honesty, academic institutions frequently have written policies that may carry consequences as serious as the student's being suspended or expelled for dishonest practices.

CASE PRESENTATION

Suspicions of Dishonesty

Sabrina and Jude have been close friends and study partners throughout their nursing program. They discuss their readings and class notes and frequently choose the same topic, sharing articles between them when writing papers. After a recent submission of papers, the instructor called them in and noted that their papers were almost identical, including mistakes in grammar, and said that it appeared that one had copied the other's paper. They each denied copying from the other.

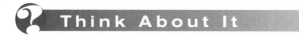

Think About It

Considering Consequences for Academic Dishonesty

- What ethical issues are involved in this situation?
- How do you feel about incidences of academic dishonesty?
- How do you think this situation should be handled? What consequences would you consider?
- In light of the standards that guide nursing practice, what is your position on allowing a student who has violated academic honesty through plagiarism, cheating, or forgery to continue in a nursing program?

RESEARCH ISSUES AND ETHICS

Nurses must be accountable for the quality of care they deliver, and research is one way of documenting the efficacy of nursing practice. Both the art and science of nursing are expanded through research. Research is necessary for the ongoing development of the unique body of knowledge that undergirds the discipline of nursing, and provides an organizing framework for nursing practice.

Participating in research can be exciting and encourage professional growth. It can also present some dilemmas for the nurse and nurse researcher in the academic and clinical realms. Seeking new knowledge and understanding is the expected motivation for conducting research. However, personal or institutional gains related to rewards like grant funds, prestige, the need to succeed, or promoting a product can be other motivating factors that may challenge principled behavior in regard to research.

A nurse who works in clinical areas where research is being conducted must be aware of principles for the conduct of research, regardless of whether the nurse has an active role with the research project. In this regard, guidelines from the American Nurses Association (ANA) state:

> A relationship of trust between nurse and patient has always been an essential element of the professional code of ethics. In research, a relationship of trust between subject and investigator requires that the investigator assume special obligations to safeguard the subject. . . . The individual has the right of self-determination concerning what will be done to his person. Each practitioner of nursing has an obligation to endorse and support self-determination as a moral and legal right of the individual. The responsibilities of safeguarding the rights of others must be fully accepted by nurses whether their roles are as practitioners, educators, or researchers. (ANA, 1985, p. 3)

Ethical Issues in Research

Many research texts focus their discussions of ethical issues in research primarily on protection of human rights. This emphasis is understandable because of violations that have occurred. The most cited violations of human rights in research are those that were perpetrated by the Nazis during World War II and that came to public awareness during the Nuremberg trials. International efforts to provide guidelines for protection of human rights have been documented in the **Nuremberg Code,** which was developed as a set of principles for the ethical conduct of research against which the experiments in the concentration camps could be judged, and the **Declaration of Helsinki,** issued by the World Medical Assembly in 1964 and revised in 1975 and in 2001 to guide clinical research. Included in the **Belmont Report,** the principles set forth in these codes serve as the basis for policies developed by the United States National Commission for the Protection of Human Subjects of Biomedical and Behavioral Research (1978).

In spite of these policies and guidelines, ethical lapses continue to occur in research with human subjects (Kaplan & Brownlee, 1999; Hilts & Stolberg, 1999; Maloney, 2000a, 2000b). These and other concerns raise questions about whether current regulations adequately protect the rights and welfare of research subjects (Moreno, Caplan, & Wolpe, 1998). In order to oversee and enforce federal regulations pertaining to research with human subjects, the United States Department of Health and Human Services recently formed an Office for Human Research Protection. Efforts to bolster protections for human research subjects focus on education and training of clinical investigators and institutional review board members, auditing records for evidence of compliance with informed consent, improved monitoring of clinical trials, managing conflicts of interest so that research subjects are appropriately informed, and imposing monetary penalties for violations of important research practices, such as informed consent (Spicer, 2000).

Principles of beneficence, respect for human dignity, and justice underlie the ethical conduct of research (Belmont Report, 1978; ANA, 1985; Newland, 2000). The principle of **beneficence** implies the right to protection from harm and discomfort, including a balance between the benefits and risks of a study. The principle of **respect for human dignity** implies the rights to full disclosure and self-determination or autonomy. The principle of **justice** implies the rights of fair treatment and privacy, including anonymity and confidentiality. A brief discussion of each principle follows. The ANA guidelines for the protection of human rights are summarized in Figure 12–1.

Beneficence. This principle derives from the maxim that says "above all, do no harm." In research situations this means that researchers need to design and conduct studies so as to protect the participants from physical, mental, emotional, spiritual, economic, and social harm. Discomfort can range from no anticipated effects to certainty of permanent damage, and include such things as fatigue, physical pain, anxiety, embarrassment, confronting meaning and purpose in life, threats to self-esteem or to values, lost earnings for time given to participate in research, and social stigma (Burns & Groves, 1997; Harrison, 1993; Wilson, 1999). If discomfort is anticipated as part of the research protocol, the participant must be willing to experience the discomfort after being given all relevant information, and the risk for harm must be balanced with anticipated benefits. In general, a minimal risk is that which is no more than would be expected within the context of routine life activities. When risks are

Figure 12–1 **Protection of Human Rights**

Right to Freedom from Intrinsic Risk of Injury

- When an individual participating in research is exposed to increased risk for social, emotional, or physical injury, the investigator must specify the degree of risk and estimate how the risk to the individual compares to the benefit to humanity through knowledge gained.

- All relevant information concerning activities that go beyond established and accepted procedures for meeting personal needs must be given to a prospective participant prior to that person's participation in the study.

- Nurses must be vigilant in their concern for persons who are unable to effectively protect themselves from harm or injury due to illness or other condition and be aware of potentials for exploiting captive populations, such as persons in institutions, students, or prisoners.

Right to Privacy

- Since an investigator cannot decide for another what is considered an invasion of privacy for that person, all proposals, protocols, investigative instruments, and procedures to be used in research activities must be specified and discussed with the prospective participant.

- The above must be discussed as well with any workers who are expected to take part in the research as data gatherers or research participants.

Right to Anonymity

- There must be safeguards against unanticipated physical, psychological, or social disadvantages occurring to participants because of their role in the research, either during the study or from dissemination of findings.

- Assurance that a participant's anonymity will be protected must be provided when the participant agrees to share personal information that might not be divulged to others in another context.

- When collected data is not to remain under the control of the investigator, mechanisms for protecting the identity of the participant and safeguarding confidentiality must be established.

- When the plan of the study or the report of the findings will sacrifice the participant's anonymity or confidentiality, specific prior consent must be obtained.

- Potential violations of human dignity from demeaning or dehumanizing situations in the research protocol require special consideration, recognizing that such violations can have long-range repercussions when significant values of the individual are involved.

Adapted from American Nurses Association (1985). *Human rights guidelines for nurses in clinical and other research* (p. 67). Kansas City, MO: Author.

greater than minimal, the researcher's aim must be to minimize risks while maximizing the benefits to participants. Since our role as nurses impels us to protect those in our care from unnecessary physical or mental suffering, if the risks of research outweigh the benefits, the study should be redesigned or discontinued.

Respect for Human Dignity. Implicit in this principle is the right to self-determination, which acknowledges the autonomy of the potential participant in research. This means that persons have the right to choose whether they wish to participate in the research; that is, participation is voluntary and free from coercion of any type. **Coercion** includes threat of harm or penalty for not participating in the research, or offering excessive rewards for participation. The right of self-determination means that the person has the right to withdraw from participation in the study at any time without imposed consequences, such as denial of health care or benefits. Voluntary participation requires **full disclosure,** that is, that the potential participant be fully informed of the nature of the study, the anticipated risks and benefits, time commitment, what is expected of the participant and the researcher, and the right to refuse to participate. This is addressed through the process of informed consent, which is discussed below.

Justice. The principle of justice includes the rights to privacy and to fair treatment. The nature of research is to gather information about that which is being studied. When persons are the focus of study, the **right to privacy** is a critical issue. Attentiveness to privacy means the participant determines when, where, and what kind of information is shared, with an assurance that information, attitudes, behaviors, records, opinions, and the like that are observed or collected will be treated with respect and kept in strict confidence. Privacy is maintained through anonymity, confidentiality, and informed consent. If even the researcher cannot link information with a particular participant, then **anonymity** exists. **Confidentiality** refers to the researcher's assurance to participants that information provided will not be made public or available to anyone other than those involved in the research process without the participant's consent. Confidentiality is maintained by using codes rather than personal identification on data collection forms and restricting access to raw data to those on the research team who need to use the data.

The **right to fair treatment** is related to the right to self-determination. Equitable treatment of participants in the selection process, during the study, and after the completion of the study is at the basis of this right. Factors to consider in fair treatment include: selecting participants based on the research needs, not on the convenience or compromised position of a group of people; equitably distributing the risks and benefits of the research among participants regardless of age, gender, socioeconomic status, race, or ethnic background; honoring any agreements made or benefits promised; treating participants with respect, providing access to research personnel or other professionals as needed; treating persons who decline to participate or withdraw from the study without prejudice; and debriefing as needed to clarify issues or when information had been withheld prior to the study.

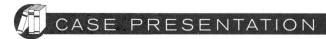

Protecting Patients Who Are Research Subjects

Annissa, a nurse in a primary care clinic, talked with her coworker Bill about his non-nursing graduate program. Bill said he has decided to study emotional attitudes of patients using a standardized instrument for his required research project. When Annissa asked about recruiting participants, he said he will have all his patients complete the instrument when he sees them for routine visits over the next few weeks. In response to Annissa's questions about the possibility of patients not wanting to participate, Bill said that he'll just tell them it's for a student project, and he's sure they'll fill out the form to help him out and keep on his good side. Annissa asked which Institutional Review Board (IRB) reviewed his proposal, and Bill replied that his school does not have an IRB, so only his advisor had to give approval.

Think About It

What Principles Guide Ethical Conduct of Clinical Research?

- What principles are involved in this situation?

- What dilemmas may arise with Bill's research project?

- What are Annissa's ethical responsibilities in this situation?

- What is the responsibility of the primary care agency related to research conducted within the agency?

Informed Consent.   As noted above, voluntary participation in a research study requires full disclosure. Informing potential participants of the research purpose, expected commitment, risks and benefits, any invasion of privacy, and ways that anonymity and confidentiality will be addressed are included in the process of **informed consent.** The researcher must ensure that the person who is agreeing to participate in the study comprehends the information included in the consent and has a chance to receive clarifications and additional information when needed. Written consent forms should be written in common language without jargon. The literacy level of the person signing the informed consent should be determined and recorded, and the person agreeing to participate in the research must be mentally and emotionally competent to make the decision.

Munhall and Boyd (1999) suggest that the process of informed consent provides a way of including the person as a collaborator in the research rather than as a mere "subject." We must, however, guard against the element of coercion. One review of nursing research protocols found more ethical concerns arising from the relationship between the researcher and study participant than from physical harm (Olsen &

Mahrenholz, 2000). When the nurse who cares for the patient is on the research team and the one obtaining the informed consent, determining whether the patient is giving consent to the "nurse" or to the "researcher" can be somewhat tricky. The nurse-researcher must determine whether the patient truly feels the freedom to refuse to participate.

The *Code of Federal Regulations* (1981) lists basic elements that need to be included in informed consent:

1. A statement that the study involves research, an explanation of the purpose of the research and the expected duration of the subject's participation, a description of the procedures to be followed, and identification of any procedures that are experimental.

2. A description of any reasonably foreseeable risks or discomforts to the participant.

3. A description of any benefits to the participant or to others that may reasonably be expected from the research.

4. A disclosure of appropriate alternative procedures or courses of treatment, if any, that might be advantageous to the subject.

5. A statement describing the extent, if any, to which confidentiality of records identifying the subject will be maintained.

6. For research involving more than minimal risk, an explanation as to whether any compensation and an explanation as to whether medical treatments are available if injury occurs and, if so, what they consist of, or where further information may be obtained.

7. An explanation of whom to contact for answers to pertinent questions about the research and research subjects' rights, and whom to contact in the event of a research-related injury to the subject.

8. A statement that participation is voluntary, that refusal to participate will involve no penalty or loss of benefits to which the subject is otherwise entitled, and the subject may discontinue participation at any time without penalty or loss of benefits to which the subject is otherwise entitled.

Nurses who are assisting with research or who work on units where research is being conducted must be familiar with these elements of informed consent. If consent forms do not contain these elements, nurses should bring this to the attention of the investigators or the institution ethics committee.

CASE PRESENTATION

Nurses, Research, and Informed Consent

Juan, a registered nurse, works in a small rural hospital clinic that has a strong commitment to the underserved population in its area, yet has been struggling financially because of the large number of indigent patients. There has been talk of possibly eliminating some positions because of the financial crisis. In a recent staff meeting he learned that a pharmaceutical company has negotiated an agreement with the physicians to use a new medication with their hypertensive patients, and gather data about side effects of this medication. A sizable financial reimbursement for the hospital is part of the agreement. As the RN, Juan will be responsible for checking patients' blood pressures and completing the side effect surveys. Juan asks about informed consent and is told that the pharmaceutical company said it is not needed because this medication has been through the clinical trials already. Juan does not feel comfortable about participating in the project, but recognizes that the money is needed by the hospital and, in fact, may make the difference in avoiding elimination of staff positions.

Think About It

Decisions About Participating in Research

- What issues do you identify in this case situation?
- What ethical principles are being violated or potentially violated?
- What ethical dilemmas do you think Juan is experiencing?
- What do you think Juan should do, and why?
- How might potential consequences affect the decision making process?

Special Considerations: Vulnerable Populations

Nurses must be especially attentive to protection of human rights in research with vulnerable populations. These populations include physically, mentally, or emotionally disabled or challenged persons; children or elderly persons; those who are dying, sedated, or unconscious; persons who are institutionalized or incarcerated; pregnant women; and fetuses. Because people in these populations are vulnerable to deception and coercion, and may have decreased ability to give informed consent, advocates or guardians who have the person's best interest in mind must be involved in decisions regarding their participation in research. An important consideration for research with vulnerable populations is that the less able the person is to give informed consent, the more important it is for the researcher to protect the person's rights (Wilson, 1999). Nurses who work with these populations need to be especially cognizant of their roles as advocates, particularly when research is proposed or being conducted in their settings.

More than Protection of Human Rights

Although protection of human subjects is a very important consideration in nursing research, other issues deserve equal attention. Wilson (1999) discusses characteristics of ethical research that go beyond the protection of human rights. These include:

Scientific objectivity—reporting all data, both supportive and unsupportive of hypotheses, and not engaging in misconduct, fraud, or acts of bad faith;

Cooperation—submitting proposals to and following recommendations of those authorized to review the research for protection of human rights;

Nobility—working actively to ensure protection of participants from harm, deceit, coercion, and invasions of privacy, even when this may inconvenience the study;

Integrity and Truthfulness—honestly describing the research process, including the purpose, procedures, methods, risks, discomforts, benefits, and findings;

Impeccability—ensuring anonymity and confidentiality of data and using discretion with information learned about people;

Illumination—publishing and presenting research findings in order to enhance nursing's body of scientific knowledge;

Equitability—noting contributions of others in publications and presentations;

Forthrightness—disclosing funding sources and sponsorship in publication and presentation of research findings; and

Courage—publicly clarifying any distortions of research findings made by others.

When nurses are working in agencies or institutions where research is being conducted, whether or not they are directly involved in the research, they must be aware of standards for ethical research in order to guard against violations of these standards.

Nurses who participate in conducting research may at times experience role conflict. A nurse is held to standards of professional practice that delineate the nurse's concern as safeguarding the health and well-being of the patient. A researcher is focused on processes and outcomes of a study in which patients may be used as sources of data. A responsible researcher is guided by humanistic values of moral concern in decisions regarding research participants (Fry, 1981). Thus, when there is a question of potential harm to a patient involved in a research study, the advocacy role of the nurse and the therapeutic imperative takes precedence over integrity of the research protocol (Fowler, 1988a; Munhall and Boyd, 1999; Namei, King, Byrne, & Proffitt, 1993). Ignorance of ethical and legal guidelines related to research is no excuse for a nurse failing to be a patient advocate in research situations. Although research is necessary for development of scientific and therapeutic knowledge, a balance between principles guiding scientific inquiry and those guiding nursing practice must be maintained.

When nurses are employed, particularly in institutions that are research focused, they need to clarify what is expected of them in regard to research. Nurses should know prior to accepting a position whether they will be required to gather data or administer treatments as part of research protocols, and whether such treatments may have potential risks to patients. Nurses in such settings need to know whether their positions will be jeopardized if they refuse to participate as part of a research team. When participation in research is expected as part of a nurse's job, the nurse must know the protocol, whether it has been approved by the institutional review board, and who to consult with any concerns about the research process and effect on patients.

Ask Yourself

What Takes Precedence—Research or Nursing Care?

Fowler (1988b, p. 354) poses some questions that are worth pondering.

- Is the good of the patient ever subservient to the acquisition of nursing knowledge?

- Does the therapeutic imperative of clinical care and the good of the patient always preempt the mandate to enlarge the nursing profession's body of knowledge?

- At what point must a nurse stop a specific nursing research project?

- When must a nurse intervene to halt a specific medical research project?

- Are there conditions under which a nurse should not include a specific subject in a study, even though consent has been secured?

ETHICAL TREATMENT OF DATA

Scholarship issues regarding data include how the data is handled during the collection and analysis process and how the data is reported. **Ethical treatment of data** implies integrity of research protocols and honesty in reporting findings. The honesty and integrity of the researcher are of utmost importance in the ethical treatment of data. Taking care to ensure that only those who are involved in the research process have access to the data and to maintain confidentiality were mentioned previously. A critical ethical obligation of qualitative nursing researchers is to present and describe the experiences of others as authentically and faithfully as possible, even when it is contrary to our own aims (Munhall & Boyd, 1999). The imperative to report the findings as accurately as possible is an ethical obligation in quantitative studies as well.

CASE PRESENTATION

Ethical Issues in Handling Research Data

A classmate and good friend is in the process of doing a research project required for graduation. You know she is frustrated because the surveys she sent out are not being returned, and the project needs to be completed soon if she is to graduate on time. She also needs to do well on this project in order to graduate with honors. In order to have a large enough sample, she tells you that she is going to fill in several forms herself and asks if you will do some for her too, noting that several other friends have already completed forms. She says that, after all, the object of the assignment is to see if one can collect and analyze the data. You are also aware that the best studies will be published in the student nursing newsletter.

Think About It

Honesty in Nursing Research

- What is your reaction to her plan and request?
- Discuss the ethical issues involved in this scenario.
- Describe the appropriate ethical stance in this situation. What factors would enable or mitigate against your taking this stance?
- What would you do with this information and what principles would guide your actions?

Nurses involved in research are accountable to professional standards for reporting findings. Principles that guide academic honesty apply as well to nurse researchers in reporting outcomes of studies. It is dishonest to exaggerate results or adjust facts of a study in order to maximize or minimize particular outcomes or hypotheses. When information from someone else is included in a report without appropriate referencing, this is plagiarism. In recent years, scientific misconduct has become a concern within the scientific community. Articles have been published in professional journals reporting studies that were never conducted, findings that were fabricated, or findings that were intentionally distorted by researchers (Burns & Groves, 1997; Chop & Silva, 1991; Friedman, 1990; Hawley & Jeffers, 1992; Parascandola, 1999). Although these reports have related more to biomedical studies than to nursing research, such reports present problems to disciplines whose clinical practice may be changed based on research findings. They also serve as a reminder to nurses to be vigilant regarding ethical reporting of research findings.

Ask Yourself

Consequences of Reporting Fraudulent Research

Pause and think about the havoc rendered by publication of fraudulent research.

- How might this affect how others view the integrity of the profession?
- How might this affect a reader's response to other research published in the same journal?
- How would this affect your ability as a nurse to determine whether you should adjust your practice based on reported research?
- Imagine that you have just read the report of a research project for which you gathered data and discovered that the process described was quite a bit different from what you had done, making the results take on a different meaning. How would you react and what would you do?

SUMMARY

Nurses are expected to exhibit principled behavior in all situations. This chapter has focused on principles related to scholarship issues facing nurses. Decisions related to academic honesty face nursing students before they ever encounter a patient. Because personal values affect professional behavior, choices made in the academic arena concerning actions such as plagiarism, cheating, or forgery may foreshadow values used to guide future professional decisions. Nurses must be familiar with principles guiding ethical practices in research and reporting of research findings. These principles guide nursing decisions about research protocols, participation, and advocacy for patients related to research issues. Ethical practices regarding scholarship are essential to the integrity of both the professional and the profession.

CHAPTER HIGHLIGHTS

- Principles of veracity and integrity are core to academic honesty and to ethical treatment of research data.

- Nursing research and researchers must adhere to nursing standards regarding the ethical conduct of research that affirm a participant's right to freedom from intrinsic risk of injury, right to privacy, and right to anonymity.

- Protection of human rights, a prime focus of research ethics, is based on principles of beneficence, respect for human dignity, and justice. These principles imply protection from physical, emotional, spiritual, economic, and social harm; voluntary participation in research; and assurance of privacy and equitable treatment of all research participants.

- Informed consent for research studies, which helps to ensure that a participant's rights are protected, must include the elements promulgated in the Code of Federal Regulations.

- When there is a question of potential harm to a patient involved in a research study, the nurse's advocacy role and therapeutic imperative takes precedence over the integrity of the research protocol. Nurses need to be especially attentive to protection of rights of vulnerable groups in clinical and research settings.

- When considering employment, nurses should clarify expectations regarding potential participation in research.

DISCUSSION QUESTIONS AND ACTIVITIES

1. Review your school's policy regarding academic honesty, and discuss ethical principles that are violated in cases of academic dishonesty.

2. Describe factors that persons reviewing cases of academic dishonesty should consider.

3. How did protection of human rights come to be required for research involving human subjects?

4. What guidance do nursing standards offer nurses who are participating in or conducting research? What principles underlie the ethical conduct of research? Discuss nursing roles related to these principles and standards.

5. Interview a nurse-researcher regarding how human rights are protected in the study. Have all the required elements been included in the informed consent?

6. Give examples of situations in which the nursing roles of patient advocate and researcher might be in conflict. Which role takes precedence and why?

7. Discuss potential effects of unethical treatment of data on patient care.

8. Compare and contrast what the American Nurse's Association (www.ana.org), the Canadian Nurses Association (www.cna-nurses.ca), and the International Council of Nurses (www.icn.ch) say about human rights in research and in nursing practice.

REFERENCES

American Nurses Association. (1985). *Human rights guidelines for nurses in clinical and other research*. Kansas City, MO: Author.

Burns, N., & Groves, S. K. (1997). *The practice of nursing research* (3rd ed.). Philadelphia: Saunders.

Chop, R., & Silva, M. C. (1991). Scientific fraud: Definitions, policies, and implications for nursing research. *Journal of Professional Nursing, 7,* 166–171.

Code of Federal Regulations. (1981, January 26). Title 45, part 46. Washington, DC.

Covey, S. R. (1992). *Principle-centered leadership.* New York: A Fireside Book.

Fowler, M. D. M. (1988a). Ethical issues in nursing research: Issues in qualitative research. *Western Journal of Nursing Research, 10,* 109–111.

Fowler, M. D. M. (1988b). Ethical issues in nursing research: A call for an international code of ethics for nursing. *Western Journal of Nursing Research, 10,* 352–355.

Friedman, P. J. (1990). Correcting the literature following fraudulent publication. *Journal of the American Medical Association, 263,* 1416–1419.

Fry, S. T. (1981). Accountability in research: The relationship of scientific and humanistic values. *Advances in Nursing Science, 4,* 1–13.

Harrison, L. (1993). Issues related to the protection of human research participants. *Journal of Neuroscience Nursing, 25,* 187–193.

Hawley, D. J., & Jeffers, J. M. (1992). Scientific misconduct as a dilemma for nursing. *Image, 24,* 51–55.

Hilts, P. J., & Stolberg, S. G. (1999). Ethics lapses at Duke halt dozens of human experiments. *New York Times,* May 13, A26.

Husted, G. L., & Husted J. H. (1995). *Ethical decision making in nursing* (2nd ed.). St. Louis, MO: Mosby.

Kaplan, S., & Brownlee, S. (1999). Duke's hazards: did medical experiments put patients needlessly at risk? *U. S. World and News Report, 126*(20), 66–68, 70.

Maloney, D. M. (2000a). Federal agency has all the legal authority it needs to suspend human subjects research. *Human Research Report, 15*(1), 1–2.

Maloney, D. M. (2000b). Court says state agency avoided usual way of reporting problems with human subjects: T. D. v. New York State Office of Mental Health (Part III). *Human Research Report, 15* (2), 7–8.

Moreno, J., Caplan, A. L., & Wolpe, P. R. (1998). Updating protections for human subjects involved in research. *Journal of the American Medical Association, 280*(22), 1951–1958.

Munhall, P. L., & Boyd, C. O. (1999). *Nursing research: A qualitative perspective* (2nd ed.). New York: National League of Nursing Press.

Namei, S. K., King, M. O., Byrne, M., & Proffitt, C. (1993). The ethics of role conflict. *Journal of Neuroscience Nursing, 25,* 326–330.

Newland, M. (1999). Questions & answers from the JCAHO. What principles guide research with human participants? *Nursing-Management, 30*(11), 24.

Olsen, D. P., & Mahrenholz, D. (2000). IRB-identified ethical issues in nursing research. *Journal of Professional Nursing, 16*(3), 140–148.

Parascandola, M. (1999). Investigator fraud in clinical research. *Research-Nurse, 5*(2), 1–9, 20–21.

Spicer, C. M. (2000). Federal oversight and regulations of human subjects research: An update. *Kennedy Institute of Ethics Journal, 10*(3), 261–264.

United States National Commission for the Protection of Human Subjects of Biomedical and Behavioral Research. (1978). *The Belmont report: Ethical principles and guidelines for the protection of human subjects of research* (DHEW Publication No. (OS)78–0012). Washington, DC: U.S. Government Printing Office.

West Virginia University. (1999–2001). *Robert C. Byrd Health Sciences Center Catalogue.* Morgantown, WV: Author.

Wilson, H. S. (1999). *Introducing research in nursing* (2nd ed.). Redwood City, CA: Addison-Wesley.

PART **IV**

GLOBAL ISSUES THAT IMPINGE ON NURSING PRACTICE

Part IV recognizes each person as part of an interrelated global population affected by many interacting forces. Focusing on nursing, this part begins by addressing challenges and changes in health care delivery. This section then explores local, national, and global issues. These chapters encourage nurses to be responsible professionals and citizens in acknowledging and participating in decisions related to various political, economic, social, gender, transcultural, and spirituality issues.

CHAPTER 13

Health Care Changes and Challenges

By Barbara Kupchak

What we remember, we can change; what we forget we always are.

(Tafoya, 1996)

OBJECTIVES

After completing this chapter, the reader should be able to:

1. Identify patterns of health care delivery from ancient times to the present.
2. Discuss historical events that have helped to shape the current system of health care delivery in the United States.
3. Examine trends in health care delivery and financing that have emerged in recent history.
4. Describe challenges facing health care delivery systems around the globe.
5. Discuss factors prompting a renewed interest in traditional healing systems worldwide.
6. Briefly describe factors affecting health care delivery for rural and urban aggregates.

INTRODUCTION

The health care delivery system and the way it is financed define the parameters within which nurses and other health care personnel function. Issues of health care delivery and the effectiveness of the health care delivery system are of concern throughout the world. In the United States and most of the Western world, delivery of health care is much like a runaway train of high technology—there is a proliferation of markets for new medications and expensive treatments. Further, the system is challenged to provide for an ever-increasing global population with decreasing resources. At the basis of this global concern is the ever-increasing cost of health care and the issue of its sustainability. Developing countries are recognizing that current and future health care systems have at their foundation expensive medicines and technologies that are imported from more developed regions of the globe. Questions arise about prioritizing health expenditures. Can countries address the health needs of their people without relying on expensive medications and treatments? Can local, existing systems of health care be utilized to provide basic health services to rural and urban poor communities? In developing countries, can traditional methods and systems of health care be utilized to promote health care and prevent disease, thus reducing the burden on the system? Has modern Western health care practice been lax in preserving and utilizing the traditional methods in favor of technology, and at what cost?

Health care systems must address global changes and challenges if they are to survive in the twenty-first century and beyond. In order to gain an understanding of these changes and challenges, we need to explore the history of various contemporary health care systems and their financing, including traditional methods of health care. In addition, we must look at rural and urban at-risk communities and factors that impede the delivery of health care in an overburdened system.

Ask Yourself

What Cultural Influences Affect Your Health Care Practices?

All persons have roots in beliefs and cultural heritage from their family of origin and place of birth.

- What do you know about the health care practices of your cultural origins?
- Have you or anyone you know ever utilized any healing modalities that are not part of what would be deemed modern health care?

A BRIEF HISTORY OF HEALTH CARE DELIVERY: THE EURO-AMERICAN EXPERIENCE

From the earliest civilizations there is evidence of some type of health care. The methods of health care were often a mixture of religious, civil, and mythological belief that combined to keep away disease, prevent wars, and ensure survival of populations in order to keep the various empires strong. In every culture there have been individuals designated to provide care to the sick. Some were formally trained as nurses and physicians, while others seemed to have a natural gift for the art of healing. Asian and Middle Eastern peoples, such as the Mesopotamians, Babylonians, Hebrews, Persians, Hindus, and Chinese, have recorded some type of system for the delivery of health care. In all of these cultures, religious or civil laws enforced systems of disease prevention in matters of hygiene and diet, some of which were connected to the various religious practices of the ancient civilizations.

Early Eras of Health Care Delivery

Achterberg notes that "the Sumerians, and not the ancient Greeks and Romans, are the parents of Western healing systems" (1990, p. 14). Archeological findings in the area of ancient Sumer, which is located in the vicinity of modern Iraq, include numerous prescriptions and two tablets that are considered to be the oldest medical text in existence (Achterberg, 1990). Sumerian knowledge of healing and theories of disease were dispersed to other areas through trade with the Phoenicians, Greeks, and Egyptians.

The ancient Greek civilization represents a major force in the systematic organization of education, both in secular and scientific fields. The most well-known name in ancient Greek medicine and health care is Hippocrates, known as the Father of Medicine. His approach of separating medicine and health care from religion, magic, and myth was considered purely scientific for his time. He diagnosed from observed symptoms, with emphasis on treating the whole patient, and he promoted continuous bedside care. His method of systematic record keeping of the patient's appearance, vital signs, and general bodily functioning became a standard for health care. Hippocrates approached medicine and health care from the highest ethical standard, believing medicine to be the noblest of arts. In addition, he believed that the physician's conduct should be of the highest quality and above reproach. Hippocrates gave the health care system organized writings of medical books that include detailed descriptive case histories, technical practices, and reports of research on various disease treatments, including treatments that worked and those that did not, in order to avoid repeating errors in care (Kelly, 1985).

As nations and populations expanded, knowledge was disseminated from culture to culture, constantly redefining the approach to health care, research, and practice. Alexander the Great, who conquered Greece in about 339 B.C.E., spread what he learned in Greece throughout the entire known world. He established medical schools in Egypt that included clinics, laboratories, and libraries. Physicians were supported by the government, and could devote their time to practice and research. Gradually, through various wars and assimilation of culture, Greek medicine supplemented or replaced practices throughout the known Western world.

The empire of Rome replaced methods of health care that were based on folklore and magic with a knowledge base developed in Greece. Within this developing culture, medicine and health care soon became a part of the necessary education of upper-class men, and women's health issues and childbearing practices regained importance. Midwives became key figures in the care of women (Kelly, 1985). Important contributions to health care delivery in the Roman Empire include public health sanitation and public health law. The Romans instituted city planning that provided for development of sewage systems, aqueducts, and baths. In addition, they can be credited for the development of hospitals with male and female attendants to care for the sick.

A new era in the care of the sick occurred after Christianity became the official religion of Rome. The Christian attitude of care for persons, based on a strong belief in the sanctity of human life, was derived from Hebrew tradition as well as the teachings of Christ. Bishops assigned individuals to care for widows, orphans, the sick, and the poor. Hospitals to care for the sick and institutions to care for the poor offered combinations of outpatient and welfare services. Monastic orders of monks and nuns, who were generally better educated than the ordinary person, controlled the health care institutions. Their writings documented the care given to the sick and techniques used, which provide early records of diseases, practices, and research for cure and care (Bullough & Bullough, 1978).

Changes from the Middle Ages to the Industrial Revolution

During the thirteenth and fourteenth centuries, the organization and founding of medical schools and universities and the advent of book binding all worked to promote a better educated health care provider. Nurses, who were not as fully established as physicians, functioned as attendants who made beds and gave baths to the sick.

As noted in Chapter 1, amidst the religious revolution that had taken place against the church of Rome (known as the Reformation) in the early sixteenth to seventeenth century, the disbanding of convents and monasteries led to severe impediments in the care of the sick. During this time, some progress was made in midwifery, medicine, and nursing. However, it was not until the mid-nineteenth century and the Industrial Revolution, when the demand for intellectual freedom brought about educational institutions for men, that the health care system as we know it began to emerge. During the nineteenth century, Florence Nightingale's leadership influenced not only nursing education and nursing care, but the health care of the world (Nightingale, 1859/1992; Bullough & Bullough, 1978; Selanders, 1998a, 1998b; McDonald, 1998; Dossey, 2000).

Ask Yourself

How Have Things Changed?

- Consider the discussion of the early era of the health care delivery system and identify problems in early civilization that might still be seen in today's world.
- Consider how Florence Nightingale's profound influence on health care systems worldwide continues to affect health care today. How can nurses continue this legacy in the twenty-first century?

Nightingale is perhaps best known for crafting the standards of Western secular nursing education and practice. Her leadership was also felt in the area of public policy and social reform. She spearheaded improvements in British military medicine, and greatly influenced public health reform in Great Britain and India. She was a pioneer in using evaluative statistics to monitor the various factors influencing health and the effectiveness of the health care system.

Changes Influencing Development of Modern Health Care in the United States

Health services in the United States developed from health care models in European countries. These systems share the products of medical innovations that took place from the late nineteenth century to the time of World War I, a time when major nations were changing from agricultural to industrial economies. Such innovations as the use of anesthesia in surgery and the recognition of bacteria as a causative factor in many widespread diseases provided the impetus that led to the development of the modern hospital as it exists today. The dissemination and incorporation of this knowledge among the large number of practicing physicians took at least a generation to accomplish. Consequently, the importance of the place of the modern hospital in society was not felt until the late nineteenth century and into the early twentieth century. At the time of this revolution of knowledge, physicians, who were the primary health care practitioners, engaged primarily in a private practice, fee-for-service system.

Physicians and Hospitals. In the United States, hospitals were generally privately funded, while European nations had both tax-supported charity hospitals and private hospitals for those patients who had the ability to pay for their own health care (Anderson, 1963). The primary purpose for hospitals built in Europe was ministry to the low-income or charity patient, while in the United States, hospitals that were built by private funding were open to charity patients as well as private-pay patients.

The development of hospitals affected European physicians by creating a class of specialists who operated in the general hospital and also had the option of treating private-pay patients. These specialists often created their own cottage hospitals, where they could treat their private-pay patients. All other physicians in that system were excluded from practicing in a hospital. In the United States, on the other hand, practitioners sought out appointments to the hospital system in order to be able to admit patients, while at the same time maintaining private offices in which to see their patients. This began a new approach to the use of the hospital system, in which resources were used more extravagantly and the system was more democratic in its care of patients than the European system. The United States health care system became immersed in greater use of technology, industrial and management skills, and scientific methods, creating by some estimates the best health care system in the world, and the most expensive (Anderson, 1963).

As an outgrowth of the development of hospitals, a greater awareness of public health problems arose. Prevention programs for the public, such as sanitation, environmental issues, control of communicable diseases, and maternity and infant care, developed. Curative programs, which were generally hospital-based, were supported by private and public funding. Hospital clinics that provided outpatient services became the primary site of health care for low-income and indigent patients. During that period, physicians provided these outpatient services free of charge and, in return, were able to participate in the hospital system, where the latest in knowledge and technologies was being introduced. This information could then be applied to the care of large numbers of both private and charity patients. Hospitals provided physicians an opportunity to develop their skills and to provide service to the public, thus fulfilling the physician's commitment to the public interest (Anderson, 1963).

Twentieth and Twenty-First Century Changes and Challenges.

The United States health care delivery system in the latter nineteenth century was affected by sources of funding (private or public), the ability of the patient to pay, and the type of control exercised by independent practitioners, which now included physicians, pharmacists, and dentists. The development of an industrialized society in the United States, the growth of the economy, and the increased capability of a growing health care system produced a healthier and more aware population. However, twentieth-century changes created new challenges for the health care system. Figure 13–1 presents some of the significant events that have influenced health care in the United States in the past two centuries.

Figure 13–1 **Selected Significant Events in Health Care History**

Date	Event
1862	William Rathbone opened a nurse training school, the Liverpool Royal Infirmary, in consultation with Florence Nightingale.
1869	The first Board of Health was established in Massachusetts.
1872	The American Public Health Association was established.
1886	The Visiting Nurse Society of Philadelphia was established.
1893	The Henry Street Settlement, under the direction of Lillian Wald, was founded to provide health promotion, disease prevention, case finding, and follow-up care. Out of this system came the first school nurse, Lina Rogers, who was assigned to the public school system.
1896	The Nurses Associated Alumnae of the United States was established, later to become the American Nurses Association.
1901	The Army Nurse Corp was established by an act of Congress.
1903	North Carolina is the first state to legislate the licensing of nursing.
1910	The Flexner Report exposed abuses in medical education and proposed reforms.
1916	The Pure Food and Drug Act was enacted.
1918	An influenza epidemic produced 500,000 deaths in the United States.

1918	The Chamberlain-Kahn Act established the Venereal Disease Division of the United States Public Health Service.
1921	The Sheppard-Towner Act was passed, providing grants-in-aid to enable states to create their own bureaus of Maternal and Child Health.
1923	The Goldmark Report was published, entitled Nursing and Nursing Education in the United States.
1925	Mary Breckinridge develops rural health care programs that become the Frontier Nursing Service.
1935	The Social Security Act authorizes grants to aid public health programs.
1940	Sister Elizabeth Kenny brings her method for treating poliomyelitis to the United States.
1946	The Hospital Survey and Construction Act, known as the Hill-Burton Act, provided for matching funds for the building of hospitals to state and local communities.
1948	The Brown Report, Nursing for the Future, was published by Esther Lucille Brown, emphasizing higher education for nurses.
1948	Eli Ginzberg's report, A Program for the Nursing Profession, recommended two levels of nursing: professional and practical.
1956	The Health Amendments Act was passed to provide traineeships for public health personnel. It gave nurses an opportunity for advanced preparation for positions in teaching, administration, and supervision.
1962	State nurses associations eliminate discriminatory membership barriers.
1965	The American Nurses Association published its "Position Paper."
1965	The Social Security Act was amended to provide funds for the health care of the elderly (Medicare–Title XVIII) and the health care of the medically indigent (Medicaid–Title XIX).
1972	Revision of the New York State Practice Act acknowledges nursing as an autonomous profession.
1977	Nurse Practitioners providing rural health care authorized to receive Medicare payment.
1978	Louise Brown, the first test tube baby, was born in England.
1981	AIDS was identified in the United States.
1982	Maryland is the first state to grant direct third-party reimbursement for nurse practitioner services without physician supervision.
1983	A prospective payment system based on Diagnosis Related Groups (DRGs) was created under Medicare.
1986	The National Institute of Nursing Research (NINR) is established at the National Institutes of Health (NIH).
1989	The Omnibus Budget Reconciliation Act (OBRA '89) phased in new Medicare payment scales for physicians. It mandated direct Medicaid reimbursement for pediatric and family nurse practitioners.

1990	The Patient Self-Determination Act and the Americans with Disabilities Act were enacted.
1992	Congressional mandate to establish the Office of Alterantive Medicine at NIH.
1993	The Omnibus Budget Reconciliation Act (OBRA '93) established an all-time record cut in Medicare funding and contained the Comprehensive Childhood Immunization Act to provide vaccines for Medicaid eligible and Native American children.
1994	President Clinton's health reform proposal, the American Health Security Act, failed.
1997	Medicare reimbursement for nurse practitioners and clinical specialists authorized by federal legislation.
1998	The NIH Office of Alternative Medicine elevated to status of the National Center for Complementary and Alternative Medicine, mandated to facilitate research on and provide public information about alternative medical treatments.
1999	NINR becomes the lead institute dealing with palliative care and end-of-life issues.
2000	Landmark legal decisions against tobacco companies related to the health hazards of tobacco use.
2000	Needlestick Safety and Prevention Act signed into law.
2000	Several states include on their ballots health care reform measures calling for universal health care.

Ask Yourself

How Do Nineteenth-Century Concepts Affect Twenty-first-Century Health Care?

- What concepts or practices regarding health care from the late 1800s and early 1900s still affect a patient's access to health care today?
- How is the health care delivery system that we know different from the system at the turn of the nineteenth century?
- What is your vision for health care for the twenty-first century?

In the early part of the twentieth century, a growing nation experienced population increases and a greater influx of immigrants, with over one million immigrants from southern and eastern Europe in 1905 alone. The need for health care and related services warranted attention. Medical schools and nursing schools expanded to provide personnel to meet the demand. Science, technology, public health services, and medicine progressed at an increased rate. Physicians and scientists began to use such diagnostic tools as x-rays. They made strides toward reduction of infectious organisms through the use of rubber gloves. They began to research the causes and cures of diseases such as yellow fever and typhoid and to use radiation to treat breast cancer. Amid such major advances as the discovery of penicillin, the proliferation of science and technology, the advancement of the professions of nursing and medicine, and the changing conceptualization about disease, a phenomenon unique to the United States emerged: the American hospital system. This phenomenon has colored the health care system in the twentieth century and into the twenty-first century as well (Stevens, 1989).

The later part of the nineteenth century and the first two decades of the twentieth century saw the transformation of hospitals from asylums for the poor to modern institutions, dedicated to science and improved patient care. Physicians expanded surgical interventions such as tonsillectomies, removal of tumors, and many gynecological operations. Nurses began to take a more active role in managing the hospital environment to control infection, and began to have more responsibility for technical management of patient care through duties such as taking the patient's pulse, temperature, and blood pressure (Stevens, 1989). Patterns that developed in the health care delivery system in the early part of the century can still be seen today. Physicians gained a new and strong identity and prestige, and the American Medical Association became a powerful force. Physicians gained increased authority in the routine workings of hospital systems, shifting the balance of power from boards of trustees to the medical decision makers (Stevens, 1989).

As a result of battlefield experiences in World War I, nurses, physicians, and other health care workers designed and set up streamlined, technically proficient, and very efficient specialized hospitals for the acutely ill or injured patient. On the home front, in response to ever-increasing numbers of immigrants, models of health care with emphasis on prevention and community interaction were developed. Prior to the war, the elite area of nursing was public health, with nurses at the forefront of campaigns for infant care and welfare, tuberculosis, and infectious disease. The war, however, emphasized the glamour of hospitals, and by 1920, more than half of the general hospitals in this country had schools of nursing attached to them. Student nurses staffed hospitals and were socialized into the hospital system. Like physicians, nurses became caught up in the culture of the acute health care environment and were reluctant to expand their professional interests into public health and the social aspect of health care (Stevens, 1989).

After World War I, the idea of group practices for physicians began to take hold, and the movement for health insurance began to develop. With the encouragement of President Theodore Roosevelt, workers' compensation was the first form of social insurance to become prominent in this country. Thirty-seven states passed laws that sanctioned workers' compensation by 1919. Through this movement, the cost of injury and damage to workers because of job-related hazards was passed on to industry. The health insurance movement entered a fast track, supported by the American Medical Association and various physicians' groups around the country. During this time, the struggle for access to care and control of fees and services escalated (Stevens, 1989).

The 1920s were years of growth and expansion of the health care industry. Consumerism flowered in direct relationship to the growth of the health care industry. As the public became aware of the availability of modern techniques, they wanted the best available. The health care delivery system developed into a middle-class entity in which many advances were taking place in private care, while the poor were increasingly underserved. By the end of this decade, there was increasing criticism of the cost and financing of the health care system, and the question of equal care for all income levels was raised. The rich and middle class were accused of having the best available to them, while the poor were viewed as manipulative of the very system that wanted to provide *charity* care to them.

During the Great Depression, government and charity hospitals were overrun with patients unable to afford health care, causing health care institutions to lose income and question their survival. The various health care professions pulled together to care for the sick, and a renewed sense of dedication kept a strained system afloat. Continually rising costs of health care led to development of plans for health insurance for everyone in the 1930s. The original Blue Cross plans were an outgrowth of the need for payment for continued growth of hospital and health care technologies. Thus, a prepayment insurance plan was born, and the health care delivery system grew by leaps and bounds. During the ensuing years major federal grant programs such as the Hill-Burton Act of 1946 funded the construction of health care facilities, and the science of medicine expanded through laboratory and clinical research. World War II prompted advances in health services that included therapy for prevention and treatment of shock, better blood replacement techniques, and research on gamma globulin, steroids, and other drugs, all of which increased the possibilities for successful treatment in surgery and internal medicine (Stevens, 1989). Expansion in the health care industry continued in the postwar years.

Think About It

How Do World Events Affect Health Care Delivery?

In reviewing history it is evident that seemingly nonrelated events can steer the course of other events, as has been noted in the development of the health care delivery system.

- How have major world events of your lifetime affected the course of health care delivery?

Between the passing of the Hill-Burton Act in 1946 and the enactment of Medicare legislation in 1966, the United States health care delivery system hit a new wave of expansion. The most widely known image of expansion in hospitals was the intensive care unit, with the greatest expansion between 1950 and 1965. In the early 1960s, coronary care units began to flourish, and by the mid-1960s premature nurseries, respiratory units, physical therapy units, and units dealing specifically with postoperative surgeries and neurosurgery were functioning in every fully operational hospital. Because of technological expansion, the cost of health care increased rapidly.

Expanding Health Insurance Coverage. Seeing a need and opportunity, the insurance industry began to compete with Blue Cross plans to provide third-party coverage for health care. These insurance plans removed the anxiety related to paying large hospital and health care bills, and also removed incentives from health care institutions to keep their costs down. Hospitals passed down increased costs to insurance companies, who in turn passed the cost on to the individual insurance subscriber. Because individual citizens had insurance, they demanded more and better service, and the system drove itself through the supply and demand cycle (Califano, 1986).

Medicare Parts A and B, which was passed in 1965 and enacted in 1966, essentially gave hospitals and other health care institutions a license to spend, and bigger and better were the watchwords. The health care delivery system was caught up in a whirlwind that has escalated to the point where the system is facing the need for serious change and the possibility of rationing at the beginning of the twenty-first century. Spiraling costs have prompted development of cost-containment mechanisms such as Diagnostic Related Grouping, case management, and managed care systems, which affect current health care delivery. Standardization and constraints of health insurance plans are more and more defining the care that patients receive in the present health care delivery system. Many people have no insurance for health care, and health care institutions have reverted to the charity care that existed in the first part of the twentieth century. The future of the system is uncertain, and continues to be influenced by political structures, economic constraints, and worldwide societal needs and demands.

HEALTH CARE PERSPECTIVES: A GLOBAL CONCERN

The challenge to provide health care for populations across the globe requires increasing effort and creativity. Many variables play a part in this challenge, including economics, cultural factors, epidemics, environment, war, and national crises. The problems are further compounded by the relationship, or lack of relationship, between modern medicine and traditional healing systems, national versus private health insurance, and preventive methods of health promotion contrasted with curative methods of treating illness. These factors all affect the functioning of health systems in various countries around the world (Bodeker, 1996).

All industrialized nations, with the exception of the United States and South Africa, have comprehensive national health care programs. The countries that operate with a nationalized system include: Australia, Austria, Belgium, Bulgaria, Canada, the Czech Republic, Denmark, Finland, France, Germany, Great Britain, Greece, Hungary, Ireland, Italy, Japan, the Netherlands, New Zealand, Norway, Poland, Portugal, Romania, Russia, the Slovak Republic, Spain, Sweden, and Switzerland. However, even with health care programs in place, all are not equal and do not function as smoothly as one would hope (Shikles, 1991).

Russia, for example, continues to suffer from a health care system that is at grave risk. Erlanger reported in 1992 a shortage of essential drugs, basic sterile equipment such as syringes, antibiotics, x-ray equipment, and basic medical supplies. Hospitals were dark and dirty, personnel were overworked, and there was a neglect of sanitation procedures. Rural areas in the former Soviet Union fared much worse. Some rural clinics had nonfunctioning or nonexistent sewage systems. Some clinics lacked piped-in water, or if water was piped in there was no system for heating it safely. Many hospital personnel, such as physicians, nurses, and technicians, had gone on strike because of poor working conditions and poor rewards for service. In this crippled health care system, there is no cohesive public health policy, and nurses are often paid less than a housemaid, and physicians less than a bus driver (Erlanger, 1992; Nursing and health in Russia, 1998). Reforms of the Russian health care system include a shift from a national system, with fairly equitable access to care, to a decentralized and fragmented variety of state systems. In the early 1990s, the Russian government mandated obligatory health insurance to replace the state-funded health care system; however, there is much dissatisfaction with the new system (Twigg, 1999). Questions arise regarding whether market-based medical insurance is the best solution to Russia's health-financing problems, given the persisting problems with overall political and economic reform (Burger, Field & Twigg, 1998; Twigg, 1999).

South Africa, while technically an industrialized nation with many natural resources, is plagued with health care problems similar to those occurring in many developing countries. The government of South Africa has as its long-term goal affordable and accessible health care for all its citizens. This goal is far from being realized, however, because the rise in urbanization and the proliferation of Third World illness is causing a deterioration in the process of organizing health care for all. In their present system, physicians and nurses are overworked, there is unequal access to public health services, hospitals are overcrowded, and much of the equipment is nonfunctioning or outdated (Bloom & McIntyre, 1998; Randolph, 1991).

The health care system of Cuba has been lauded by both the World Health Organization (WHO) and the United Nations as a major achievement for the citizens (Shikles, 1991). This system provides services from primary care to the most sophisticated procedures, available free to urban and rural citizens alike. Upheld as a model for other developing nations, the Cuban system greatly reduced rates of infant mortality and communicable diseases such as diphtheria, malaria, polio, and whooping cough. Primary-care clinics abound in rural areas and are open around the clock. Nurses and physicians make house calls to older or very ill residents. However, over the past fifteen years a shortage of medical supplies has threatened this model health care system (Barry, 2000). Factors affecting the supply shortage include the U. S. embargo and absence of aid from the former Soviet Union. Barry cites examples of lye ingestion in toddlers related to very limited availability of soap, and blindness related to decreased access to necessary nutrients, as some of the profound effects of the shortages on nutrition and overall health of vulnerable populations.

As was mentioned earlier, most industrialized nations have some type of universal health coverage. These systems vary in regard to the amount of government and private pay insurance, and some countries have a combination of several methods. Germany, France, and Japan have systems of health care coverage that mandate benefits coverage, the cost of which is shared by employees, employers, and government tax revenues. These health care delivery systems share three traits with the system in the United States. Medical care is offered through private physicians and through private and public hospitals. Patients may choose their providers. Most people in these countries have health insurance coverage through their place of employment. Health insurance is offered to the citizens of these countries through multiple third party insurance agencies.

In Germany, France, and Japan, reimbursement rates are standardized for physicians and hospitals through a negotiation system between hospitals, physicians, third-party payers, and the government. Similar problems to those existing in the United States exist, such as high costs and increased spending for technology. However, every citizen has some type of health care coverage. In an attempt to hold down rising health care spending, all have instituted direct controls on the price of health care. The controls apply to all of the health care systems in the respective countries, and policies are strictly enforced to comply with the set limit on health care spending (Shikles, 1991).

Canada and Great Britain have developed national health care systems that provide health care for their citizens. The government-run plans provide cradle-to-grave services that are financed through taxes. These plans enable patients to receive services free, and to choose their own hospitals and physicians. The plans pay salaries to physicians and operate their own hospitals.

There are both champions and critics of the national health insurance systems in Canada and Britain. Some say the systems are sound, while others say they are flawed. In Canada, for example, citizens can go to physicians or hospitals of their choice when they need care. Physicians bill the province for patient care. Patients do not pay for services, nor are they required to fill out endless forms. Negotiations for fees, cost-containment measures, and salaries take place between the provinces and the health care system.

Citizens of Canada and Great Britain consider health care to be one of their basic rights, and they value and respect their health care systems. Major political parties in these countries support the systems, and physicians and hospitals seem generally satisfied as well, since they receive a guaranteed payment. Businesses applaud the programs because payment is spread across society, and they do not have to carry a large part of the payment burden for employees (Beatty, 1991).

The national health insurance system in these countries have their critics. Some say the system is flawed, and that being insured in this way sets up a system of rationing because of insufficient funds for specialized health care. It has been said that waiting for care in these systems sometimes means death. Access to certain procedures and technologies is limited. Waiting lists are getting longer. Critics say that there is an unequal access to health care from province to province, depending on the affluence of the province. Some Canadian citizens who can afford to pay out-of-pocket come to the United States for specialized care and surgeries. In all instances, the increase in health care spending due to the high cost of technologies and research is having an impact on these systems in much the same ways as it is across the globe (Walker, 1992; Farrell, 1998; Katz, Verrilli, & Barer, 1998).

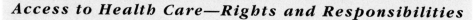

Ask Yourself

Access to Health Care—Rights and Responsibilities

Much of the discussion regarding the health care delivery systems of the United States, as well as those of many countries in the world, is a commentary on access to what is termed *modern medical care.*

- How does access to health care affect an individual's participation in the health care system?

- What is our individual responsibility in the big picture of these vast health care systems?
- Do you consider health care a basic right? If it is a right, what are our individual responsibilities in ensuring this right for all citizens?

ALTERNATIVE TRADITIONS OF HEALTH CARE

Indigenous populations in cultures throughout the world have traditional forms of health care that view humanity as connected to the wider dimensions of the earth and nature. In developing countries, these forms of traditional healing systems provide comprehensive approaches to prevention of illness and promotion of health that go beyond the scope of modern medical care. The World Health Organization (WHO) refers to these systems as holistic—that is, viewing a person in totality within a vast ecological spectrum, and emphasizing the notion that illness or disease occurs as a result of an imbalance between the person and his or her ecological systems (WHO, 1978).

An important component of traditional systems of health care is their basis in models that take into account mental, spiritual, physical, and ecological factors in assessing health and well being. A basic concept of all traditional health care systems is that of balance between mind and body, function and need, and individual, community, and environment. Illness or disease is thought to be a breakdown in the balance in one or more of these areas. Treatments are designed to restore health and balance between the individual and his or her internal and external environments. While these models of traditional health care systems have been considered primitive and unsophisticated by modern practitioners, an increasing number of developing countries are showing a new interest in program development toward revitalizing these traditional systems. There are several factors at work in promoting this resurgence of interest.

The majority of rural populations of developing countries cannot afford Western types of medical health care. Rural people have to travel many days to reach the larger health care centers, resulting in loss of wages in addition to money spent for travel and medicines. In Asia, the traditional systems are being incorporated into other, more formal health care systems to provide for care and ease the burden of cost. India has over 200,000 traditional practitioners. In Thailand, the Ministry of Health promotes the use of traditional medicinal plants in primary health care, state-run hospitals, and health service centers. In Korea, 20 percent of the national health care budget is directed to traditional health care services. Health insurance coverage is available for Oriental medical treatments and traditional health care methods (Bodeker, 1996).

In Africa, the governments are facing huge bills for the exploding AIDS crisis. These governments are exploring their traditional indigenous medicinal treatments for inexpensive and effective ways to relieve the suffering of AIDS patients. Health care providers in Uganda have been active in promoting research into traditional medicine for treating people with AIDS.

China has had a policy of integrating traditional health care into the national health care policy for over forty years. The Chinese are trying to combine the modern and the traditional as formal components of health care provision. In China, the traditional health care providers perform the majority of care to the poor and rural communities.

The country physicians are educated in a three-year program that includes a combination of traditional medicine and modern medicine. Modern Western medicine is being strongly pursued at great financial cost to the government, but at the same time hospitals and health care systems offer a choice to patients. Persons who take advantage of these choices are often the older and the less affluent. As the country is opening up to capitalist beliefs and free enterprise, some Chinese citizens who now have the financial means to make different choices are choosing Western methods of treatments, and often ignore the tried and true Oriental methods for status reasons. The younger generation of Chinese seem to believe that what is Western is always better. In observing some of the health care delivery in China, there is evidence that the government, while allowing the practice of the ancient Oriental medicine, is putting a strong emphasis on a belief that technology is the answer to health care in this heavily-populated country. This is especially disconcerting, in view of the fact that Oriental medicine and the tradition of health care with alternative choices have been functioning well for two thousand years, and Western health care providers are beginning to research and utilize these traditional systems of care in order to offer them to their patients.

Ask Yourself

What Do You Know About Traditional Healing?

Traditional methods of healing and health care have kept indigenous populations healthy and functioning for thousands of years. Many countries are trying to reinstate these practices to promote health and reduce the cost of health care and health care delivery.

- How do you think traditional and modern healing systems should relate to each other?
- What traditional methods of health care are available in your community or nearby area?
- With what traditional or folk health practices are you familiar? Have you or persons you know utilized these practices?

CHALLENGES FOR RURAL AND URBAN AGGREGATES

Problems in the delivery of health care to populations around the world occur not only because of expensive technology or lack of money to pay for insurance, but also because of geographic barriers. Rural populations in the United States and abroad often have to do without services because of lack of providers and facilities within a reasonable distance from their homes. Health care for persons in these populations requires a day off of work for travel and waiting in crowded waiting rooms. Many rural areas lack health care personnel, and emergency care is often nonexistent. In one mid-Atlantic state, all counties boast of an access to a 911 emergency number, but for some, the switchboard and EMT vehicle is three counties away and travel is over narrow mountain roads. Patients often delay treatment or do not become involved with prevention or health education plans because they require so much effort to accomplish. In addition, many rural citizens tend to be older persons for whom travel and finances are a great consideration in health care services.

The urban poor face similar access problems, not because care is geographically distant, but because access requires trips to places they cannot afford or free clinics, where lines are long and workers are few. Individuals are often required to take time from work, like their rural counterparts, in order to see a provider. Medications may be unaffordable. Large immigrant populations live in overcrowded situations in the urban setting. In addition to financial constraints, there may be language and cultural barriers and lack of knowledge about how to access the system.

Think About It

Health Care Changes and Challenges

The challenges and changes in health care can seem insurmountable and overwhelming. It seems as though only the very wealthy will be able to have health care services. Some sociologists say that the middle class is disappearing and that this country, as well as other world countries, will have only the rich and the poor. Health care costs are rising, and there seems to be no end to it.

- How should these issues be addressed? How should nurses respond to these issues?
- What issues have you encountered in accessing health care providers for you and your family?
- Are you able to afford a comprehensive health plan? If not, what do you do when you become ill?

SUMMARY

Historical awareness enables us to have a more informed view of circumstances in the present. Contemporary issues and concerns regarding health care delivery and financing are related to the historical interplay of advances in scientific and medical knowledge, social and political climate, and waxing and waning of economic and other resources. Current parameters in which health care providers function are changing. Acute-care hospitals are changing the focus of, and in some cases limiting, services; and many people are looking to the traditional healing systems of various cultures to provide needed health care services. Although some countries ensure access to basic health care services for their citizens, many individuals throughout the world have limited or no access to basic health care. Questions regarding access to and availability of resources are not new, but they must be addressed anew in light of the various currents within contemporary society. The future of the system is uncertain, and we must consider whether issues of the past are destined to repeat themselves. Perhaps we can take what is positive from the past, and blend this with both traditional and modern healing approaches in order to rescue a flawed health care system in this country and around the world.

CHAPTER HIGHLIGHTS

- Systems of health care, which have existed to address societal needs for healing from early civilization to the present, have been influenced by cultural, political, economic, religious, and scientific factors throughout history.

- Scientific and medical innovations, coinciding with the shift in Western nations from agricultural to industrial economics in the latter nineteenth and early twentieth centuries, provided a basis for modern day health care. Societal changes such as wars, women working more outside the home, and the influx of immigrants have raised new issues and concerns for health care delivery at various times in United States history.

- Skyrocketing health care costs can be traced to the advent of health insurance (1930s and later) and the enactment of Medicare and Medicaid (1960s), which removed incentives from health care institutions and physicians to keep costs down, and to public awareness of the availability of medical interventions, which prompted consumers to demand the best care and services available.

- Expansion of hospital and other health care services has reached a point of crisis in which out-of-control health care costs have prompted imposition of external controls on institutions and health care providers. Many people have no means of paying for expensive services.

- Some nations provide basic health care services for their citizens, while people in many areas suffer from limited access to or availability of such services. People in both developing and industrialized countries are exploring ways to incorporate traditional and modern healing practices into contemporary health care systems, in an effort to utilize the benefits of both systems in meeting the health care needs of society.

- Problems of access to and payment for health care services are of special concern among rural populations and the urban poor.

DISCUSSION QUESTIONS AND ACTIVITIES

1. Interview or read a biography of a person who worked as a nurse during or within the decade following World War II, and discuss nursing roles and duties, types of health concerns for which patients were hospitalized, and what was considered new therapies at the time. Compare the information you obtain to your experience of health care today.

2. Review nursing and medical journals and texts from the earlier part of the twentieth century regarding issues of concern in practice and to the profession. Compare and contrast these issues to issues of current concern.

3. Imagine that it is the year 2040 and you are being interviewed by a nursing student about factors that affected health care delivery and financing in your early days in nursing. What would you say?

4. Discuss global issues related to health care delivery. Which of these issues would have the greatest impact on your nursing practice and why? Use the Internet to investigate health care issues in a non-industrialized country. Share with classmates how these issues might affect your nursing practice.

5. Describe the impact of health delivery and financing on patient care and outcomes. Identify potential ethical dilemmas related to current systems of delivery or financing.

6. How should traditional and modern healing practices and practitioners relate to each other?

REFERENCES

Achterberg. J. (1990). *Woman as healer*. Boston: Shambhala.

Anderson, O. W. (1963). Medical care: Its social and organizational aspects. Health services systems in the United States and other countries—critical comparisons. *The New England Journal of Medicine, 269,* 839–843.

Barry, M. (2000). Effect of the U. S. embargo and economic decline on health in Cuba. *Annals of Internal Medicine, 132*(2), 151–154.

Beatty, P. (1991). Canada's health care system is sound. In G. McCuen, ed., *Health care and human values* (pp. 162–176). Hudson, WI: GEM Publications.

Bloom, G., & McIntyre, D. (1998). Towards equity in health in an unequal society. *Social Science and Medicine, 47*(10), 1529–1538.

Bodeker, G. C. (1996). Global health traditions. In M. S. Micozzi, ed., *Fundamentals of complementary and alternative medicine* (pp. 279–290). New York: Churchill Livingstone.

Bullough, B., & Bullough, V. (1978). *The care of the sick: The emergence of modern nursing*. New York: Prodist.

Burger, E. J., Field, M. G., & Twigg, J. L. (1998). From assurance to insurance in Russian health care: The problematic transition. *American Journal of Public Health, 88*(5), 755–758.

Califano, J. A., Jr. (1986). *America's health care revolution: Who lives? Who dies? Who pays?* New York: Random House.

Dossey, B. M. (2000). *Florence Nightingale: Mystic, visionary, healer*. Springhouse, PA: Springhouse Corporation.

Erlanger, S. (1992, May). Cuts gut Russian health care. *The New York Times*.

Farrell, M. (1998). Trends in the global healthcare environment: The developed countries. *Contemporary Nurse, 7*(4), 180–189.

Katz, S. J., Verilli, D., & Barer, M. L. (1998). Canadians' use of U.S. medical services. *Health Affairs, 17*(1), 225–235.

Kelly, L. Y. (1985). *Dimensions of professional nursing* (5th ed.). New York: Macmillan.

McDonald, L. (1998). Florence Nightingale: Passionate statistician. *Journal of Holistic Nursing, 16* (2), 267–277.

Nightingale, F. (1859/1992). *Notes on nursing: What it is and what it is not* (Commemorative ed.). Philadelphia: Lippincott.

Nursing and health in Russia. (1998). *International Nursing Review, 45*(3), 89–93.

Randolph, E. (1991, November). Soviet hospitals besieged by filth, shortage of drugs. *Washington Post.*

Selanders, L. C. (1998a). Florence Nightingale: The evolution and social impact of feminist values in nursing. *Journals of Holistic Nursing, 16*(2), 227–243.

Selanders, L. C. (1998b). The power of environmental adaptation: Florence Nightingale's original theory for nursing practice. *Journal of Holistic Nursing, 16*(2), 247–263.

Shikles, J. L. (1991, November). Health care spending: The experience of France, Germany and Japan. *U.S. General Accounting Office Report.*

Stevens, R. (1989). *In sickness and in wealth.* New York: Basic Books.

Tafoya, T. (1996, May). *Embracing the shadow: Mending the sacred hoop.* Paper presented at the South Texas AIDS Training (STAT) for Mental Health Providers: The Human, Transcultural, and Spiritual Dimensions of HIV/AIDS, San Antonio, TX.

Twigg, J. L. (1999). Obligatory medical insurance in Russia: The participant's perspective. *Social Science and Medicine, 49*(3), 371–382.

Walker, M. (1992). How they don't do it in Canada. *Reason, 35*–42.

WHO (1978). *Traditional medicine.* Geneva: WHO Publications.

SUGGESTED READINGS

Bullough, B., & Bullough, V. (1994). *Nursing issues.* New York: Springer.

Castro, J. (1994). *The American way of health.* Boston: Little, Brown.

Dauner, C. D. (1994). *The health care solution.* Sacramento, CA: Vision.

Kalisch, P., & Kalisch, B. (1989). *The advance of American nursing* (2nd ed.) Boston: Little, Brown.

Knowles, J. H., ed. (1977). *Doing better and feeling worse.* New York: Norton.

Kovner A. (1995). *Health care delivery in the United States* (5th ed.). New York: Springer.

Long, R. E., ed. (1991). *The crisis in health care.* New York: Wilson.

Rosenberg, C. E. (1987). *The care of strangers.* New York: Basic Books.

Wekesser, C., ed. (1994). *Health care in America: Opposing viewpoints.* San Diego, CA: Greenhaven Press.

CHAPTER 14

Health Policy Issues

To leave the world a bit better,
whether by a healthy child, a garden patch
or a redeemed social condition;
To know even one life has breathed easier
because you have lived;
This is to have succeeded.
(Ralph Waldo Emerson, *What Is Success?*)

OBJECTIVES

After completing this chapter, the reader should be able to:

1. Describe the process by which issues become "political issues."

2. Distinguish between the terms political and partisan.

3. Give examples of specific political issues related to health care.

4. Discuss your personal stand on various political issues in relation to ethics.

5. Describe the health policy process.

6. Discuss the role of ethics in policy making.

7. Explain the role of nurses in the policy making process.

8. Describe various methods of influencing public policy.

INTRODUCTION

We can view health policy and politics in a number of different ways. Some perceive health policy as a political process, strongly influenced by ideology and party politics. Others see the health policy-making process as a thoughtful one, by which decisions are based on data and the rational analysis of needs, outcomes, and costs (Donley, 1996). In reality the health policy process is a combination of both informed rational judgments and ideological partisan politics.

Nurses have become more involved in the political process, particularly in the realm of health policy. Nurses view health, at least in part, as dependent upon various environmental factors that can be altered by health policy decisions. Recognizing our role as advocates for patients' health, and acknowledging the importance of being involved in regulatory processes, we are assuming more responsibility in the political arena. This chapter features examples of selected political issues in the discussion of the process of creating health policy, and describes specific methods that nurses can utilize to influence policy.

POLITICAL ISSUES

The term **political** relates to the complex process of policy making within the government. Government is an essential element of society, and politics is inherent in government. **Political issues** are those that are created, affected, or regulated by decisions within either the executive, judicial, or legislative branches of government. **Political parties** are organized groups with distinct ideologies that seek to control government. When political parties take opposing positions on an issue, the different opinions and subsequent decisions are said to be **partisan**. Though individuals may genuinely and independently agree with the position of a particular party, partisanism is sometimes portrayed in a negative light—that is, consisting of blind, prejudiced, and unreasoning allegiance to a party. Because many people think that every problem in society can be solved by passing a law, legislatures make more and more laws to satisfy demands. Depending upon the existence of legitimate need or the interest or whim of society at large, special interest groups, individuals, or government, any issue can become a political one.

? Think About It

Abortion—A Moral and Political Issue

Abortion, a moral issue, raises questions about basic beliefs regarding life and death, sanctity of life, the beginning of life, and a woman's individual rights. Over time, abortion has become a political issue. Examples of this change include legal arguments over women's choice versus right to life, as in *Roe v. Wade*; congressional discussions regarding public funding of abortions, including debate related to the level of coverage; and the definition of acceptable circumstances surrounding conception and abortion. Within the last two decades, the two major

American political parties have polarized on the issue. One party supports the freedom of a woman to make her own decision, while the opposing party advocates the fetus's right to life. As a result, abortion has become a partisan issue.

- What is your moral stand on abortion?
- How did you develop this stand?
- How is your opinion about abortion related to the position of the political party to which you belong?
- Would you support a particular party based solely upon one issue?
- What is the government's role related to moral issues? Explain your position.
- How does your opinion influence your ability to give quality care?

An issue can become "political" in a number of ways. As discussed in Chapters 7 and 8, the administrative branch of government is involved in the operation of government agencies. State boards of medicine, nursing, and health, for example, are administrative agencies that are charged with regulating the activity of specific groups of professionals or particular aspects of health care. Rules and regulations promulgated by these groups can have a profound effect upon health care delivery. Because positions on these boards are often granted through the process of political appointment, decisions are occasionally viewed as partisan. Examples of political issues occurring within the administrative branch include prescriptive authority for nurses in advanced practice and implementation of mandatory standards of care.

The judicial branch of government influences health care professions and health care delivery through the common law system. As was noted in Chapter 7, judicial precedents take on the force of the law. Consider, for example, the profound effect on the American health care system of the landmark Supreme Court decision in *Roe v. Wade*. Although the Supreme Court is considered to be a nonpartisan entity, partisan politics plays a tremendous role in judicial appointments. Supreme Court appointments are particularly important to political parties, because of the potential to further party ideology through the unusual power granted the Court in the United States by virtue of the common law system, the small number of justices, the durability of Supreme Court decisions, the Court's relative freedom from special interest groups, and the fact that Supreme Court justices are appointed for their lifetime.

Ask Yourself

Is the Supreme Court Partisan?

Supreme Court justices are appointed by the president of the United States, with the advice and consent of the Senate. The Senate Judiciary Committee holds a series of hearings, during which the appointee is questioned on judicial and legal matters. The committee makes a recommendation on the suitability of the appointee; the entire Senate then votes to confirm or reject the president's appointment. Try to recall the confirmation process of nominees for the Supreme Court within the past fifteen years.

- Were the prospective justices questioned about issues with moral/ethical implications?
- Were they questioned about their position on specific partisan issues?
- Why do you think it is important to political parties that judges with certain beliefs are appointed to the Supreme Court?
- What role does the Supreme Court have in shaping the country's health policy?

As nurses we are most familiar with political issues in the legislative arena. These issues are the ones decided through the passage of federal or state laws. Within the legislative forum, nurses can influence the outcome of various political issues. Examples of well-publicized legislative issues with health care implications include: Medicare and Medicaid revisions, health insurance reform, and issues related to advanced practice nursing, such as prescriptive authority, scope of practice, and third-party reimbursement.

Nurses function in a variety of roles. They are citizens, knowledgeable consumers of health care, professionals whose practice is regulated by government, and advocates for patients. Responsible political involvement is an important function of each of these roles. Because nurses are individuals with a variety of backgrounds, experiences, beliefs, and values, opinions about political issues are diverse. This diversity, when coupled with sensitivity to moral and ethical implications, provides a foundation for productive and fair political discussion.

Political issues of particular interest to nurses fall into four distinct categories: those involving moral values; those involving professional regulation; those involving the health of individuals in society; and those involving distributive justice. Nurses' positions on these issues are based upon personal experience, ethical orientation, religion, cultural bias, and a number of other factors. Naturally, there is a healthy diversity of opinion among nurses on most issues—particularly those involving moral values. Figure 14–1 shows examples of selected political issues of interest to many nurses.

HEALTH POLICY

Because health plays a critical role in the physical, psychological, and economic condition of individuals, it affects society in general. The central purpose of health policy, therefore, is the improvement of the overall health of the population. Health policy is far reaching; it influences the behavior and decisions of people in relation to their environment and living conditions; it affects lifestyle and personal behavior; and it affects

Figure 14–1 **Selected Examples of Political Issues**

Issues Involving Moral Values

Beginning of Life Issues

- Abortion
- Use of Fetal Tissue
- Genetic Testing
- Contraception and Sterilization

Health Care Issues

- Medically-Assisted Pregnancy
- Deciding for Infants and Children
- Distributing Harvested Organs
- Use of Animal Organs for Research and Treatment
- Informed Consent
- Patient's Bill of Rights
- Health Records Privacy

End of Life Issues

- Active and Passive Euthanasia
- Physician-Assisted Suicide
- Patient Self-Determination
- Organ Procurement

Issues Involving Professional Regulation

Nursing Education

- Entry into Practice
- Funding for Nursing Education and Research

Workplace Issues

- Safety, such as needlestick legislation
- Americans with Disabilities Act

Advanced Practice Issues

- Third-party Reimbursement
- Prescriptive Authority
- Scope of Practice

Issues Involving the Health of Individuals in Society

Environmental Health

- Clean Indoor Air
- Clean Groundwater
- Air Pollution Control

Public Health
- Treatment and Reporting of STDs
- Family Planning Programs and Regulations
- Tobacco Legislation
- Childhood Immunizations
- Gun Control
- Seatbelt and Helmet Laws
- Food and Product Labeling

Issues Involving Access to Care
- Social Security
- Medicare and Medicaid
- Regulation of Private Insurance
- Managed Care Legislation
- Health Care Reform
- Mental Health Insurance Parity

---

availability, accessibility, and quality of health care services. Health-related issues receive considerable attention in the policy-making forum.

Different people define health in different ways. The most popular definition of health affects the investment society is willing to make in health care programs and the programs that are eventually funded. For example, if our society defines health narrowly in terms of illness, policymakers might choose to fund programs that focus on treatment of illness, but neglect programs that support health-promoting behaviors. In contrast, a society that defines health positively, in terms of wellness, would place more emphasis on funding programs to prevent illness or maximize health potential.

Health policies are formal and authoritative decisions focusing on health. Health policies are made in the legislative, executive, or judicial branches of government, and are intended to direct or influence the actions, behaviors, or decisions of others. Policy is comprised of a very large set of decisions. Examples of health policy include legislation, rules and regulations established for the purpose of implementing legislation, rules and regulations established to operate the government and its various programs, and judicial decisions related to health. **Statutes** or **laws** are pieces of legislation that have been enacted by legislative bodies and approved by the executive branch of government. **Rules** or **regulations** are policies that are established to guide the implementation of laws and programs. **Judicial decisions** are authoritative court decisions that direct or influence the actions, behaviors, or decisions of others. In addition to these different types of policies, there are also two broad categories of health policies.

Although there is significant potential for overlap, health policies fit into two basic categories: allocative and regulatory. **Allocative policies** determine what programs are funded—that is, where the resources are allocated. This is the area in which we see distributive justice in practice. Allocative policies are essentially economic in nature. In most countries, these policies are geared toward guaranteeing access to goods and services for the disadvantaged. Allocative policies are based upon fundamental beliefs about which distinct group or class of individuals or organizations should receive the benefits. Policymakers realize that some will receive benefits, some will not, and others will bear the expense. Ideally, these decisions are based upon public objectives (Longest, 1995). The most well-known examples of allocative health policies are those of Medicare and Medicaid. The American Nurses Association is active in lobbying for various allocative policies. For example, ANA supports legislation to require insurance plans to offer the same coverage for mental illness that they offer for physical illness. Labeled "Mental Health Parity," this issue has been hotly debated in Congress (Legislative Branch, 2001).

Regulatory policies are those designed to direct the actions, behavior, and decisions of individuals or groups. These policies place rules on health care delivery. Longest (1995) lists five basic classes of regulatory policies:

1. market entry restrictions;

2. rate or price-setting controls on providers;

3. provider quality controls;

4. market-preserving controls; and

5. social regulation (geared toward such socially desired ends, such as safe workplaces and nondiscriminatory provision of health care).

As with all policies, the purpose of regulatory policy is to ensure that public objectives are met. Many nurses do not realize the impact regulatory policies have on nursing practice. Following are selected examples of recently debated regulatory policies: policies that would allow women unrestricted access to their choice of ob-gyn providers, including advanced practice nurses; policies to require health records privacy; and policies to protect workers from accidental needlestick (Legislative Branch, 2001).

The Health Policy Process

Health policies are those that affect health in any way, either directly, as with immunization programs, or indirectly, as with statutes that describe scope of practice of health care providers. The process of health policy includes three distinct phases. These phases are both consecutive and circular. The first phase is that of **policy formulation.** This phase includes such actions as agenda setting and the subsequent development of legislation. The second phase is that of **policy implementation.** This phase follows enactment of legislation, and includes taking actions and making additional decisions necessary to implement legislation, such as rule making and policy operation. The final stage is **policy modification.** The purpose of this stage is to improve or perfect legislation previously enacted. This might entail only minor adjustments made in the implementation phase, or it may involve major changes or the elimination of particular statutes (Longest, 1995).

Policy Formulation. The first phase of policy making is policy formulation. This phase is divided into two distinct sequentially related sets of activities: agenda setting and legislation development (Longest, 1995). At any point in time, there is a complex mix of three variables: health related problems, possible solutions and alternatives, and diverse political interests. As agenda setting progresses, the emerging issues can proceed to the development of legislation.

Problems. The existence of real or perceived problems is the impetus for the policy formulation phase of policy making. Problems may become evident in a number of ways. Some problems occur as the result of the interaction of certain variables related to previous policy. For example, it is likely that the predicted shortfall of Social Security is related to a policy that did not take into account inequities between program budget and rapidly escalating expenditures. Other problems may gain attention as they reach unacceptable levels. Growth in the numbers of people with AIDS is an example of this type of problem. Other problems emerge as a result of some specific event that forces public attention. Examples of this type of problem include the discovery of medical waste products washing up on beaches and the development of a new drug for treating AIDS that is so expensive few people can afford to purchase it (Longest, 1995). Nevertheless, the mere existence of problems is not always sufficient to ensure the formulation of legislation. There must also be feasible solutions to the problems and the political will to enact legislation.

Solutions. Someone must come up with an idea to solve a problem before legislation as initiated. The process of offering solutions to problems involves generating ideas for solving the problems, refining the ideas, and selecting from among the options (Longest, 1995). *Nursing's Agenda for Health Care Reform* (American Nurses Association [ANA], 1991) is an example of the profession's attempt to formulate specific solutions to problems in health care delivery.

Political Circumstances.

Even if we identify a serious problem and offer feasible solutions, we may not be able to influence legislation. Legislation can only progress through the process with the sponsorship of influential policymakers who believe in the issue and invest time and energy. Potential sponsors are sensitive to political will. Factors that influence political will include: public attitudes, concerns, and opinions surrounding an issue; the preferences and relative ability to influence political decisions; the positions of key political leaders on the issue; and the other competing items on the policy agenda. Longest (1995) believes that creating a political thrust forceful enough to cause policy makers to formulate and implement new policy is often the most difficult problem. Nurses are a significant percentage of the voting population. We are in a good position to influence political decisions collectively and enhance the political will essential to formulate health policy.

Think About It

Failure of the Health Care Reform Initiative

Whatever happened to health care reform? On September 22, 1993, President Bill Clinton introduced the American Health Security Act. Following months of high-level negotiation and planning, this reform package included many of the ideas presented in at least eleven separate proposals made within the preceding five years. Administration officials thought the public and many special-interest groups were demanding a radical reform of the health care system. Leah Curtin, nursing leader and ethicist, predicted in May of 1991 that there would be a universal access system within three to eight years (Curtin, 1996, p. 225). Yet Clinton's proposal, along with all of its predecessors, failed. Universal access did not become a reality, and it does not appear that it will happen anytime soon.

- A great deal of time and energy was invested in the policy formulation phase. How effective do you believe leaders were in this phase?
- What was the problem being addressed? How clear was the problem?
- Were the proposed solutions realistic and acceptable? Discuss specific solutions.
- Do you think the political circumstances were favorable for passage of a health care reform proposal? Why or why not?
- Do you think the influence of special-interest groups affected the eventual outcome of the proposal? Explain your thinking.
- At what point in the policy making process do you think the proposal failed?

Policy Implementation. Policy implementation immediately follows the enactment of legislation. Because legislation seldom contains explicit language on how it is to be implemented, details are left to the process of rule making. A formal part of the implementation phase, the promulgation of rules is accomplished by specific implementing organizations. For example, the various states' boards of nursing are the organizations responsible for promulgating rules related to nursing practice. Generally, these organizations accept input from affected groups during the rule making process. Thompson (1991) calls the interaction between the implementing organizations and affected interest groups "strategic interaction." Interest groups routinely seek to influence rule making, because they are so often the targets of rules established to implement health policies. Lobbying is one of the major means by which interest groups attempt to influence policy makers. Lobbying is especially intense when various interest groups disagree upon the formulation of a particular policy.

Policy Modification. As the third phase of the policy making process, policy modification occurs when outcomes, perceptions, and consequences of existing policies indicate that either the original problems still exist, or new problems have arisen from unforeseen circumstances or from the policy itself. The policy modification phase is intended to spiral backward, with feedback, into the agenda-setting and legislation-development stages of the formulation phase—potentially creating new legislation—and spiral forward into the rule making and policy operation stages of the implementation phase, stimulating changes in rules or operations. Many programs are routinely amended, some of them repeatedly, over a period of many years. These modifications may reflect, among other things, the development of new technologies, changing economic conditions, and public demand (Longest, 1995). Newly proposed changes in Medicare and Medicaid programs are examples of the policy modification process (Legislative Branch, 2001).

Ethics in Policy Making

Because policy affects people's lives and relationships and is often part of the distributive justice process, policy making is an inherently ethical endeavor. The outcomes and consequences of most health policy affect large groups of people. There are two equally important functions of ethics in public policy making. In the policy formulation phase, ethics can guide the original development of new policies. Ethics is also useful in the policy modification phase as a means to legitimately criticize policies that are already implemented (Thompson, 1985). There is, however, some practical difficulty in adhering strictly to specific ethical principles during the policy making process. Discussing the complexity of policy making and ethics, Beauchamp and Childress (1994) write:

> Policy formation and criticism involve more complex forms of judgment than merely invoking ethical principles and rules. The ethics of public policy must proceed from impure and unsettled cases, in which there are profound social disagreements, uncertainties, different interpretations of history, and imperfect procedures to resolve the disagreements. Obviously, no body of abstract principles and rules can dictate policy, because it cannot contain enough specific information or provide direct and discerning guidance. The specification and implementation of moral principles and rules must take account of problems of feasibility, efficiency, cultural pluralism, political procedures, uncertainty about risk, noncompliance by patients, and the like. Principles and rules provide background moral considerations for policy evaluation, but a policy must also be shaped by empirical data and by special information available in relevant fields of [nursing], medicine, economics, law, psychology, and so on. In this process, moral principles and various uses of empirical data are often closely connected. (p. 10)

Thus, Beauchamp and Childress suggest that health policy is so complex as to prohibit the strict and exclusive use of specific rules or principles in guiding policy formulation; rather, the authors suggest that ethical considerations must be accompanied by the rational use of empirical data.

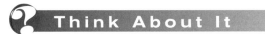

Think About It

Ethics and Politics of Tobacco Sales

The sale and distribution of tobacco products has become a highly publicized political issue. The tobacco industry is increasingly affected by legislative and judicial decisions regarding the health effects of tobacco.

- What are the ethical issues of which the policy makers should be aware?
- Can you think of ethical arguments in favor of regulating the production and sale of tobacco products?
- Can you think of ethical arguments in favor of allowing the industry to operate on the free market, unrestricted?
- There are judicial precedents that assign at least some responsibility for the health problems of smokers to the tobacco companies. Is this a legal, ethical, or political issue, or some combination of these?
- Is this an issue in which nurses should be interested? What factors determine whether nurses should be interested in this issue?

Research Data In Policy Making

In order to prevent policies based upon unsubstantiated beliefs or personal values, when we are interested in an issue, we must furnish officials with important and reliable information. If they have reliable facts and research findings, policy makers are able to identify problems, make comparisons, confirm trends, and establish policy based on evidence (Donley, 1996). Because time is a precious commodity, officials are often more interested in research findings than unsubstantiated personal opinion. Pender (1992) suggests that nurses who plan to discuss policy with officials carefully review research findings that pertain to the issue and be ready to quote a few particularly attention-getting statistics. Cost savings often gets attention when other facts elicit little response.

The federal government recognizes the importance of health care research in the development of policy. Established by Congress as part of the 1989 Omnibus Budget Reconciliation Act, the Agency for Health Care Policy and Research is one of eight agencies of the United States Public Health Service. Seeking answers to some of the most pressing health concerns facing our population, this agency serves as a bridge between researchers, clinicians, and policy makers (Bavier, 1995).

NURSING, POLICY, AND POLITICS

Not since the days of Lavinia Lloyd Dock have nurses been so actively involved with policy making and politics. It is through the perspective of knowledge, experience, and intimacy with the health care needs of the population that nursing is in the unique position to bring balance to the policy making process (Murphy, 1992). Moreover, professional codes of ethics identify the goals and values of the profession, and explicitly call for nurses to be involved in policy formulation. For example, the ICN *Code of Ethics for Nurses* (2000) calls for nurses to share with society the "responsibility for initiating and supporting action to meet the health and social needs of the public, in particular those of vulnerable populations." The ANA *Code of Ethics for Nurses* (2001) clearly describes nurses' responsibility for health policy participation as follows:

The nurse collaborates with other health professionals and the public in promoting community, national, and international efforts to meet health needs. The nurse has a responsibility to be aware of . . . broader health concerns such as world hunger, environmental pollution, lack of access to health care, violation of human rights, and inequitable distribution of nursing and health care resources. [The nurse] participates in legislative and institutional efforts to promote health. In addition, the nurse supports initiatives to address barriers to health, such as homelessness, unsafe living conditions, and lack of access to health services. Nurses can work individually as citizens or collectively through political action to bring about social change. It is the responsibility of a professional nursing association to speak for nurses collectively in shaping and reshaping health care within our nation, specifically in areas of health care policy and legislation that affect accessibility, quality, and the cost of health care. Here the professional association maintains vigilance and takes action to influence legislators, reimbursement agencies, nursing organizations, and other health professions. In these activities, health is understood as being broader than delivery and reimbursement systems, but extending to health-related sociocultural issues such as homelessness, hunger, violence, and the stigma of illness.

The formulation of health policy requires strong nursing leadership and an understanding of the nature of local and national policy making. Calling for the political empowerment of nurses, Batra (1992) charges that if we are serious in our efforts to promote health, we must understand the crucial role of public policy. To do this, we must develop the ability to think, teach, research, and act in ways that are relative to policy; we must be aware of the impact that policies have on health and on our clinical practice; we must conduct research on health policy issues; and we must find strategic ways to influence state and national policy agendas. Recognizing health problems as policy issues allows nurses to move into the realm of policy formulation.

Nursing's Political Strengths.   There are notable strengths with which nursing enters the political arena. First, the most sizable group of health care providers, the nursing profession boasts an extremely large number of political constituents. Acting together, the nation's nurses have the potential to be a formidable political force. Second, nurses have traditionally been perceived in a favorable light. Nurses are viewed as much less self-interested than any of the other major health-related interest groups (Hadley, 1996). Third, once nurses become involved in health policy, they usually continue to be active (Gebbe, Wakefield, & Kerfoot, 2000).

Nursing's Political Weaknesses.   The profession also has a number of political weaknesses. First, relatively new to the political arena, many nurses are not astute or comfortable in policy making or lobbyist roles. Second, there has historically been a lack of ideological and political unity within the profession, a weakness Hadley

(1996) believes stems from the lack of uniform educational requirements and titles. Third, though nurses comprise the largest number of professionals, there are fewer dollars in nursing coffers specifically earmarked for intense lobbying than in those of many other special-interest groups.

Policy Goals for Nursing

How do nurses become aware of the issues that are important and require energy and focus? Each of us has the responsibility to reflect upon problems and potential solutions. In addition, one of the major functions of professional organizations is to provide leadership and assistance to members in political and other matters. Congruent with the *Code of Ethics for Nurses*, the American Nurses Association has developed a specific agenda for nurses interested in policy making. Nursing's legislative and regulatory agenda, as devised by the American Nurses Association, encompasses four basic goals: to maintain nursing control of nursing practice; to have a positive impact on health care policy; to advocate on behalf of the client; and to institute workplace reforms (deVries & Vanderbilt, 1992).

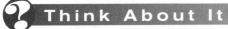

Think About It

Nurses Take Positions on Political Issues

The American Nurses Association has been a powerful lobbying force for many years. Issues of interest to members of the organization are freely accessible through ANA's website at http://www.nursingworld.org/ This site includes ANA legislative position statements, fact sheets, and transcripts of congressional testimony. It also includes transcripts of some pertinent legislation. ANA has been active in advocating policy for many issues including the following: campaign finance reform, child and elder care, civil rights, collective bargaining, domestic violence, drug control policy, family and medical leave, gun control, homelessness, malpractice/liability reform, migrant and seasonal farm worker health issues, pay equity, rural health care, and sexual harassment. These are but a few of the issues ANA has been involved in over the past decade.

- Why do you think the professional organization published these position statements?
- Why are nurses concerned with issues such as campaign finance reform and gun control?
- What impact do you think the profession could make if each nurse became familiar with all of the issues and promoted them to policy makers?
- Can you identify any issues within your state that affect the health of your patients or your practice?
- How could you begin the process of health policy formulation for this issue?

LOBBYING

Sometimes nurses are privileged to be legitimate members of governmental or institutional policy making bodies. More often, the nurse's role in policy formulation, implementation, and modification is that of lobbyist. "**Lobbying** is the art of persuasion—attempting to convince a legislator, a government official, the head of an agency, or a state official to comply with a request—whether it is convincing them to support your position on an issue or to follow a particular course of action" (deVries & Vanderbilt, 1992, p. 1). Though many special-interest groups employ lobbyists, every nurse can be a lobbyist and should lobby on issues of concern. Lobbyists have a powerful voice in determining the policymaking process, from agenda setting to policy modification. In fact, some nurses believe it is a nurse's duty to participate in political **activism**. Hagerdorn defines activism as "a passionate approach to everyday activities that is committed to seeking a more just social order through critical analysis, provocation, transformation, and rebalancing of power" (1995, p. 2). Activism promotes "exposing, provoking, and unbalancing the social power that maintains people in a state of disease, while simultaneously nurturing caring" (1995, p. 2). There are others who believe that constrained, subtle, and persistent political activity is more effective in the long term than overt activism.

To be effective in the political domain, nurses are charged to become politically astute. According to Jennings, "most decisions at the policy table and in the halls of Congress are politically driven. . . . one can have the best policy proposal on the table but if he or she doesn't know how to play the political game, all will be lost. Nurses must be very adept at discerning who has the power in the policy arena and how to link to that source" (1996, p. 4). Knowing the "power players" in the political arena is one of the most important steps in the lobbying process.

Methods of Lobbying

The most familiar type of lobbying is the face-to-face approach. This process involves either meeting directly with a policy maker to request a desired action, or testifying at a hearing. When possible, both paid and volunteer lobbyists should utilize the face-to-face method of lobbying. A second form of lobbying is **grassroots lobbying.** Grassroots lobbying involves mobilizing a committed constituency to influence the opinions of policy makers. Different types of grassroots lobbying include organized letter writing and implementing campaigns designed to mobilize public opinion.

One of the most important facets of lobbying is knowing whom to lobby. In seeking help to promote a particular legislative agenda, nurses want to begin by enlisting policy makers who have the following characteristics: (1) legitimate power, (2) an interest in the problem, (3) an affinity for nursing or for health care issues in general, (4) time and energy to invest in the process, (5) the respect of colleagues, and (6) committee or other positions that are appropriate to the particular legislation. Finding an official with all of these characteristics will greatly improve the probability of legislative success. New lobbyists waste time and energy lobbying officials who are uninterested, have conflicting loyalty, are powerless, or are not respected by their colleagues. The first step in lobbying is to connect with the appropriate policy makers.

The Lobbying Campaign. Once nurses have identified the appropriate policy making officials and are familiar with the issues and the legislative and regulatory process, the lobbying campaign can begin. There are two basic types of lobbying: direct and indirect. Indirect lobbying strategies are geared toward influencing public opinion, which in turn will influence policymakers. Methods of indirect lobbying include: media broadcasts; newspapers and other written materials; dissemination of the results of opinion polls; paid advertisements; educational campaigns; and organizations' agendas. Direct methods include party platforms, political elections, influence of committees, agency regulations, face-to-face lobbying, letter writing, and contact with policy makers during social events (deVries & Vanderbilt, 1992).

Letter Writing. Handwritten, personal, mass letter writing is a powerful grassroots lobbying technique. Certain letter writing techniques that have been found to be more effective. Here are some practical tips for letter writing:

- Whenever possible, individualize and legibly handwrite or type letters on personal stationery. Though more effective than no letters at all, form letters are much less likely to be read by officials than individualized letters.
- Write the letter in your own words, using your own thoughts and logic and drawing pertinent inferences.
- Identify yourself as a nurse and state your reason for writing in the first paragraph, including the title and number of the legislation in which you are interested.
- Be specific and include key information and examples supporting your position.
- Be explicit. Tell the official exactly what you want. If you are writing to ask for cosponsorship or a vote for or against a bill, say so.
- Be brief but informative. Keep your letter to a maximum of one to two pages.
- Include only one topic in each letter.
- Never threaten or use hostility. This immediately destroys your chances of developing a cooperative relationship.
- Offer your assistance as a resource.
- Promptly thank the official for favorable votes.

Personal Visits. A personal visit is usually a more powerful lobbying tool than letter writing. Whenever possible, nurses should seize the opportunity to meet with policy makers face to face. Following are a few suggestions for personal visits with policy making officials:

- Be prepared. Develop your plan of action and know what you intend to say.
- Be on time for your appointment and be patient if the official is late.
- Be courteous and greet the official with a firm handshake, introduce yourself, and present your business card.
- Identify the subject of the meeting and present your facts in an orderly, succinct, and direct fashion.

- Support your position with personal experiences and anecdotes; use valid research and statistics when appropriate.

- Keep your presentation simple. Avoid technical language and professional jargon. Your goal is to inform and influence, not to impress.

- Close the meeting strongly and effectively, asking for the official's support.

- Leave a short fact sheet summarizing the issue and your position. Include the names and telephone numbers of contact people.

- Send a letter within a few days thanking the official for the meeting, restating your position, and including any information requested during the meeting.

Think About It

Be Careful of Your Wording

Nurses must be careful in choosing words to use when lobbying. One nurse relates a story of her first experience testifying before a state legislative committee. Feeling her presentation was well prepared and would be effective, the nurse decided at the last minute to substitute the words *nurse voters* for the word *nurses*. There were many people giving testimony that day. Following the completion of the testimony phase, the legislators were given an opportunity to make comments or ask questions. There were no questions. Every comment was directed toward the nurse, who was surprised to learn that the legislators perceived the term *nurse voters* to indicate a veiled threat. They did not hear the substance of the presentation, but rather the perceived threat, "If you do not support our position, we will vote you out of office." By unintentionally giving this impression, the nurse ruined a productive relationship with these legislators. The legislation that the nurses were supporting failed.

- Why do you think the nurse changed the wording of her presentation in the first place?

- What words would you have used?

- Describe similar circumstances in which you were speaking and the reaction of the listeners was based upon their inferences from your choice of words rather than their intended meaning?

- How can nurses avoid mistakes of this sort?

Political Campaigns

One very effective direct lobbying technique is for nurses to become involved in either supporting candidates or themselves running for elective office. According to Wakefield (1990), nurses are encouraged to get involved in lobbying for specific legislation, not realizing that the ability to influence decisions occurs long before the issues are revealed to the public. Wakefield suggests that nurses become involved in campaigns and elections. This can be done in any number of ways. First, nurses should become involved in political party organizations. Political party activity serves as a vehicle for developing important relationships with elected officials. Involvement in a political party is essential to building a political network. Second, nurses can become involved through district and state nurses' associations. These organizations provide an opportunity to meet candidates, form relationships, and offer candidates forums. Forums remind a candidate that nurses are an organized group interested in politics and public policy and acquaint nurses with the candidate's position on important issues. Third, nurses can become actively involved in campaigning for candidates who support their positions on various health care issues. This may take the form of campaigning door to door, stuffing envelopes or publicly endorsing candidates. Actively supporting candidates for public office helps to forge relationships with officials and elect candidates to public office who will sympathize with issues important to nurses. Involvement with political parties and the consequent relationships with public officials can also lead to either nurses' candidacy and election to public office, or nurses' appointments to important policy making positions. The ANA offers assistance to nurses wanting to seek public office. Their web site includes links to candidate schools and other Internet resources. The address of the ANA Legislative web site is: http://nursingworld.org/gova/index/htm

SUMMARY

There are many political issues that are important to nurses. Most issues for which nurses are actively concerned are related to health policy: issues of a moral nature; issues related to professional regulation; issues related to public health; and issues related to distributive justice. Fulfilling the role of advocate, nurses are challenged to become politically active: to know and become involved with important issues; to learn the political process; to form relationships with public officials; and to become astute in methods of influencing health policy.

CHAPTER HIGHLIGHTS

- The term *political* relates to the policy making process within the government.
- Political issues are those that are created, affected, or regulated by any of the government branches.
- Political parties are organized groups with distinct ideologies that seek to control government.
- Partisan issues are those issues for which the political parties have distinct ideology.
- Health policies influence the actions, decisions, and behaviors of people in the domain of health.

- Society's definition of health reflects the extent to which society is willing to go toward maximizing the health of citizens.
- Allocative health policies are designed to provide benefits to a distinct group.
- Regulatory policies are designed to influence others through directive techniques.
- The process of health policy includes the phases of policy formulation, policy implementation, and policy modification.
- There are two important functions of ethics in public policy making—guiding the original development of policy and criticizing previously implemented policy.
- Nurses are able to affect health policy through various political means.

DISCUSSION QUESTIONS AND ACTIVITIES

1. Explore the ANA's website at http://www.nursingworld.org/ Review the legislative and policy news found at the link to the *Legislative Branch*. Read the news on *NursingInsider*. Are all the issues presented supported by the American Nurses Association? Discuss the up-to-date list with your classmates. How do the various issues relate to nursing ethics?

2. Discuss the issues listed in Figure 14–1 in class. How do classmates' positions compare to those of the major political parties? Are each student's opinions politically consistent from issue to issue?

3. Discuss the following question in class: What purpose do political parties serve?

4. Compile a list of political issues and classify them as to the branch of government with which the issue is most closely aligned—administrative, judicial, or legislative.

5. Discuss methods for influencing health policy in the administrative and judicial domains.

6. Compile a list of at least five political issues related to health that have been decided within the judicial domain. How have the judicial decisions affected health care delivery?

7. Compile a list of political issues related to moral values. Discuss the role of the professional organization in guiding members' actions related to these moral issues.

8. Discuss popular definitions of health and determine how each definition, if adopted by government, would affect health care delivery.

9. Discuss the role of ethics in policy making.

REFERENCES

American Nurses Association. (1991). *Nursing's agenda for health care reform*. Kansas City, MO: Author.

American Nurses Association. (2001). *Code of ethics for nurses*. Washington, DC: Author.

Batra, C. (1992). Empowering for professional, political, and health policy involvement. *Nursing Outlook, 40*(4), 170–176.

Bavier, A. (1995). Where research and practice meet: Opportunities at the Agency for Health Care and Policy and Research. *Nursing Policy Forum, 1*(4), 20–38.

Beauchamp, T. L., & Childress, J. F. (1994). *Principles of biomedical ethics* (4th ed.). New York: Oxford University Press.

Curtin, L. (1996). *Nursing into the 21st century: Health care reform, restructuring, practice, leadership.* Springhouse, PA: Springhouse.

deVries, C. M., & Vanderbilt, M. W. (1992). *The grassroots lobbying handbook: Empowering nurses through legislative and political action.* Washington, DC: American Nurses Association.

Donley, R. (1996). Shaping health policy. *Nursing Policy Forum, 2*(1), 12–19.

Emerson, R. (1995). What is success? In W. Bennett, ed., *The moral compass: A companion to the book of virtues.* New York: Simon & Schuster.

Gebbe, K. M., Wakefield, M., & Kerfoot. (2000). Nursing and health policy. *Journal of Nursing Scholarship, 32*(3), 307–315.

Hadley, E. (1996). Nursing in the political and economic marketplace: Challenges for the 21st century. *Nursing Outlook 44*(1), 6–10.

Hagerdorn, S. (1995). The politics of caring: The role of activism in primary care. *Advances in Nursing Science, 17*(4), 1–11.

International Council of Nurses (2000). *The ICN code of ethics for nurses.* International Council of Nurses, Geneva Switzerland. Retrieved January 23, 2001 from the World Wide Web: http://icn.ch/indes.html/

Jennings, C. (1996). Politics and nursing do mix! *Nursing Policy Forum 2*(3), 4.

Legislative Branch (2001, January 24). Washington, DC: American Nurses Association. Retrieved January 24, 2001 from the World Wide Web: http://www.nursingworld.org/

Longest, B. B., Jr. (1995). *Health policymaking in the United States.* Ann Arbor, MI: AUPHA Press/Health Administration Press.

Murphy, N. (1992). Nursing leadership in health policy decision making. *Nursing Outlook 10*(4), 158–161.

Nagelkerk, J. (1994). Policy making. *JONA 24*(5), 14–15.

Pender, N. (1992). Making a difference in health policy. *Nursing Outlook 40*(3), 104–105.

Roe v. Wade, 410 U.S. 113 (1973).

Thompson, D. (1985). Philosophy and policy. *Philosophy and Public Affairs 14*(2), 205–218.

Thompson, F. J. (1991). The enduring challenge of health policy implementation. In T. J. Litman & L. S. Robins, eds., *Health politics and policy* (2nd ed., pp. 148–169). Albany, NY: Delmar.

Wakefield, M. (1990). Political involvement: A nursing necessity. *Nursing Economics 8*(5), 352–353.

CHAPTER 15

Economic Issues

I begin with the assumption that suffering and death
from lack of food, shelter, and medical care are bad.
I think most people will agree about this. . . .

(Singer, 1972, p. 229)

OBJECTIVES

After completing this chapter, the reader should be able to:

1. Describe the role of economics in health care.

2. Explain the concept of distributive justice.

3. Discuss utilitarian, libertarian, communitarian, and egalitarian theories.

4. Discuss basic questions related to the distribution of health care resources.

5. Describe recent trends in health care economics and the relationship of economic trends to the delivery of health care.

6. Discuss ethics in relation to managed care systems of health care delivery.

INTRODUCTION

Nursing, other health care professions, and the overall health care delivery system exist to deliver health care to society. Over the past several decades, dynamic forces have worked together to create a complex system that has been called the best in the world. From advances in knowledge and technology to changes in health care financing, the system has experienced rapid and drastic changes. It is not unusual to hear the term crisis used to describe the state of the current health care system. This "crisis" relates to problems with cost, quality, and access to health care services. Current debates about social justice are fueled by inequalities in access to health care and health insurance, combined with dramatic increases in the costs of care. Thoughtful, systematic consideration of ethics is necessary for the process of devising solutions to the current problems. This chapter discusses particular aspects of health care economics, distributive justice, and emerging trends.

OVERVIEW OF TODAY'S HEALTH CARE ECONOMICS

Though given its own twists, the history of economic thought is closely associated with the utilitarian movement in the last century (Honderich, 1995). One of the main assumptions in traditional economics is that we should judge the institutions of a society by the preferences of the people that those institutions affect. There are different ways to judge the total preference of society. One method claims that one arrangement is better than another only if it satisfies the preferences of some people and does not frustrate the preferences of any others. This idea is at the center of what is known as welfare economics. Another method suggests that one arrangement is better than another only if it would be preferred by people allowed to make a collective choice. Given that institutions are only properly judged according to the preferences of the people they affect, the institution of health care should be judged by the people it serves. Discussion and debate about the current state of health care economics is integral to the process of evaluating the present system and formulating one that is more just.

Today's problems in the health care system have a long history, with many intervening factors. Partially a result of lawsuits, we have produced a system with progressively higher standards that require the most and the best care for a large segment of the population, regardless of cost. This spiraling pattern is combined with irresponsibility caused by a third-party reimbursement system that (in the past, at least) did not require the providers or patients to be careful of cost. This has led to a skewed model that focuses heavily on technology and personal autonomy, and ignores basic principles of social responsibility and distributive justice. Except for newer managed care programs, this system features an odd split between those who make the spending decisions (patients and physicians) and those who must actually pay for those decisions (third-party payers such as insurance companies, business corporations, or government) (Morreim, 1995). Moreover, there are staggering contrasts within this system. In some instances, hundreds of thousands of dollars are spent on what is recognized as futile care, yet much of the population has no access to even basic health care services.

Within the traditional fee-for-service system, ethics is predominantly driven by codes of ethical behavior and patients' rights statements, with a strong focus on the principle of autonomy. This model focuses on the individual patient, protects physician autonomy, promotes treatment that offers potential benefit or prolonged life, and assumes unlimited resources. Clearly, there are ethical problems associated with this model, including both overutilization and rationing on the basis of financial means (Biblo, Christopher, Johnson, & Potter, 1995).

Ask Yourself

Paying for Futile Care

One often hears stories about elderly patients with terminal illness, and even "no code" status, who remain in intensive care settings for extended periods of time, often because of family members who insist that everything be done for their loved one.

- Is the expenditure of expensive health care resources appropriate for these types of situations? Explain your position.
- Who should bear the financial burden for futile care?
- What are the ethical principles that conflict in situations of this sort?

In an essay on reforming American health care, deBlois, Norris, and O'Rourke (1994) discuss the problems with our health care financing system. Though most people agree that modern health care in America is highly sophisticated and technologically advanced, they also recognize that there are many deficiencies in the system. First, health care services and resources are inaccessible to nearly 20 percent of the population. Second, health care costs are accelerating at an unsustainable annual rate, consuming a huge portion of the gross domestic product. Third, the high cost of health care threatens the competitiveness and profitability of business and industry. Fourth, the benefits to the individual and corporate providers within the system are often pursued at the expense (and sometimes harm) of persons who are in need of health care. DeBlois et al. propose that the real problems with the current system are related to its priorities and the values and commitments that support them, the most significant of which are:

1. an extreme form of individualism that routinely prefers individual interests over concerns about the community of persons;

2. an endorsement of profit making as a primary motive for providing health care services; and

3. an uncritical acceptance of technology as morally neutral and as unambiguous in the service of human goods and goals. (p. 55)

DeBlois et al. charge that the health and well-being of people subjected to a system under the influence of these values are often threatened by the kinds of services offered, the manner in which they are provided, and the priorities that determine both.

Further, if improvements in the system are intended to promote health and well-being of people, efforts need to be ethically grounded and challenge the values that drive the present system.

DISTRIBUTIVE JUSTICE

The ethics of **justice** relates to fair, equitable, and appropriate treatment in light of what is due or owed to persons, recognizing that giving to some will deny receipt to others who might otherwise have received these things (Beauchamp & Childress, 1994; Honderich, 1995). The "others" may be those living in a person's community, or those in other communities, or even those yet to live. For example, if Social Security becomes bankrupt through excessive expenditures in the present, "others" who would have received benefits in the future (even if they are not yet born) will be denied these benefits. As mentioned in Chapter 3, the relevant application of the ethical principle of justice within the health care system focuses on the fair distribution of goods and services. This application is called **distributive justice.** Beauchamp and Childress (1994) define distributive justice as fair, equitable, and appropriate distribution of diverse benefits and burdens such as property, resources, taxation, privileges, and opportunities. Because there is a scarcity of resources and competition for resources and services, it is impossible for all people to have everything they might want or need. One of the primary purposes of government is to formulate and enforce policies that deal with distribution of scarce resources.

Three areas of health care are relevant to questions of distributive justice: Which population groups should be the recipients of health care resources? What percentage of society's resources is it reasonable to spend on health care? Recognizing that health care resources are limited, which aspects of health care should receive the most resources? These are important questions, both practical and ethical in nature.

Entitlement

In deciding questions of distributive justice, we must ask, "Who are entitled to these services?" As with all of ethics, there is no universally accepted answer. Distribution of limited resources is the function of various levels of governing bodies. In attempting to distribute limited resources fairly, leaders will seek systematic means of deciding. Historically, these questions have been answered by such **material rules** as: to each person an equal share, to each person according to need, to each person according to merit, to each person according to social contribution, to each according to the person's rights, to each person according to effort, to each person according to ability to pay, or to each person according to the greatest good to the greatest number. Most societies will utilize several of these principles in establishing public policies. We find many of these principles in effect in the United States where, for example, welfare payments and many health care programs are distributed on the basis of need; jobs and promotions in many sectors are awarded on the basis of demonstrated achievement and merit; comparably high incomes of some are awarded on the basis of superior effort, merit, or potential social contribution; and the opportunity for basic education is distributed equally to all citizens (Beauchamp & Childress, 1994).

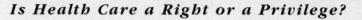

Ask Yourself

Is Health Care a Right or a Privilege?

- Discuss whether you think health care is a right or a privilege. Explain your thinking.
- Should all people have access to the same health care services regardless of ability to pay? How should ability to pay influence access to health care services?
- If you believe health care is a right, to how much health care is each person entitled?

Right to Health Care.   In examining who should receive care, we ask questions about the basic right to health care. Is health care a right, or a privilege? This is a question that is debated fiercely in the media, in the professional and political arenas, and around the dinner table. Is society responsible for providing health care for all citizens, and if so, to what degree? Should each person be eligible for minimum basic health care, or should everyone be allowed to have everything there is to offer, from organ transplants to tummy tucks? Would the public benefit from a strict free-market system that would provide health care services only to those who can pay, or should the government be responsible for the health care needs of all citizens? If health care is a right and health care resources are scarce, what resources are allocated to which group of people? These and other questions fuel the debate about the right to health care.

Discussion of health care as a right is not new. On December 10, 1948, the General Assembly of the United Nations adopted the Universal Declaration of Human Rights, which identifies medical care as a necessary social service ensuring the right to a standard of living adequate for health and well-being (Giesen, 1994). In 1983 the President's Commission for the Study of Ethical Problems in Medicine and Biomedical and Behavioral Research concluded that society has a moral obligation to ensure that everyone has access to adequate care without being subject to excessive burdens. The commission made a clear distinction between society and government, recognizing that a collective or societal obligation does not imply that government should be the primary institution involved in making health care available but, rather, that government should participate with the private sector.

The issue of health care as a right has some basis in constitutional law. The commission reported that neither the Supreme Court nor any appellate court has found a constitutional right to health care, but many federal and state statutes have been interpreted to provide statutory rights in the form of entitlements to some vulnerable groups. As a consequence, these groups have benefited from many legal decisions. Bandman and Bandman (1978) argue that the common welfare clause of the Constitution implies the protection of basic needs, including a right to the protection of health.

Health care as a right is not a universal belief. There are those who believe that health care is a privilege to be enjoyed by some, but beyond the common advantage of all citizens. The entrepreneurial model of libertarianism declares that health care is not a right, but a commodity that must be purchased on the open market like any other service. This model compares the health care professional's right to conduct a practice and charge fees with other business's right to do likewise. It can be argued that this model provides health care only for those who can pay, or for those who are given health care services as a gift. It is hypothesized that, as a result of a free market system of health care delivery, supply-and-demand and pricing competition would result in lower health care costs. This in turn would result in health care services becoming more accessible to a larger portion of the population. Except for the fact that professionals can choose to provide services free of charge, this model makes little allowance for children and the very poor (Bandman & Bandman, 1978; Beauchamp & Childress, 1994).

How Much and to Whom?   If one accepts that health care is a right or that society has an ethical obligation to provide health care services to vulnerable populations, then one is required to examine the question of how much health care is to be provided, and to whom. There are two broad views about the right to access to health care: some believe all should have equal access to health care, while others believe the right extends only to a decent minimum of health care. Consider the following case.

CASE PRESENTATION

Should Public Funds Pay for Extraordinary Procedures?

There was a recent court case in which a middle-aged indigent woman, who suffered from insulin-dependent diabetes mellitus, demanded that Medicaid pay for a pancreas transplant. This patient was reported to be uncooperative in her previous diabetic regimen and disliked giving herself insulin injections. Even though Medicaid in that state has a fiscal policy that denies payment for this surgery to all program recipients, the state supreme court ruled that this woman had a right to the surgery because other people with insurance or adequate funds have access to the surgery. The decision was based on the principle of nondiscrimination.

Think About It

Decisions About Entitlements

- Do you think the patient had a "right" to this surgery? Why or why not?
- Should society (through taxes) pay for the surgery, even though the patient was known to be nonparticipative in her previous regimen? Why or why not?

- Should the government make arbitrary decisions permitting or prohibiting certain therapies? Explain.
- Do you think there were others who might have received benefits but were subsequently denied them because extraordinary funds were used for this patient?
- What are the ethical implications of the court decision?
- What are ethical arguments for and against the court decision?

Fair Distribution

The court's decision to require public payment for the pancreas transplant in the previous case study raises questions about restricting health care services. Few people would argue that there are enough resources to pay for all services. Think about your household budget. If you have only $300 to spend on Christmas gifts for your three sisters and you also need to purchase groceries for the week and antibiotics for yourself, it would be foolish to spend $150 on one gift. By doing that, you would ensure that your sisters would not be treated equitably, that you probably would not be eating very well for the next week, and that you would not feel well anyway, since you could not afford your prescription medication. The same principle applies to health care dollars. The limited public budget must be divided among many interests. In order to maintain a functioning infrastructure, the government must ensure that public schools, highways, police, national defense, social security, and other services in the public domain have a proportionate share of the total budget. Policy makers are charged with the difficult task of making equitable decisions about distribution of resources. These decisions must balance health care spending with other programs, and must carefully avoid both extravagant excess spending and frugality that threaten the health of citizens.

Distribution of Resources

Limited health care dollars must be spent wisely. There are several different criteria that have been proposed to make distributive justice decisions. One method involves making judgments about cost in relation to predicted benefit. For example, we could question the practice of allowing patients in the last stages of terminal illness to monopolize limited and expensive intensive care beds, thus utilizing the most expensive kind of health care for the least benefit. Some propose that the best way to avoid making arbitrary decisions in these kinds of situations is to set mandatory guidelines. For example, some suggest that expensive therapies, such as dialysis or organ transplant, be reserved only for those below a certain age. A second method involves making judgments about the usefulness of given therapies. Immunizations, for example, are cost effective and benefit a large percentage of the population. Some would suggest that the most utile therapies (the ones that are less costly and nearly guaranteed to help a large number of people) are the ones that should have priority.

Theories of Justice

Distributive justice is based upon common morals and ethics. Several theories have been proposed to determine how resources and services should be distributed. Utilitarian, libertarian, communitarian, and egalitarian theories are examples of popular theories of justice. Because of society's fragmented beliefs about social justice, no single theory can be expected to bring coherence to the situation. Beauchamp & Childress discuss the current system in the United States:

> We seek to provide the best possible health care for all citizens, while promoting the public interest through cost-containment programs. We promote the ideal of equal access to health care for everyone, including care for indigents, while maintaining a free-market competitive environment. These desirable goals of superior care, equality of access, freedom of choice, and social efficiency are difficult to render coherent in a social system. Different conceptions of the just society underlie them, and one goal is likely to diminish another. (1994, p. 335)

Recognizing that no single theory will satisfy society by fulfilling all principles, we suggest that several theories of justice be used to understand competing social goals.

Utilitarian Theories. Based, in general, upon the rule that it is good to maximize the "greatest good for the greatest number," **utilitarian theories** favor social programs that protect public health and distribute basic health care equally to all citizens. This is based on the belief that the outcome of these programs maximizes utility. Although these theories are the basis of many social programs, there are problems in their application. For example, because utilitarianism places aggregate social good before individual rights, social utility might be maximized by denying access to health care for some of society's sickest and most vulnerable populations (Beauchamp & Childress, 1994).

Libertarian Theories. **Libertarian theories** propose that the just society protects the rights of property and liberty of each person, allowing citizens to improve their circumstances by their own effort. Libertarian theories support a private citizen or group's right to own and manage a health care business. Libertarian theory does not classify health care as a right, but rather as a commodity that operates on the material principle of ability to pay either directly or indirectly through insurance. Strict libertarians view taxation as an unjust redistribution of private property, but do not oppose other methods of distribution if they are freely chosen. Market strategies and managed competition are proposals in the United States that are influenced by libertarianism (Beauchamp & Childress, 1994).

Communitarian Theories. **Communitarian** theories place the community, rather than the individual, the state, the nation, or any other entity, at the center of the value system. Less fully developed than utilitarianism or libertarianism, communitarianism emphasizes the value of public goods and maintains that values are rooted in communal practices. Communitarians believe that human life will go better if collective and public values guide peoples' lives. They have a commitment to facilities and practices designed to help members of the community develop their common and hence their personal lives (Honderich, 1995). Modern communitarian writers disagree on the application of these theories to health care access. Some propose a federation of interlinking community health programs that are democratically administered by citizen-members. In this model, each individual program would determine which benefits to provide, which care is most important, and whether expensive services will be included or excluded. Another communitarian theory holds that community tradition includes commitments of equal access to health care, and suggests that as long as communal funds are spent, services must be equally available (Beauchamp & Childress, 1994).

Egalitarian Theories. Egalitarian theories are related to the concept of equality, in which people who are similarly situated should be treated similarly, though much depends on what kinds of similarity count as relevant and what constitutes similar treatment (Honderich, 1995). Promoting ideals of equal distribution of social benefits and burdens, egalitarian theories recognize the social obligation to eliminate or reduce barriers that prevent fair equality of opportunity. These theories are cautiously formulated to avoid requiring equal sharing of all possible social benefits. A leading proponent of egalitarianism, John Rawls suggests that in making decisions of justice, one should examine the situation behind a veil of ignorance. In this hypothetical situation, "no one knows his place in society, his class position or social status, nor does anyone know his fortune in the distribution of natural assets and abilities, his intelligence, strength, and the like" (1996, p. 567). This veil of ignorance ensures that no one is able to design principles to favor his or her particular condition. Supporters of Rawls's theory recognize a positive social obligation to eliminate or reduce barriers that prevent fair equality of opportunity, and suggest that health policy formulated according to egalitarian principles would guarantee a safety net or minimum floor below which citizens would not be allowed to fall (Beauchamp & Childress, 1994).

Ask Yourself

Making Fair Decisions

- Which theory of distribution appeals to you as the most fair and equitable? Why?
- Do you think the theory you chose would be fair to all people in all circumstances? Discuss your thinking.
- Could you combine two or more theories to make a system that is fair and equitable?

RECENT TRENDS AND HEALTH ECONOMIC ISSUES

Questions of ethics and distributive justice began to be discussed well before the mid-1990s. Claims that the United States was experiencing a crisis in health care economics escalated in the last two decades. Skyrocketing expenditures and a general tightening of health care dollars resulted in fiscal scarcity. Both government and business responded by attempting to gain control over expenditures. This tightening assumed a variety of forms, including managed care systems, prospective payment, and utilization review. Sacrificing, in part, the traditional focus on the welfare of patients, health care corporations devised ways to cut costs, improve profits, increase efficiency, and branch out into more profitable ventures such as landscaping, catering, and laundry service.

Government was the prime mover of cost containment during the early 1980s. Having experienced virtually no incentives for cost controls up to this point, in the 1980s hospitals were unprepared when the government instituted the payment system based on Diagnosis Related Groups (DRGs). This shift represented the first major change in the way hospitals were paid for Medicare patients, and placed the responsibility for efficiency and cost savings on hospitals and physicians. Certificate of Need programs were established to restrain the building or purchasing of unnecessary and expensive technologies and capital construction. Organizations such as Professional Standards Review Organizations (PSROs) and Peer Review Organizations (PROs) were established to require physicians to develop more efficient practice standards (Sherrill, 1995). By the early 1990s, the system was in a state of disequilibrium. While large hospital corporations were finding ways to cut costs (utilizing such methods as eliminating support services and reducing nursing staff) and many small rural hospitals were closing as a result of the financial strain, inherent problems were unsolved—care remained excellent, though expensive, for some but inaccessible to many.

Economic influences also arose from outside the health care system. Two of the major outside influences were increased malpractice litigation and employment-negotiated health insurance plans. Malpractice litigation resulting in huge awards and the subsequent birth of defensive medicine added to the expense of the system. Califano (1986) attributes this to dynamic forces that included elements from many distinct programs and entities. The system moved from one that traditionally called for community standards to one in which scientific invention, medical technology, specialization, Medicare and Medicaid, and regional heart, cancer, and stroke centers required nationalized standards of care for physicians. This resulted in the routine practice of ordering batteries of diagnostic tests to meet new, stricter standards. Fearing malpractice litigation, physicians began to lose a measure of the autonomy that would allow them to choose only the diagnostic tests they thought were appropriate.

Employment-negotiated insurance plans fueled the practice of overspending and added to these pressures. Negotiated as part of employment contracts, many health insurance plans featured first-dollar, 100 percent coverage of health care costs. As a result, a large percentage of patients did not pay directly for any health care services; thus, the cost of the doctor or hospital was rendered irrelevant (Califano, 1986). Everyone expected the most and best. Being indifferent to the costs of the medical services, patients were much more likely to buy more of them, even those that were of marginal utility or duplicative (Gordon, 1992). Hospitals and physicians were more than happy to participate. For hospitals and doctors alike, maximizing services resulted in increased cash flow and consequent lessening of financial problems. This trend contributed to the even higher standards of care that required very aggressive diagnosis and treatment, resulted in greater costs, and opened the door for more malpractice litigation.

Health Care Reform

Recognizing these problems in the health care delivery system and sensing a groundswell of public support, the Clinton administration devised a health care reform proposal. Unveiled in the fall of 1993, this proposal called for universal access to health care through managed competition. It also described a system of financing that would be accomplished primarily through mandated coverage at places of employment, with employers required to pay a large percentage of the premiums. Subsidies were planned for small businesses, and the federal government assumed the employer responsibility for persons who were not covered by employer-based plans (Drake, 1994).

After months of highly publicized debate, the Clinton health care reform proposal was defeated. Examining the defeat in terms of ethics, Jean deBlois (1995) attributes the failure to four fundamental factors: lack of social consensus on the question of a right to basic health care for all persons; strength and energy of those who argued on behalf of individual rights and liberties over the needs of the community or the nation; unconstrained powerful interest groups; and little or no recognition that substantive reform required a significant challenge to the values that inform and drive health care.

Having lost features intended to ensure integrity within the new system, managed care was the only piece that emerged unscathed from Clinton's health care reform proposal. Existing as a small part of the United States health care system for several decades, managed care gained prominence as a preferred method of delivery and financing of health care services (deBlois, 1995).

At the beginning of the twenty-first century, the United States continues to experience a crisis of health care access. Health care insurance is a critical factor in access to health care. The uninsured population is growing rapidly. In 1982 there were an estimated 32 million uninsured. In 2000 the number is estimated at 44 million, with over 70 million lacking insurance for at least one month each year (Smith-Campbell, 2000; ANA, 1999; Bennefield, 1998; Campbell, 1999; Shearer, 1996). One study estimated that the uninsured may reach over 60 million by 2008 (Custer & Ketsche, 1999). Piecemeal, incremental efforts have been made toward solving the health care access problems. A network of free clinics serves the indigent in all fifty states. The Children's Health Insurance Program provides health insurance for uninsured indigent children who do not meet the Medicaid guidelines. Nevertheless, lack of access to health care services is a serious problem. We will see efforts on many fronts to solve the problem. Similar to the original *Nursing's Agenda for Health Care Reform* (1992), the ANA currently supports proposals for a single-payer system to ensure basic health care to all citizens (ANA, 1999).

Managed Care

Though there is no one accepted definition, Chang, Price, and Pfoutz define **managed care** as a "health care system willing to be held accountable both clinically and financially for the health outcomes of an enrolled population for a capitated (fixed) payment" (2001, p. 299). It is an integrated form of health care delivery and financing that represents attempts to control costs by modifying the behavior of providers and patients. Managed care moves away from a system based on patient and provider autonomy. According to supporters, managed care lowers costs through the elimination of waste and excess. The lower costs result in benefits to each patient and the membership as a whole. Aiming toward lower premiums and preventive care benefits, managed care organizations claim that members receive appropriate, quality care. In this regard, managed care is attentive to the needs of the membership as a group, as well as the needs of individual patients. As a result of the goal of lower costs, some propose that patients in managed care plans can be saved from unnecessary tests and treatments, which are viewed as a risk inherent in the traditional system (Biblo et al., 1995).

Raising questions about the ethics of managed care, Fiesta (1996) discusses four notable legal cases that have resulted in significant financial losses for managed care organizations. These cases involved patients who experienced unfavorable outcomes as a result of managed care providers' efforts to follow program policy in cutting costs. One case involves an infant who was febrile, moaning, panting, and flaccid when the parents consulted the managed care emergency line. Even though there were closer hospitals, the parents were instructed to take the child to a hospital that was nearly an hour away because it offered reduced cost to the managed care plan. The infant suffered a cardiac arrest en route. After resuscitation, both of the child's hands were amputated as a result of extraordinary complications. The family was awarded a $45 million verdict in a malpractice suit against the health maintenance organization.

In another case, the court concluded that, by limiting enrollees' choice of provider to those on a specified panel, there is an unreasonable risk of harm to members if the selected clinicians are incompetent or unqualified. Another case involved the refusal of a physician assigned to a particular patient to admit the patient to the hospital. Although assigned by the managed care organization as the primary care provider for the patient filing suit, the physician argued that a physician-patient relationship did not exist because he had never seen the patient. Refused admission to the hospital as a result of this disagreement, the patient experienced a stroke in the hospital's parking lot. The court held that the plan's designated physician owed the patient a duty of care as a result of an implied physician-patient relationship inherent in the plan's enrollment agreement. In another case, the court rendered a $90 million verdict based upon the

Ask Yourself

Ethical Problems in Managed Care

- What ethical problems can you foresee with managed care economics?
- How do you think nurses will be affected by managed care?
- How do you think nurses can influence the resolution of ethical problems in managed care?

managed care organization's refusal to cover a bone marrow transplant. The court held that the managed care organization's internal utilization review decisions were unduly influenced by financial incentives to minimize care. Each of these cases illustrates ethical problems associated with balancing utilitarian views of cost-effective care with a respect for persons and the traditional view of a duty to care.

Ethics in Managed Care. We must pay particular attention to the potential for ethical abuses that occur as a result of managed care organizations' unique role of both payer and provider of health care services. Like American society as a whole, the ethics community was slow in recognizing the profound ethical implications of managed care. Based upon the assumption that the basic ethical criterion for the planned allocation of resources in a managed care setting at the policy level is the well-being of the entire group for whom the decisions are being made, balanced by the requirement of respect for individual health care needs, the Midwest Bioethics Center developed a list of considerations to be used by managed care organizations for ethically rationing care:

1. Caring is an ethical imperative for health care providers because it is an essential benefit.

2. The first duty or obligation of any health care professional is to provide treatment that is clearly of benefit.

3. It is never ethically defensible to ration palliative care.

4. Futile treatment is of no benefit and should not be provided. However, care must be taken when defining a treatment as futile that the point of view of the patient is considered.

5. Treatment of marginal benefit needs to be carefully evaluated so that decisions are not inappropriately influenced by concerns such as subjective quality of life judgments of anyone other than the patient, cost constraints, or defensive medicine.

6. Individuals should make for others only those rationing decisions they are willing to impose upon themselves.

7. Populations that are especially needy or vulnerable should be given special consideration in order to be able to compete for the benefits society has to offer.

8. In rationing decisions, people ought not to be discriminated against without cause.

9. Lifestyle choice in and of itself is not a reason for denying care. However, it is ethically justifiable to provide positive incentives to support the development of healthy lifestyles. (Biblo et al., 1995, pp. 19–20)

SUMMARY

Because health care is a scarce resource, citizens rely upon social institutions to make fair and equitable distributive justice decisions. There is little consensus on basic ethical questions such as: Who should receive health care resources? Is there a right to basic health care? How much should be spent on particular health care services? What percentage of the society's overall resources should be invested in health care? Utilitarianism, libertarianism, communitarianism, and egalitarianism are theories that attempt to describe fair means of distributing resources. Recent focus on problems related to the economic aspects of the health care delivery system of the United States has prompted debate on practical issues of distributive justice. Emerging from the struggle to reform the health care system, managed care is becoming a major component of the health care system. Moving from a traditional system that valued patient and provider autonomy to a system that values the economic delivery of health care to a particular population, close attention must be paid to ethical standards in health care.

CHAPTER HIGHLIGHTS

- The history of economic thought is closely associated with the utilitarian movement in the last century.

- The traditional health care system in the United States is fee-for-service.

- Within a fee-for-service system, there is a strong focus on the principle of autonomy.

- Justice relates to fair, equitable, and appropriate treatment in light of what is due or owed to persons, and recognizes that giving to some will deny receipt to others who might otherwise have received these things.

- Distributive justice is the fair, equitable, and appropriate distribution of benefits and burdens. Theories of distributive justice seek to render diverse principles coherent.

- Utilitarian theories are based upon the rule that it is good to maximize the greatest good for the greatest number.

- Libertarian theories propose that the just society protects the rights of property and liberty of each person, allowing citizens to improve their circumstances by their own effort.

- Communitarian theories place the community, rather than the individual, the state, the nation, or any other entity, at the center of the value system.

- Egalitarian theories are related to the concept of equality in which people who are similarly situated should be treated similarly.

- Scarcity of health care resources has led to a rethinking of the structure of health care economics.

- Managed care gives rise to ethical problems associated with balancing utilitarian views of cost-effective care with a respect for persons and the traditional view of a duty to care.

DISCUSSION QUESTIONS AND ACTIVITIES

1. Visit the American Association of Health Plans on-line to find out the managed care perspective on various economic and policy issues. http://www.aahp.org/

2. Discuss current problems in health care economics with classmates. Is there a consensus regarding root causes, right to health care, or the role of the government as a payer for health care services?

3. Go to the library and find a basic economics text. How does the health care system differ from other free-market systems?

4. Discuss the influence of utilitarian theory on the economics of the current health care system.

5. Why do patient and provider autonomy affect health care delivery and financing?

6. Define distributive justice. In class, discuss the material rules of distributive justice. Which material rule is most popular among classmates?

7. What method of distributing goods and services do you think is fair and equitable? Do your classmates agree with your theories?

8. Discuss health care ethics as related to managed care.

REFERENCES

American Nurses Association. (1999). *Achieving access for all Americans*: A proposal from the American Nurses Association for health coverage 2000. Washington, DC: Author. Retrieved June 10, 1999 from the World Wide Web: http://www.nursingworld.org/readroom/rwjpaper.htm

Bandman, E. L., & Bandman, B. (1978). *Bioethics and human rights: A reader for health professionals*. Boston: Little, Brown.

Beauchamp, T., & Childress, J. (1994). *Principles of biomedical ethics* (4th ed.). New York: Oxford University Press.

Bennefield, R. (1998). Current population reports: Health insurance coverage: 1997 (P60-202). Bureau of Census. Retrieved from the World Wide Web: http://www.cencus.gov/hhes/www/hlhin97.html

Biblo, J. C., Christopher, L. J., & Potter, R. L. (1995). *Ethical issues in managed care: Guidelines for clinicians and recommendations to accrediting organizations*. Kansas City, MO: Bioethics Development Group.

Califano, J. A., Jr. (1986). *America's health care revolution: Who lives? Who dies? Who pays?* New York: Random House.

Campbell, J. A. (1999). Current population reports: Health insurance coverage 1998 (P60-208). Bureau of Census. Retrieved from the World Wide Web: http://www.census.gov/hhes/www/hlthin98.html

Chang, C. F., Price, S. A., & Pfoutz, S. K. (2001). *Economics and nursing: Critical professional issues*. Philadelphia: Davis.

deBlois, J. (1995, Autumn). Ethical issues and managed care: Asking the right questions. *Health Care Ethics, USA 3*(4), 6–7.

deBlois, J., Norris, P., & O'Rourke, K. (1994, Autumn). *A primer for health care ethics: Essays for a pluralistic society,* pp. 5–6. Washington, DC: Georgetown University Press.

Drake, D. (1994). *Reforming the health care market: An interpretive economic history.* Washington, DC: Georgetown University Press.

Fiesta, J. (1996). Legal update, 1995: Part 2. *Nursing Management, 27*(6), 24–25.

Giesen, D. (1994). A right to health care?: A comparative perspective. *Health Matrix 4*(2), 277–295.

Gordon, J. S. (1992, May/June). How America's health care fell ill. *American Heritage*, 49–65.

Honderich, T., ed. (1995). *The Oxford companion to philosophy.* New York: Oxford University Press.

Morreim, E. H. (1995). *Balancing act: The new medical ethics of medicine's new economics.* Washington, DC: Georgetown University Press.

President's Commission for the Study of Ethical Problems in Medicine and Biomedical and Behavioral Research. (1994). Securing access to health care. In B. L. Beauchamp & L. Walters, *Contemporary issues in bioethics* (4th ed., pp. 683–689). Belmont, CA: Wadsworth.

Rawls, J. (1996). A theory of justice. In J. Feinberg, ed., *Reason and responsibility: Some readings in basic problems of philosophy* (pp. 567–572). Belmont, CA: Wadsworth. (Reprinted from J. Rawls, *A theory of justice,* 1971, Cambridge, MA: Harvard University Press)

Shearer, G. (1996, April 15). Health care check-up: Consumers at risk. Washington, DC: Consumers Union.

Sherrill, R. (1995, January 9–16). Medicine and the madness of the market. *The Nation,* 45–72.

Singer, P. (1972). Famine, affluence, and morality. *Philosophy & Public Affairs 1,* 229–243.

Smith-Campbell, B. (2000). Access to health care: Effects of public funding on the uninsured. *Journal of Nursing Scholarship, 32*(3), 295–300.

CHAPTER 16

Social Issues

By Mary Jo Butler

In the deserts of the heart let the healing fountain start. . . .

(W. H. Auden, p. 986)

OBJECTIVES

After completing this chapter, the reader should be able to:

1. Explain how social conditions such as poverty, homelessness, domestic violence, an increasing elderly population, and racism affect health.

2. Apply the concept of justice to vulnerable populations, elaborating on the implications for society and the health care system.

3. Discuss the application of beneficence and nonmaleficence to vulnerable groups in light of today's health care system.

4. Identify the pros and cons of promoting autonomy for health care decision making among vulnerable populations.

5. Analyze evidence of victim blaming within the health care system.

6. Illusrate application of the concepts of advocacy and nonviolence to care of vulnerable populations.

7. Examine current research for application to culturally diverse groups.

INTRODUCTION

Health is unquestionably a product of the person and environment interchange. Thus, social conditions that alter the person and environment interchange process are critical concerns for nurses and nursing students. Nurses confront social issues that shape the health and health care management of individuals on a daily basis. These social issues may create conflicts in values and ethical dilemmas that must be addressed in order to determine appropriate health care interventions for involved individuals. The purpose of this chapter is to help elucidate the principles inherent in decision making when social issues create ethical dilemmas for the nurse.

SOCIAL ISSUES

Many pervasive social issues are of special concern to health care providers today. Poverty, homelessness, domestic violence, an increasing elderly population, and racism are examples of some of these very important concerns. Each of these issues is reviewed briefly in this chapter, along with the dominant guiding principles for related ethical decision making.

Poverty

Poverty and homelessness continue to be prevalent in the United States as a consequence of changes in government assistance programs and taxes. Health care is influenced more and more by poverty, as increasing numbers of people lack health insurance due to limitations in employment-based health insurance. Due to welfare reform, a publicly financed health care system for the medically indigent is becoming available to fewer people, and meets only a fraction of the needs of enrolled individuals. Without health care coverage, the poor often postpone needed health care, or cope with public clinics that are often degrading and impersonal.

Federal programs for the indigent cover only about half of all individuals living on incomes below the poverty level. Individuals without coverage must find health care systems that will provide free care, or do without. For this reason, many people below the poverty level do not participate in basic preventive care programs.

Poverty, growing worldwide, is known to have a negative impact on both the health of individuals and the receipt of health care services (Catley, 1992). Poorer people are sicker than people with adequate financial resources. While poverty is detrimental to the health of all individuals living with inadequate resources, it produces a next generation of citizens with more health problems than usual. Children living in poverty have a higher incidence of conditions associated with trauma, drugs, burns, mental illness, and HIV infection (Wessell, 1992). Children living in poverty are more likely to experience poor nutrition, inadequate exercise, and diseases from environmental factors such as vermin or lead. They are more likely to grow up with chronic illnesses that require extensive health care resources. Overall, poverty and health are inextricably enmeshed.

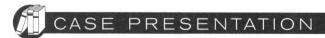

CASE PRESENTATION

Socioeconomic Influences on Health

Martha D is a sixty-nine-year-old African-American woman who lives in a substandard third-floor walk-up, cold-water apartment in a housing project with a high crime rate. She draws a small Social Security check that does not cover living expenses. Her income is supplemented by food stamps, housing assistance, and by working as a nanny for three small children for twenty hours a week. Ms. D earns minimum wage for her job as a nanny, and accepts cash for her work to avoid any interference with her Social Security check. She uses public transportation to go to and from her job, spending $2.00 each working day on bus fare.

Ms. D helps her alcoholic single daughter, age forty-seven, with two teenage children, especially when the daughter is experiencing a drinking binge. The children frequently stay with Ms. D and rely on her for food, shelter, and love. Mr. D is an alcoholic and has not been home for two years; however, he does occasionally call from a homeless shelter or treatment facility. Neither the daughter nor Mr. D contribute to household expenses, but Ms. D is very devoted to her family, especially her two grandchildren.

Martha D is 5'8" tall and weighs 285 pounds. She has hypertension, with her blood pressure ranging from 200/90 to 250/110. She is on medication for her blood pressure, and the physician has linked her with a county home health nurse to encourage a diet and simple exercise regime for her obesity and hypertension. Ms. D is beginning to show signs of Type II diabetes and has been encouraged to lose weight and adhere to a diabetic diet. In addition, Ms. D has some small ulcerations on her left ankle.

The home health nurse visits Ms. D and instructs her in the care of her ulcers, advising her to keep her left foot elevated as much as possible. The nurse spends considerable time explaining a 1200-calorie diabetic diet with moderate sodium restriction to Ms. D, and talks with Ms. D about the need to begin walking as soon as the ulcers on her foot heal. Ms. D lets the nurse know she used to attend a weight control group and understands low fat and diabetic diets. However, she says coming home to a nice pot of beans with fried chicken and biscuits is her only daily pleasure. "I've lived sixty-nine years on this diet, don't wish to change, and have nothing to lose if I remain on it the rest of my life." She also points out that it is not safe to walk in her neighborhood, so she stays inside. In addition, she indicates that she is too tired to exercise after working all day.

Think About It

Who Decides What Is Best for a Patient?

- Consider Ms. D's decision to ignore recommendations regarding diet, exercise, and, perhaps, care of her ankle ulcerations in relation to autonomy, beneficence, and nonmaleficence.

- Since the principle of beneficence requires actively doing good for Ms. D, who decides what is good?

- Discuss implications of justice and health care for Ms. D.

Homelessness

Homeless individuals, although not a homogenous group, are increasing in society. While good census data are hard to obtain, estimates suggest that between 250,000 and 3,000,000 people are homeless in the United States. The homeless are not all mentally ill or substance abusers. The new homeless are often families, single women with children, and the elderly. Like those living in poverty, homeless people suffer from acute and chronic health problems. Burg (1994) categorizes their health problems as those resulting from limited access to care, those coincident with homelessness, and those associated with the psychosocial burden of homelessness. Health problems resulting from limited access to care include exacerbated or advanced conditions that would have responded to early and thorough intervention. Health problems coincident with homelessness include illnesses resulting from living with inadequate nutrition, warmth, hygiene, safety, and other basic needs. Health problems associated with the psychosocial burden of homelessness are primarily mental illnesses, suicide, assault, and substance abuse which can dull the anxiety of homelessness. The percentage of homeless children who have a chronic health problem is well above the rate for children who are not homeless (National Association, 1989). The homeless, like those living in poverty, have few options for health care, limited access to care, and difficulty with follow-up treatment or compliance. This is due, in part, to the typical model of health care delivery in the United States.

Mondragon (1993) describes the pervasive assumptions that undergird the government's health promotion model. These assumptions view health as the absence of disease and associate common diseases with controllable risk factors. Thus, the key to improved health is deemed to be the provision of knowledge and skills to individuals. It is assumed that people will use self-determination, individualism, and responsibility to secure adequate housing, employment, and proper nutrition. While this model may benefit people with good education, a continuum of options, and resources to elicit change, it is less applicable to those with limited choices who are not in charge of their destinies. It can be hypothesized that poverty and homelessness will contribute to the poor health of American citizens as long as the dominant models for health care delivery inhibit patient participation in care.

CASE PRESENTATION

No Home to Go To

Ms. Brown comes into the emergency room to secure treatment for a head injury, plus minor bruises and abrasions that she reportedly received during an assault that happened about twenty hours ago. Ms. Brown is thirty-four years old and accompanied by her boyfriend, Roy. She indicates they were sleeping in a protected entrance to an elevator in the city parking garage when two young men began beating and kicking them. The two men took Ms. Brown's purse, a sack of food she and Roy had accumulated, and Roy's wallet which contained $5.00. Ms. Brown indicates she has been homeless for over a year. She occasionally stays in city shelters but spends most of her time roaming the city and walking to secure meals at the various programs that feed the poor. She is tall and thin, with a variety of skin lesions. She came to the hospital due to dizziness that prevented her from walking to the church where she could eat. She and Roy occasionally work odd jobs, but use the bulk of their income to support Roy's drug habit. She is trying to get Roy to quit using.

The physician has the nurse clean Ms. Brown's scalp and tape the traumatic lesion. A contusion is expected, and the physician suggests Ms. Brown rest for a few days and go to the neurological clinic if the dizziness worsens. The nurse points out that Ms. Brown has no place to rest and cannot get to the clinic without access to public transportation. The physician realizes this but indicates it is beyond her control.

Think About It

When Resources Are Lacking

- Apply the concepts of justice, nonmaleficence, and beneficence to Ms. Brown's care.
- Does society have any responsibility for Ms. Brown? If so, what?
- Can thorough treatment be denied if a client has no resources? If not, who pays for the treatment?

Domestic Violence

A third common social condition affecting health and health care delivery is domestic violence, the most common but least reported crime in the United States. Estimated numbers of battered women range from two to twelve million per year. Domestic violence flows from a historical position of sexism. Eisler (1987) describes how select tenets of Judaism, Christianity, and Islam support patriarchy, the inferiority of women, and women as the property of men. In the United States it was legal for a husband to beat his wife to maintain his authority until 1899 (Diehm & Ross, 1988). Remnants of these beliefs are still threaded through society, affecting the way families socialize their children and the way communities tolerate gender inequity. Butler and Weatherley (1992) and Roberts (2000) indicate that women have long been defined by the mothering role and dependence on men in American society. While these role definitions are changing, daily events in society continue to perpetuate gender inequity. As long as gender inequity exists, domestic violence will remain a social problem.

The vast majority of abused women eventually leave their abusive partners. However, leaving is a process that takes time, energy, and resources. Many abused women will leave and return to their abusive partners several times before permanently terminating the relationship. Esposito (1993) attributes this to the inability to find housing or suitable jobs; the fear, loneliness, or poverty that results from being out on their own; concern for children who are experiencing relocation and other difficulties; relentless pressure from family and friends to try harder to make the relationship work; or poor support from the criminal justice system. It is sometimes easier to return to a familiar though unpleasant situation than to start over and deal with numerous unknowns.

Since sex is the risk factor, domestic violence affects women of all socioeconomic, racial, and ethnic groups (Esposito, 1993; Ewing, 1987; MMWR, 2000). All women living in violent relationships will experience poorer health. Women living in abusive situations experience acute traumatic injuries and chronic physical and emotional problems (Butler & Weatherley, 1992; Kernie, Wolf, & Holt, 2000). They are especially vulnerable to battery during pregnancy and at a higher risk than nonbattered women for poor pregnancy outcomes (Bohn, 1990). The health care system may add insult to abused womens' injuries. The women often feel humiliated by and blamed for the abuse by a health care system that minimizes the abuse, makes insufficient referrals, and fails to acknowledge abuse as the culprit (Campbell, Pliska, Taylor, & Sheridan, 1994). As a result, women leave health care settings without having the domestic violence addressed, remaining isolated and uninformed about their options (Fishwick, 1995).

CASE PRESENTATION

Suspicions of Abuse

Maria P is a twenty-five-year-old Hispanic woman who made an initial visit to the clinic for prenatal care when she was eighteen weeks pregnant. She has returned for a second prenatal visit at twenty-two weeks gestation. Maria has a four-year-old son and a two-year-old daughter. Her record indicates she had several bruises, lacerations, and a black eye during her last pregnancy that she attributed to clumsiness. Her two-year-old weighed four pounds, eight ounces at birth and was seventeen inches long.

As part of routine prenatal care for the most recent pregnancy, Maria was tested for HIV antibodies. The test was positive, and the physician and nurse conveyed this information to Maria during her second prenatal visit. Maria, of course, was quite upset. She admits that her spouse has been physically abusing her for some time and that both have used intravenous drugs in the past. She has had no sexual partners other than her spouse.

The nurse encourages Maria to tell her spouse that she is HIV positive so that he can be tested for antibodies. She also encourages use of condoms during sexual intercourse to help avoid transmission to her spouse should he not be infected.

Maria insists that her husband refuses to use condoms as they interfere with his pleasure. In addition, she says he would kill her if he knew she was HIV positive.

The nurse encourages Maria to go to a shelter for abused women and links her to both a counselor and a social worker who help her devise a safety plan. However, Maria ultimately decides to go home because she cannot abandon her children, and she does not want them in a shelter. She knows she cannot make it on her own, as she has neither income nor job skills. She requests that the clinic not interfere and that they allow her to decide if, when, and how she will notify her spouse about her HIV status.

Think About It

When Patient Choices Place Them at Risk for Harm

- Consider the principle of autonomy when determining the appropriate decision in this situation. Remember that confidentiality is an inherent part of autonomy.
- Who is the patient in this situation?
- If Maria's husband is notified by the clinic of her HIV status and he does significant harm to Maria, would liability become an issue?
- If Maria's husband discovers he is HIV positive in the future, blames Maria, and discovers the clinic has known she was HIV positive for some time, is there any liability? Explain.

Increasing Elder Population

In addition to poverty, homelessness, and domestic violence, the elderly are a growing population worldwide (Catley, 1992). By the year 2050, Stark (1991) predicts that sixty-nine million Americans will be over age sixty-five. People are living longer due to healthier diets, vaccines, and improvements in the environment (Windom, 1988). Certainly advances in health care knowledge have contributed to greater longevity. However, many elderly, especially from minority populations, live without pensions and on incomes below the poverty level (Hall, 1993). Vast numbers of the elderly are socially isolated, in need of work to survive, and susceptible to economic hardship. Chronic illnesses, pain, especially from arthritic processes, frailties, and disabilities occur with increasing frequency as people age (Tebb, 1995). Health problems contribute significantly to the social isolation, financial burden, and general discomfort that may accompany aging.

The assumption in current prevailing health care models is that the frail elderly will be cared for at home by friends and family to alleviate strain on the health care system. In reality, family members may be unable to provide needed support due to geographical distance from the frail elderly family member or personal responsibilities. Skaff and Pearlin (1992) describe how caregivers of the elderly experience emotional and financial strain. The caregivers often have to help with finances of the elderly, since their fixed incomes cannot cover the basic cost of living as well as health care expenses. Reliance on friends and family for health care of the frail elderly is especially problematic for the elderly without the necessary social or financial resources. Even though the elderly are known to be vulnerable and at risk, one proposal to control health care costs in the United States is the rationing of care to the aged and a shift to more home care (Arcangelo, 1994).

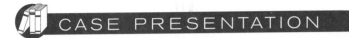

CASE PRESENTATION

Aging, Poverty, and Illness

Mr. Chang is a sixty-five-year-old widower with chronic kidney disease. He is supposed to receive dialysis three times a week but frequently misses his appointments due to no transportation or not feeling well. His only hope for a cure is a kidney transplant, which Mr. Chang really wants. Mr. Chang is very frail with many health problems. He lives alone in a small garage apartment. The landlord is threatening to evict Mr. Chang because he is behind in his rent payments. Mr. Chang lives on a small pension and Medicare. His prescription costs are excessive.

A home health nurse used to transport Mr. Chang to dialysis occasionally, as Mr. Chang lives outside the township limits and is unable to access public transportation services. The clinic, which does not believe Mr. Chang is a candidate for a transplant, has revised their policies regarding home visits due to changes in reimbursement mechanisms. The home health nurse can no longer visit Mr. Chang unless there is a reimbursable need such as a dressing change; and for liability reasons, she can no longer transport Mr. Chang to dialysis.

Think About It

What Health Care Should Society Provide for Its Citizens?

- Consider the principle of justice in deciding if health care is a right or a privilege that comes with the ability to pay. If health care must be rationed, who decides what services an individual will receive?

- Is society prepared to pay health care costs for all citizens?

- Is there a level of care that society should provide to all citizens, with private financing providing all care beyond the set level? Explain.

- What is fair for Mr. Chang?

Racism

Racism is another social concern that affects health. The term race generally refers to an attribute that allows classifications of human beings on the basis of certain biological characteristics (Melville, 1988). Although no racial group of people ascribes to the same cultural beliefs and practices, it is often race that stereotypes a group of people or engenders ethnocentric beliefs and moral conflicts in values. Brown (1991) believes racism is an ethical problem based on inadequate respect, violation of personal boundaries, and an imbalance of power.

Mondragon (1993) and Fowler and Risner (1994) describe how race affects health. African Americans, Hispanics, and Native Americans have the worst health status of American groups according to all public health indicators. In addition, they have the highest rates of risk behaviors for disease. Hunger has increased among these three racial groups. They have poorer cancer survival rates and higher incidences of stroke, hypertension, diabetes, and other problems. In addition, African-Americans and Hispanics have the lowest levels of health insurance and the most inappropriate use of expensive emergency rooms. While socioeconomic conditions contribute to these health conditions, it is easy to discern possible racial influences on health.

There is evidence that the health care system itself is racist (Breton, 2000; Fowler & Risner, 1994; Funkhouser & Moser, 1990; Roberts, 2000; Spigner, 1994). Problems of access and inequity of treatment are frequently cited as evidence of racial bias. In addition, traditional solutions to health problems, such as health education and health promotion programs, do not seem to be programmed for minority groups (Breton, 2000; Mondragon, 1993). More importantly, minority groups tend to demonstrate poorer health outcomes in some areas revealing inadequate health care; for example, the infant mortality rate of African Americans is twice that of the European American population (Hogue & Hargroves, 1993).

There is significant interface of poverty, homelessness, domestic violence, an increasing elderly population, and racism. Poverty underpins homelessness. In addition, the African American living in poverty is more likely to face homelessness (Davis & Winkleby, 1993). African Americans, Native Americans, and Hispanics are overrepresented among the homeless. Women experiencing domestic violence move frequently and often deal with homelessness and poverty as they try to improve their situations (Kanna, Singh, Nemil, & Best, 1992). Goodman (1991) provides data that poverty and homelessness are linked to a high abuse rate, and Campbell (1993) indicates that violence and poverty are linked, at least among African Americans. The elderly are often made homeless as they face mounting health care and living costs on a fixed income. Persons experiencing poverty, homelessness, aging, domestic violence, and racism are vulnerable to poor health and inadequate health care delivery. Often these vulnerable groups are the least powerful and vocal persons in society, yet they are the groups most affected by ethical decisions regarding health (Wessell, 1992).

These social situations represent examples of classism, sexism, and racism. Each indicates prejudice or discrimination against a particular class, gender, or racial group. The implication is that one group of people is held to standards espoused by another group. Statistical data on these social situations, and the health of persons experiencing the social situations, explain why a feeling of helplessness may emerge when social situations are so intrinsically intertwined with health. Yet treating a person's symptoms without attending to the root causes of the problem may be viewed as inadequate health care.

ETHICAL PRINCIPLES APPLIED TO SOCIAL ISSUES

Ethical dilemmas involving classism, sexism, and racism are difficult to resolve. The common principles most essential in unraveling ethical dilemmas encompassing social issues include justice, nonmaleficence, beneficence, and autonomy. A brief discussion of each principle follows.

Justice

Justice is the duty to treat all people fairly without regard to age, socioeconomic status, race, or gender. This implies a fair distribution of the benefits and burdens among members of a society, with equal treatment to all or to those most in need. This could mean extending necessary treatment to those in need, even though they may not have the requisite means to pay for the treatment. A frail elderly gentleman, beloved by his family, might receive an expensive but desired transplant procedure based on justice, even though there is only a moderate chance that the extensive surgery will prolong life or improve the quality of life.

Ask Yourself

Who Should Receive Limited Health Care Resources?

- In this day of declining health care resources, should those with the greatest need or those who have contributed to society receive expensive restorative procedures? Or should these procedures be available to all? Support your position.

Nonmaleficence

Nonmaleficence is the duty to prevent or avoid doing harm, whether intentional or unintentional. This could mean refusing to discharge an abused woman to her home if there is a possibility of further injury. It might also entail ensuring a safe, hygienic environment before hospital release of a newborn infant and mother suffering from poverty or homelessness.

Beneficence

Beneficence is the duty to actively do good for patients. This principle is described by the Council on Ethical and Judicial Affairs of the American Medical Association (1992) as healing, with attention to the psychological, social, and spiritual dimensions of disease or injury as well as the physical problems. Thus, the homeless lady with leg ulcers and diabetes who walks all day and stands in lines in poor shoes and all types of weather to secure free meals and safe sleeping quarters will receive treatment for the leg ulcers that will ensure adequate diet and rest, elevation of the legs, and proper hygiene. Treatment would have to go beyond the usual prescriptions for drugs and address the social conditions contributing to the physical problems.

Autonomy

Autonomy is the patient's right to self-determination without outside control. Related to this principle are the principles of veracity, privacy, confidentiality, and respect for all persons. Little (2000) reminds us that we must develop our sense of autonomy. She suggests that autonomy involves a set of skills that people possess to greater or lesser degrees. These skills often require someone to help us cultivate them, a context that sustains them, and help in exercising them when we are in a vulnerable position. One of the skills is the capacity to think through different options and imagine possibilities. Our social context, however, can get in the way of seeing our options. Autonomy would direct us to work with the abused woman to develop a stronger sense of herself and to help her to see various options and available support. Autonomy would also honor her choice to return home, even if her safety is a concern, continuing to

Think About It

The Impact of Social Conditions on Vulnerable Groups

Consider how social conditions affect other vulnerable groups such as children, people who are mentally or physically disabled or challenged, and people who are institutionalized or incarcerated.

- Discuss the factors that make these populations vulnerable.
- Describe the issues related to these populations that give you concern as a nurse.
- Discuss the ethical concerns related to the needs and care of people in these groups.
- How would you apply principles of justice, nonmaleficence, beneficence, and autonomy to health care concerns with people in each of these groups?

offer support as she struggles with difficult decisions. We must always consider how factors, such as the chronic stress of living with abuse, affect a person's ability to act autonomously (Limandri & Tilden, 1993).

PERSONAL IMPEDIMENTS TO INTERVENING WITH VULNERABLE GROUPS

Working with people who are poor, homeless, experiencing domestic violence, aged, or of a different race requires exploration of personal values to ensure that negative attitudes do not interfere with health care. Price, Desmond, and Eoff (1989) caution that victim blaming is a real phenomenon that can color attitudes and interactions.

Victim Blaming

Victim blaming tends to hold the people burdened by social conditions accountable for their own situations and responsible for needed solutions. Victim blaming is often evident in language. If there is evidence of personal or systemwide victim blaming, a new world view is needed. A desirable world view would see all persons as autonomous beings who deserve to be treated with dignity and fairness. Of interest, the health care system may not be designed to extend the needed degree of autonomy to all people. Nurses and other health care providers are generally educated to take charge and make decisions. Sines (1994) describes how prominent power relationships interfere with therapeutic practice and desirable client outcomes. To respect others by allowing them to make choices and decisions, when they are capable of doing so, requires an attitude of caring with a focus on advocacy. This implies guarding patient rights, preserving patient values, championing social justice in health care, and serving as the conservator of the patient's best interests (Sines, 1994). Reeducating nurses and other providers to enhance the advocate role and foster the needed world view may improve care within a health care agency.

Ask Yourself

How Does Language Reflect One's Values?

How do the values reflected in the language of the following statements imply victim blaming?

- Most young, single, poor women get pregnant to increase their welfare benefits.
- If poor, homeless people would take more responsibility for themselves, they could improve their situation. There are jobs out there for people who want to work.
- The highest calling for a woman is to be the family nurturer.
- If an abused woman wanted help, she would just leave the abusive relationship.

- An important part of assessing for domestic violence is to ask what the woman was doing or if she was drinking right before she was hit.
- Resistance to change is a normal part of aging.
- All five senses tend to decline as a person ages.
- Since most low-income women do not comply with therapies, it is not cost-effective to spend too much time with them on health education.
- What did you expect? Look at how her mother behaved.
- People can get ahead if they take advantage of life's opportunities.

Language of Violence

Another possible impediment to intervention, specifically with the social situation of violence, is the violence mode that colors speech and actions. Ewing (1987) describes how the health care system uses metaphors of violence such as "attacking" germs, "battling" disease, "plotting strategies" against or "defeating" invasive cells and unwanted organisms, and, ultimately, "suffering defeat" or "achieving victory." The prevailing mind set behind this strategy of confrontation is the antithesis of a needed compassionate approach that values nonviolence. This is especially true for women experiencing domestic violence. Language that supports violence can inadvertently lead to victim blaming, or covertly encourage futile and dangerous retaliation. Indeed a first step in effective intervention with those experiencing violence is to create a milieu that emphasizes nonviolence. The message has to be clear that violence of any form is wrong and, generally, illegal. This may necessitate a change in how health care providers approach and work therapeutically with people experiencing violence.

SOCIAL ISSUES AND SCHOLARSHIP

Many health care interventions are based, properly, on research; however, nurses need to ask if the underlying research, and therefore the determined therapy, may create problems based on classism, sexism, and racism. For example, growth and development knowledge is based largely on studies of the experiences of white heterosexual men (Gilligan, 1982). Thus, application of growth and development theory to both genders and to other races requires prudence. Campbell (1993) provides excellent data that knowledge of the abuser in domestic violence situations is based on sex role socialization in European American families and therefore does not explain the violence in African American families. Violence in the African American family, according to Campbell, may be better explained by role conflict, discrimination, isolation, financial stress, and other variables. Demi and Warren (1995) and Vasquez and Eldridge (1994) explore the issues of valid research for vulnerable populations, pointing out that the way family is defined and the systems for recruiting and retaining families contribute to the inability to generalize research findings. In addition, so many of the research instruments in use are not designed for diverse and vulnerable populations.

Spigner (1994) points out that African Americans do not participate as readily in research as European Americans due to the way they are represented in the social structure. Their socioeconomic status and the professional hierarchy often impede African American participation in research studies. Certainly, many intelligence tests are under scrutiny for cultural bias. In addition, research that is less than twenty-five years old has viewed women as inferior to men and nonwhite groups as inferior to whites (Vasquez & Eldridge, 1994). These historical roots have contributed to a dearth of scholarly studies on women and minority populations. This means that classroom teachings and clinical knowledge may be based on inadequate research for minority populations.

There is an ethical responsibility to teach how to provide nursing care to diverse cultural groups. Thus, faculty and students must be cognizant of the benefits of selected interventions for all population groups. In addition, they must be vigilant in generalizing research findings to diverse population groups. Research on vulnerable populations needs to be done to ensure an adequate data base for working with those growing populations that are experiencing social issues such as poverty, homelessness, domestic violence, unhealthy aging, and racism.

SUMMARY

This chapter focused on ethical dilemmas that emerge when health care is considered for vulnerable population groups. Ethical decisions related to health care for vulnerable populations confront nurses who work with those experiencing the social conditions of poverty, homelessness, domestic violence, unhealthy aging, and racism on a daily basis. Since values affect professional behavior, nurses must analyze personally held values as well as those of the health care agency where they are employed for appropriate consideration of justice, beneficence, nonmaleficence, and autonomy. Nurses who work with vulnerable groups need to utilize these principles in ethical decision making. Nurses must consider the impact and validity of health care interventions and research on vulnerable populations, and ensure that what nurses teach both in the classroom and to patients is based on research applicable to the populations being served and studied.

CHAPTER HIGHLIGHTS

- Poverty, homelessness, domestic violence, aging, and racism affect health in a negative fashion. Limited choices and inappropriate treatment options often interfere with the best health care for these vulnerable populations.
- Applying the concept of justice to vulnerable populations can change the way society and the health care system provide health care. Addressing the social conditions of the individual with an illness or disease is basic to health care.
- Nonmaleficence and beneficence may clash with autonomy when providing care for vulnerable populations.
- Victim blaming, evident in covert or overt beliefs that all people are accountable for their own situations and responsible for solutions, interferes with health care delivery for vulnerable populations and is evidence of sexism, classism, or racism.
- Advocacy and caring, which are ways to avoid delivering health care that is

grounded in sexism, classism, and racism, require letting go of the power relationships that often dominate health care delivery.

- Clearing speech patterns and other behaviors of words and actions that are based on violence is a step toward therapeutic interventions with those who experience violence in their lives.

- Findings from research studies may not be applicable to vulnerable populations if the vulnerable are not part of the study population.

DISCUSSION QUESTIONS AND ACTIVITIES

1. Visit a homeless shelter or shelter for abused women. Interview residents about their health and ability to access health care.

2. Spend a few afternoons volunteering in a soup kitchen. Talk with people who come in for free meals about their health problems and ability to secure health care.

3. Spend some time with a home health nurse or Meals-on-Wheels, making contact with the elderly who live at home alone. Explore with them their perceptions of quality of life, health dilemmas, and needs.

4. Work with classmates to develop a "health fair" for the homeless, discussing the value of typical activities and materials made available at traditional fairs, while designing a more relevant approach.

5. How many examples of toys, advertisements, acting roles, literature, childrearing practices, and the like can you identify that continue to perpetuate the woman's role as one of caregiver or sexual object? Discuss how the examples contribute to gender inequity for women.

6. Investigate racial and ethnic disparities in health at: http://www.cdd.gov/nccdphp/cvd/womensatlas and http://www.4woman.gov/minority/index.htm

REFERENCES

American Medical Association. (1992). *Diagnostic and treatment guidelines on domestic violence.* Chicago: Author.

Arcangelo, V. (1994). Should age be a criteria for rationing health care? *Nursing Forum, 29,* 25–29.

Auden, W. H. (1986). In memory of W. B. Yeats. In C. Bain, J. Beaty, & J. P. Hunter, eds., *The Norton introduction to literature* (4th ed.) New York: Norton.

Bohn, D. K. (1990). Domestic violence and pregnancy: Implications for practice. *Journal of Nurse Midwifery, 35,* 86–98.

Breton, J. H. (2000). Treating beyond color: Health issues in minority women. *Advance for Nurse Practitioners,* (November), 65–66, 68, 101.

Brown, L. S. (1991). Antiracism as an ethical imperative: An example from feminist therapy. *Ethics and Behavior, 1,* 113–127.

Burg, M. A. (1994). Health problems of sheltered homeless women and their dependent children. *Health and Social Work, 19,* 125–131.

Butler, S. S., & Weatherley, R. A. (1992). Poor women at midlife and categories of neglect. *Social Work, 37,* 510–515.

Campbell, D. W. (1993). Nursing care of African-American battered women: Afrocentric perspectives. *AWHONNS Clinical Issues in Perinatal and Women's Health Nursing, 4,* 407–415.

Campbell, J. C., Pliska, M. J., Taylor, W., & Sheridan, D. (1994). Battered women's experiences in the emergency department. *Journal of Emergency Nursing, 20,* 280–288.

Catley, C. M. (1992). Global considerations affecting the health agenda of the 1990s, *Academic Medicine, 67,* 419–424.

Council on Ethical and Judicial Affairs, American Medical Association. (1992). Physicians and domestic violence. *Journal of the American Medical Association, 267,* 3190–3193.

Davis, L. A., & Winkleby, M. A. (1993). Socio-demographic and health related risk factors among African American, Caucasian, and Hispanic homeless men: A comparative study. *Journal of Social Distress and the Homeless, 2,* 83–101.

Demi, A. S., & Warren, N. A. (1995). Issues in conducting research with vulnerable families. *Western Journal of Nursing Research, 17,* 188–202.

Diehm, C., & Ross, M. (1988). Battered women. In S. Rix, ed., *The American woman, 1988–1989* (pp. 292–302). New York: Norton.

Eisler, R. (1987). *The chalice and the blade.* San Francisco: Harper & Row.

Esposito, C. N. (1993). Abuse: Breaking the cycle of violence: The victim's perspective. *Trends in Health Care, Law, and Ethics, 8,* 7–11.

Ewing, W. A. (1987). Domestic violence and community health care ethics: Reflections on systemic intervention. *Family and Community Health, 10,* 54–62.

Fishwick, N. (1995). Getting to the heart of the matter: Nursing assessment and intervention with battered women in psychiatric mental health settings. *Journal of the American Psychiatric Nurses Association, 1,* 48–54.

Fowler, B. A., & Risner, P. B. (1994). A health promotion program evaluation in a minority industry. *ABNF Journal, 5,* 72–76.

Funkhouser, S. W., & Moser, D. K. (1990). Is health care racist? *Advances in Nursing Science, 12,* 47–55.

Gilligan, C. (1982). *In a different voice.* Cambridge, MA: Harvard University Press.

Goodman, L. A. (1991). The prevalence of abuse among homeless and housed poor mothers: A comparison study. *American Journal of Ortho Psychiatry, 61,* 489–500.

Hall, C. (1993). Long term care and the minority elderly. *Pride Institute Journal of Long Term Health Care, 12,* 3–8.

Hogue, C. J. R., & Hargroves, M. A. (1993). Class, race and infant mortality in the United States. *American Journal of Public Health, 83,* 20–33.

Kanna, M., Singh, N., Nemil, M., & Best, A. (1992). Homeless women and their families: Characteristics, life circumstances, and needs. *Journal of Child and Family Studies, 1,* 155–165.

Kernic, M. A., Wolf, M. E., & Holt, V. L. (2000). Rates and relative risk of hospital admission among women in violent intimate partner relationships. *American Journal Of Public Health, 90*(9), 1416–1420.

Limandri, B. J., & Tilden, V. P. (1993). Domestic violence: Ethical issues in the health care system. *AWHONNS Clinical Issues in Perinatal and Women's Health Nursing, 4,* 493–502.

Little, M. (2000). Introduction to the ethics of care. Presentation at *New century, new challenges: Intensive bioethics course XXVI,* Kennedy Institute of Ethics, Georgetown University, Washington, DC, June 10, 2000.

MMWR morbidity and mortality weekly report (2000). Prevalence of intimate partner violence and injuries—Washington, 1998. (July 7, 2000), 49 (26), 589–592.

Melville, M. B. (1988). Hispanics: Race, class, or ethnicity? *The Journal of Ethnic Studies, 16*(1), 67–83.

Mondragon, D. (1993). No more "Let them eat admonitions": The Clinton administration's emerging approach to minority health. *Journal of Health Care for the Poor and Underserved, 4,* 77–82.

Price, J. H., Desmond, S. M., & Eoff, T. A. (1989). Nurses' perceptions regarding health care and the poor. *Psychological Reports, 65,* 1043–1052.

Roberts, D. (2000). Race, gender, justice, and reproductive health policy. Presentation at *New century, new challenges: intensive bioethics course XXVI,* Kennedy Institute of Ethics, Georgetown University, Washington, DC, June 9, 2000.

Sines, D. (1994). The arrogance of power. A reflection on contemporary mental health nursing practice. *Journal of Advanced Nursing, 20,* 894–903.

Skaff, M. M., & Pearlin, L. J. (1992). Caregiving: Role engulfment and the loss of self. *Gerontologist, 32,* 656–664.

Spigner, C. (1994). Black participation in health research: A functionalist overview. *Journal of Health Education, 25,* 210–214.

Stark, P. L. (1991). Health care under seige: Challenge for change. *Nursing and Health Care, 12,* 26–30.

Tebb, S. (1995). An aid to empowerment: A caregiver well-being scale. *Health and Social Work, 20,* 87–92.

Vasquez, M. J. T., & Eldridge, N. S. (1994). Bringing ethics alive: Training practitioners about gender, ethnicity, and sexual orientation issues. *Women & Therapy, 15,* 1–6.

Wessell, M. L. (1992). Said another way: An ethical issue for a profession for all seasons. *Nursing Forum, 27,* 29–33.

Windom, E. (1988). An aging nation presents new challenges to the health care system. *Public Health Reports, 103,* 1–2.

CHAPTER 17

Gender Issues

By Sandra L. Cotton

The women must learn to dare to speak,
The men must learn to bother to listen.
The women must learn to say I think this is so.
The men must learn to stop dancing solos on
*   the ceiling.*

(Marge Piercy, 1982)

OBJECTIVES

After completing this chapter, the reader should be able to:

1. Describe historical bases of gender issues in nursing.
2. Discuss the relationship between issues of gender and race.
3. Describe factors associated with and the impact of sex discrimination in nursing.
4. Discuss sexual harassment within a nursing context.
5. Discuss communication issues related to gender.
6. Describe nursing issues related to modern sexism.

INTRODUCTION

In a perfect world, people would consistently relate to each other with mutual respect and empathy. Unfortunately, the reality of our lives is that our interactions are sometimes clouded by prejudice or lack of understanding. The workplace is a common arena for many societal issues to manifest. Issues such as pay equity, employment opportunities, sexual harassment, role strain, and race relations are but a few examples of gender-influenced conflicts that may be encountered in professional relationships. There are two basic approaches to dealing with these social justice issues. We can simply pretend that these issues do not exist. This approach may result in increased frustration as unresolved feelings and issues play out on the job. Alternatively, we can become aware of the issues and define ways to deal with the realities of our society head-on. This chapter focuses on the latter approach and explores issues concerning gender in the nursing workplace.

HISTORICAL PERSPECTIVES AND OVERVIEW OF GENDER-BASED ISSUES

The American Nurses Association (ANA) expanded its definition of nursing from "the diagnosis and treatment of human responses to actual or potential health problems" to include the "application of scientific knowledge, integration of objective data, inclusion of the full range of human experiences, and provision of a caring relationship that facilitates health and healing" (ANA, 1995, p. 6). While some authors contend that most have come to accept the term *nurse* as "a person who cares for or tends to the needs of the sick" (Ellis and Hartley, 1995, p. 6), controversy remains concerning exactly what a person who provides nursing care should be called, and how this relates to the gender of the person providing the care (Bernardi, 1996).

In her comprehensive work, *Woman as Healer,* Achterberg chronicles the journey of women in healing professions. Citing the masculinization of American medicine as one of many issues that challenge nurses, Achterberg states that, although nursing has gained professional status, it suffers because of issues of "nurses' functioning subordinate to multiple layers of authority" (1990, p. 177).

Lewenson (1996) notes that nurses have constantly had to struggle with paternalistic ideology that continues to permeate the profession. **Paternalism** has been defined as "the system, principle, or practice of managing or governing individuals, businesses, or nations, etc. . . . in the manner of a father dealing benevolently and often intrusively with his children" (*Webster's*, 1995). Lewenson contends that paternalism coupled with **nursism**, "a form of sexism that specifically maligns the caring role in society [has led to] discrimination in nursing by virtue of the role undertaken, regardless of gender" (1996, pp. 226, 228).

Societal Expectations

As nursing continues to be a predominantly female profession, societal issues that have affected women have also been reflected in nursing. In a turn-of-the-century commentary entitled *The Hospital Hotel*, nurses were noted for being "well-bred, well-educated specimens of womanhood" (JAMA, 1996, p. 324). Women have been socialized to achieve or be less than they are capable of becoming. This reluctance to achieve is evident in the lack of women in positions of power, especially in the political arena (Hamilton, 1996). Although more recent societal influences have had a positive impact in this regard, nursing is still a female-dominated profession, which unfortunately has a history of oppression that many believe it has yet to overcome.

Ask Yourself

Is There Gender Stereotyping in Nursing?

Survey data indicate that many Americans would approve of nursing as a career choice for their sons (Begany, 1994). Of those opposed to having their sons in nursing, "a nurse should be a woman" was cited as the most frequent response for opposition to the profession.

- In what ways do you think nurses can help dispel this declining but continuing stereotype?
- How would you respond if your son or daughter chose nursing as a profession? Would you encourage him or her? Why or why not?

Authors such as Achterberg (1990), Baldwin (1995), Kane & Thomas (2000), Kavanagh (1996), Lewenson (1996), and Stromberg (1988) believe that nurses have been forced to work within a framework that focuses on societal expectations of women and what is considered women's work. In what has been termed the medicalization of American society, nursing has been forced to overcome the prejudices of a society that has historically embraced the biomedical curative model of health care. As diversified consumers of health care are demanding more sophisticated and culturally congruent care, nurses are in a prime position to provide cost-effective, high-quality care. If nursing is to be successful in this and other arenas, it must concomitantly address issues of territoriality, power, and authority within its own ranks as well as with other health care professionals. A model of interdependence that seeks to create a positive situation for all providers and consumers of care may be most desirable (Baldwin, 1995).

GENDER AND RACE

Issues concerning race are closely linked to gender as they relate to access to educational preparation, employment opportunities, and wage inequities (Amott & Matthaei, 1996; Kavanagh, 1996; Lewenson, 1996). Amott and Matthaei additionally discuss class as it relates to gender and race in their extensive review of *A Multicultural Economic History of Women in the United States*. Based on their conceptual framework that race, gender, and class are intrinsically interconnected, Amott and Matthaei believe that the explanatory power of each concept, in itself, is limited, but together may broaden our understanding of the lives of women who enter nursing. Both Achterberg (1990) and Amott and Matthaei concur that the the takeover of medicine by white men, who forced midwives and other women healers out of health care coincided with the development of nursing.

An increasing number of persons from diverse racial and ethnic backgrounds are joining the nursing profession (National League of Nursing [NLN], 1995). A rich history of the African American nurse experience in the United States is depicted by Lewenson (1996) as she describes the establishment of educational programs for African American nurses in the late 1800s and the forty-three-year history of the National Association of Colored Graduate Nurses (NACGN) (1908–1951). The NACGN eventually integrated with the American Nurses Association (ANA), because the ANA did not discriminate as many state organizations did when African American nurses tried to join.

Racism, the assumption that members of one race are superior to those of another (Kavanagh, 1996) was an everyday experience for African American nurses at the turn of the century. Despite Title VII of the Civil Rights Act of 1964, many African Americans continue to experience racism today. African American nurses are disproportionately employed in institutions that serve African Americans and in public as opposed to private organizations (Stromberg, 1988). Discussion related to transcultural nursing is raising the awareness of nurses working with culturally diverse populations and will potentially improve patient outcomes. Foolchand notes that research efforts need to "move beyond the view that it is sufficient to understand Black people's cultural practices in order to improve service delivery" (1995, p. 104). Foolchand expresses the caution of another educator that too much emphasis placed upon culture may divert "attention away from the central issue of racism in professional institutions and training" (1995, p. 102). Strategies Foolchand identifies for improving racial equality in the nursing profession include incorporating race equality issues in school of nursing curriculums, educating staff in equal opportunities and antiracist strategies, and the recruitment, selection, and career progression of African American faculty. If nursing is a reflection of society at large, issues related to racial inequalities within the broader context of society must also be examined.

SEX DISCRIMINATION IN NURSING

Historically, women have worked for lower pay than their male counterparts. Pay equity is generally protected by state laws. However, issues of comparable worth, which have long been associated with traditionally female-dominated professions such as nursing, have not had the same protection. Salaries in nursing remain low compared with other professions that require comparably high levels of skill, education, and responsibility. Some suspect that men in nursing are raising salaries; however, other economic considerations, such as nursing shortages, fair labor-related legislation, and collective bargaining, may be responsible (Ellis & Hartley, 2001). Although a disparity in earnings, known as a *pay gap*, exists between men and women of many occupations, the gap is considerably narrower for nurses (Reskin & Padovic, 1994). When compared to other occupations, the fact that nurses have historically earned less may account for this lack of difference (Stromberg, 1988). However, the fact that a gap exists at all is striking in that men make up only a small percentage of the nursing profession (Benokraitis & Feagin, 1995). As Gilloran (1995) notes, the development of a patriarchal structure within nursing, with fewer women in senior management positions, may account for this.

According to sociologist Christine Williams (1995), issues of comparable worth are a real concern for nurses. Williams identifies several hidden advantages to being a man in nursing, particularly related to hiring and promotion. Williams's work supports Gilloran's (1995) assertions of gender disequity, as men are typically *tracked* into higher paying and more prestigious positions. Even in a predominantly female profession, women may be experiencing a form of economic gender discrimination.

Gender Issues in Women's Health

Although men may have hidden advantages in nursing, some areas, primarily in women's health, have remained closed (Ketter, 1994). California bans prices based upon gender, for example, for services such as haircuts, dry cleaning, or tailoring ("California Bans Prices," 1995). At the same time the state exempts labor and delivery rooms from state job discrimination laws by upholding a hospital's ban on employing nurses who are men in these areas (Letizia, 1994). California's Fair Employment and Housing Commission cited "invasion of a woman's privacy" as justification for the exemption, but one nurse called it "the most outlandish ruling" she had ever encountered (Thompson, 1995, p. 9).

In court proceedings that addressed this issue, the fact that most obstetricians are male was not deemed analogous to the situation of the nurse who is male (Ketter, 1994). Most courts cited that the doctor was chosen by the patient, while the nurse was not. Several state courts addressed this aspect of gender discrimination; however, none sided with the nurse. Section 703(e)(1) of the Civil Rights Act allows for gender-based discrimination if gender "is a bona fide occupational qualification reasonably necessary to the normal operation of that particular business or enterprise" (Ketter, p. 24). Many men in nursing believe this form of discrimination is reinforced in educational settings when faculty members seek the permission for male student nurses to observe or participate in procedures with female patients, but do not seek the permission of male patients when female students are involved. Some postulate that women are more universally accepted by patients because they are viewed as nurturers (Ellis & Hartley, 2001). Although no data support these assumptions, institutions continue to promote this form of gender discrimination when they proactively provide for the modesty and privacy of their female patients. Some nurses agree with this position, while others do not (Spancraft, 1995; Thompson, 1995).

Expanding Numbers of Men in the Profession

Although the number of men in nursing has increased steadily, men still comprise a relatively small number of all practicing RNs (NLN, 1995). Sullivan (2000) stresses the value of gender diversity in nursing, noting that men play an important role in the profession. Citing societal stereotyping as one of the major limiting factors for men in nursing, Squires (1995) may be categorizing men further when he asserts that health care reform that increases responsibility and autonomy will attract more men to the nursing profession. Perhaps what Williams (1995) perceives as hidden advantages for men in nursing adds some credence to Squires's assertions. Despite these and other stereotypes, Squires considers the lure of nursing to be universal regardless of gender. Noting the challenge, variety, and excitement of nursing, Squires is quick to acknowledge that the road men in nursing have traveled thus far has not been without controversy. One professional organization formed in 1974, the American Assembly for Men in Nursing (AAMN), addresses these issues, with a goal to "encourage men to become nurses, support those men already in nursing, and educate society as to the benefits of male nurses" (AAMN, 2001).

Gender and Caring

Men now comprise over 12 percent of students entering schools of nursing (NLN, 1995). Nursing graduate degree programs also report a steady increase in the number of male students entering their programs (NLN). As the number of men in nursing increases, research directed toward gender-related issues in the profession has begun to emerge (Ekstrom, 1999; Fisher, 1999; Gilloran, 1995; Paterson, Crawford, Saydak, Venkatesh, Tschikota, & Aronowitz, 1995). For example, many authors have focused nursing research on caring as it relates to gender. Although much of this work is in its infancy, research questions related to possible differences in the learning or expression of caring as it relates to the gender of the student, educator, or recipient of care demonstrate the attention these and other issues in nursing has commanded. Recognition of the need to explore gender became evident for Peter and Gallop (1994) in their comparative study designed to examine whether caring uniquely reflected the moral orientation of nursing students. They discovered that differences in caring noted between medical and nursing students appeared to be related to gender differences. A study exploring the relationship between nurse gender and both nurse and patient perceptions of caring found no significant difference in actual caring according to nurse gender (Ekstrom, 1999). However, from both nurse and patient perspectives, expectations of certain nurse caring behaviors were lower for male nurses.

Ironically, a gender bias may already exist in the literature that focuses on caring. Reverby (1987) offers an historical perspective of caring as it relates to women, but does not address any possible implications in relation to the addition of men to the profession. Chinn (1991) devoted an entire anthology to caring, but did not explore gender in relation to caring, except as it related to economic gains (or lack thereof) for male faculty members in male-dominated academic centers. The exclusion of men by Grigsby and Megel (1995) as they explored the caring experiences of nursing faculty is another example of current nursing research that does not include men.

Despite an increased interest in the caring aspect of nursing, Begany (1994) perpetuates a nursing stereotype by equating the positive attribute of caring to images of nurturer or handmaiden. Some men in nursing may already experience a form of gender discrimination with regard to the stereotypical belief that all men in nursing are homosexuals. This stereotype is rooted in gender-based role assumptions, such as Begany's, related to the caring attributes that many perceive as feminine. Because nursing has historically been viewed as "woman's work," men in nursing have been categorized as feminine, and have subsequently been labeled as homosexuals. Even though Williams (1995) found there were hidden advantages in nursing for men, she also discovered that, ironically, these "opportunities . . . may extend only to those who exhibit conventional masculine characteristics, including a heterosexual orientation" (p. 65).

Think About It

Do Men and Women Express Caring in Different Ways?

- What do you think of Begany's (1994) images of caring? What does caring mean to you?
- Williams (1995) believes that organizations are gender biased in how they regard masculine behaviors versus *feminine* ones. She suggests the development of gender-sensitive evaluation tools that would acknowledge women's contributions to the profession. If you were appointed to develop such an evaluation tool, what attributes would your tool reward and recognize as unique to women? What justice issues may be involved in using gender-sensitive evaluation processes?
- Goals of the American Assembly for Men in Nursing include supporting men already in nursing and educating society about the benefits of male nurses. What do you think are the benefits of nurses who are men? How do these differ from the benefits of nurses who are women?

As more men enter the profession, additional gender issues may be identified. For example, once in the workforce, men in nursing may experience difficulty when cross-gender mentoring relationships exist (Feist-Price, 1994). Feist-Price notes several potential adversities in cross-gender mentoring relationships, mainly related to communication differences between men and women (Tannen, 1990). Feist-Price further notes that cross-gender mentoring relationships have successful outcomes, especially when formal mechanisms are in place to deal with issues as they arise. One implication for nursing may be in the area of caring. If differences in the development or expression of caring in male nurses indeed exist, these and other differences need to be recognized and utilized to improve the practice of nursing.

SEXUAL HARASSMENT IN NURSING

Bullough (1990) describes Florence Nightingale's encounters with harassment and the prevailing strategy of the day "to gain respect" through being a lady (Nightingale,

1859). Bullough contends that sexual harassment has been a dominant theme in American nursing. The Equal Employment Opportunity Commission (EEOC) has defined **sexual harassment** as "all unwelcome sexual advances, request for sexual favors, and other conduct of a sexual nature when (1) submission to such conduct is made a condition of a woman's employment or academic advancement; (2) submission to or rejection of such conduct by a woman is used as a basis for employment decisions or academic decisions affecting the individual; or (3) such conduct has the purpose or effect of unreasonably interfering with a woman's work or academic performance or creating an intimidating work environment" (Benokraitis & Feagin, 1995, p. 73). Nurses may not immediately recognize or label behaviors as sexual harassment, and often have difficulty finding appropriate words to describe the experience concisely (Madison & Minichiello, 2000). Indicators of sexual harassment identified by these authors include:

- Invasion of space—the harasser enters your personal space or corners you
- Lack of respect—the harasser's past or present behavior is deemed disrespectful
- Overtly friendly behavior—that which feels too friendly
- Deliberative nature of behavior—that which is planned or intentional
- Confirmation—your suspicions of harassment are confirmed by another
- Perceived power or control—physical or organizational power that supports or protects the harasser while limiting the options of the harassed
- Sexualized workplace—where explicit jokes, innuendos, pictures are common

Bullough suggests that nurses need to employ specific strategies to combat sexual harassment. The National Organization for Women (NOW) recommends being assertive, seeking support from other workers, keeping a diary to document each incident, filing a complaint or grievance, keeping performance documents, seeking counseling, initiating legal action, and seeking a new job as strategies to deal with sexual harassment on the job (NOW, 1993).

Ask Yourself

Women's Rights

The National Organization for Women (NOW) is the largest women's rights organization in the country, actively working to achieve full and meaningful equality for all women.

- How do issues of women's rights relate to nursing?
- What issues remain for women in the nursing profession?
- How do these issues differ from issues that may impact men in the nursing profession?

We do not need to venture far to find images that reinforce the view that nurses are sexual objects. A quick tour of the *get well* section at your local greeting card shop graphically illustrates this point. Although sexual harassment does not recognize gender boundaries, clearly sexual harassment has historically been the bane of women. As more men enter the nursing profession, issues concerning sexual harassment directed toward them or from them may emerge. Research is needed that is directed toward understanding issues concerning sexual harassment in nursing, how best to address the needs of men in nursing, and implications for the women with whom they work.

COMMUNICATION ISSUES RELATED TO GENDER

How nurses communicate with each other, their patients, and their colleagues has long been discussed in the nursing literature (Campbell-Heider & Hart, 1993; Sweet & Norman, 1995; Corser, 1998). Nurses need to address how changing societal roles and expectations relate to the practice of nursing, and what research is needed to promote and bring about positive change.

The Doctor-Nurse Game

A gender division of labor has been a significant factor in how nurses, who are primarily women, and physicians, who are primarily men, relate to each other in health care settings. Initially described as the *doctor-nurse game* (Stein, 1967), issues regarding communication with physicians remain an area of primary concern for many nurses (Anderson, Maloney, Oliver, Brown, & Hardy, 1996). Favorable patient outcomes have been positively associated with successful nurse-physician communication (Shortell, Zimmerman, Rousseau, Gillies, Wagner, Draper, Knaus, & Duffy, 1994; Zimmerman, Shortell, Rousseau, Duffy, Gillies, Knaus, Devers, Wagner, & Draper, 1993).

Many nurses still use less than straightforward methods to manage conflict among themselves or between nurses and physician colleagues (Valentine, 1995). Valentine indicates that staff nurses are most comfortable using avoidance, while nurse managers tend to use compromise as their primary method of conflict management. These methods may be reinforced by nursing educators, whom Valentine found also employed avoidance as their primary conflict management tool. According to Tannen (1990), the primary reason for these and other communication conflicts relates to identifying and understanding gender differences in communication. Previously linked to societal roles and expectations of women, the "doctor-nurse game" was re-examined by Stein, Watts, and Howell (1990). The authors found that a more humanistic public image of physicians and the increasing numbers of female physicians and male nurses have generally improved physician-nurse relations.

Think About It

Do Men and Women Communicate Differently?

Tannen (1990) asserts that men and women communicate from such differing frames of reference that their communication could be considered a cultural clash of sorts.

- What has your experience been in this area?
- What communication concerns with fellow students, faculty, patients, or physicians have you experienced in your program of study?
- How would you rate the nurse-physician communication in your clinical agencies? Describe why.
- Describe potential gender based differences in communication.

With females comprising nearly 50 percent of students entering medicine, and males comprising 12 percent of students entering nursing school, perhaps the patriarchal system of health care will shift. The implications this may have for nursing remain unknown. Several studies focus on the traditional nurse-doctor relationship. None to date have examined the interactions of nurses, male or female, with physicians who are female.

Communicating with Patients

Through informal dress and communications, nurses may in fact be sending powerful negative messages to their patients and medical colleagues (Campbell-Heider & Hart, 1993). The bedside manner of nurses is discussed by these authors, who note that the tone of familiarity expressed by nurses who use their first names with patients may translate sociologically into persistent stereotypic themes and become a mechanism of social control. While superior nursing care may reduce these stereotypes, Campbell-Heider and Hart discuss the role of deliberative communications strategies, both verbal and nonverbal, in accelerating professional recognition.

Successful interpersonal communications with patients is central to the practice of nursing. In relation to sensitive issues and sexuality, Propst (1996) found that registered nurses' communication practices are lacking. Only half of the respondents in her sample of women's health nurses discussed issues concerning sexuality with their patients. Even in a specialty practice area, such as women's health, nurses are not immune to communication issues when sensitive topics are involved.

Gossip

Another area of communication related to gender involves the use of gossip. Laing proposes that gossip, as viewed from a feminist perspective, plays an important role in the socialization process of nurses. Discussed as a legitimate form of communication, gossip has many purposes and serves many functions. In the context of nurses, Laing believes that gossip may be a critical variable when defined as a "healing form of communication derived from trust which only develops over time" (1993, p. 40). Laing does not explore implications for men in nursing; she is quick to note that, although gossip is primarily associated with women, both sexes engage in gossip, often about similar topics.

MODERN SEXISM

Even though women have made tremendous inroads in the workplace, Benokraitis and Feagin (1995) report that sex inequality is still a major problem. In fact, it may be on the rise in some areas. **Sexism** is "the assumption that members of one sex are superior to those of the other" (Kavanagh, 1996, p. 296). In our predominantly male-oriented health care system, issues concerning sexism may evidence themselves in power struggles for reimbursement, as nurses take on advanced practice roles (Baldwin, 1995). Unfortunately, even within the nursing profession, issues of sexism related to men in nursing are present. An example of this is the male colleague who feels he has a hiring edge over women in nursing, because he never needs to be off for maternity leave or stay home from work to care for sick children.

Ask Yourself

Are Male Nurses Perceived as More Competent?

Benokraitis and Feagin (1995) interviewed male nurses. The authors report that physicians view male nurses as more competent than their female counterparts. They also found that female nurses were often ignored, whereas male nurses' opinions were valued.

- Have you observed this behavior in your clinical or classroom settings?
- How could you best deal with this form of modern sexism?

Heterosexism is "the assumption that everyone is or should be heterosexual, and that heterosexuality is superior and expectable" (Kavanagh, 1996, p. 296). We must be alert for this form of sexism directed toward patients and some nurses (Stevens, 1995; Williams, 1995). Van Ooijen and Charnock (1995) note that very little attention is given to addressing this and other gender issues within the nursing curriculum, despite the belief that developing an understanding of these issues may have a tremendous effect upon nursing care.

SEXUAL ORIENTATION

Lesbians and gay men may be the largest minority group in nursing. Although nobody knows exactly how many of the nearly 2 million nurses in America are lesbian or gay, there are probably between 100,000 and 200,000 (Zurlinden, 1997). These nurses are likely to be practicing in every state and working in every hospital. Fearing sexual harassment and discrimination from coworkers, superiors, and bureaucratic systems, many remain reluctant to have their sexual orientation known.

Sexual harassment and bigotry is a fact of life for many lesbians and gay men. Twenty-five years after the birth of the modern gay rights movement, a poll in *Time* magazine revealed that 52 percent of respondents consider same-gender relationships between consenting adults to be morally wrong (Henry, 1994). This culturally prevalent attitude can range from prejudice to homophobia. Prejudice that is operationalized on the institutional level leads to discrimination. More extreme forms of bigotry include harassment and physical violence. Zurlinden (1997) writes, "Unmasked, homophobia is really hatred, willful ignorance, mean-spiritedness, and narrow-mindedness. People suffering from homophobia do not run screaming in terror when they encounter a lesbian or gay man. Instead, they assume they are justified to be cruel; to discriminate in housing, employment, and education; and to pass laws to prevent gay men and lesbians from enjoying the civil liberties that other Americans take for granted" (p. 11).

Within institutions, bigotry can be insidious, damaging, and difficult to change. Some employers systematically discriminate against lesbians and gay men through hiring, promotion, and disciplinary practices. This may be the result of institutional policy (as in the military), discriminatory administrative practice, punitive supervisors, or discrimination by coworkers (Zurlinden, 1997). Discrimination may also take the form of absence of employment benefits available to heterosexuals. Though a few university hospitals have agreed to extend spousal benefits such as health insurance, life insurance, and maternity leave to same-gender couples, these are not available in most institutions.

There are also legal implications for nurses who are gay or lesbian. Nearly half of all states still have laws that forbid particular types of sexual relationships, including same-gender sex. In some states, lesbian and gay men may risk losing their nursing licenses. Being accused of a felony is enough to lead to suspension of a nurse's license in some states; conviction can lead to permanent loss of license (Zurlinden, 1997). Additionally, a number of state boards of nursing have provisions that require "good moral character" to retain a nursing license (National Council of State Boards of Nursing, 1992). This policy is potentially troublesome, in that many consider same-gender relationships to be morally wrong.

Though discriminatory practices remain, most health care professions have publicly endorsed a nonjudgmental attitude toward sexual orientation. The American Nurses Association (ANA), American Psychiatric Association, American Psychological Association, National Association of Social Workers, and the American Medical Association all include statements related to nonjudgmental recognition of sexual orientation (Zurlinden, 1997). Additionally, the ANA *Code of Ethics for Nurses* (2001) promotes the nondiscriminatory practice of nursing.

SUMMARY

Nursing has been faced with gender issues since the early days of the profession. Nursing role and status has been colored by societal expectations of women and paternalistic ideology permeating the health care arena. Considerations of gender can be related to lower salaries for nurses compared with primarily male professions, communication patterns with physicians and patients, perceptions of abilities to carry out nursing's caring imperative, and stereotypical expectations of how nurses should look and act. While men in the profession face the challenge of dealing with societal stereotypes, they are also often tracked into higher paying and more prestigious positions. Issues concerning discrimination based on sexual orientation occur on many fronts and may be underrecognized. Awareness of these issues enables nurses of both genders to be alert for inequities and to develop strategies for change.

CHAPTER HIGHLIGHTS

- Controversy exists regarding how the title of the person caring for the sick relates to the gender of the person providing care. Both women and men in nursing must deal with social stereotyping regarding expected roles and behaviors.

- Societal expectations of women and paternalistic ideology throughout history have led to discrimination in nursing, though gender discrimination may exist for both women and men in different nursing settings.

- Issues concerning race and gender are closely related and must be addressed in nursing.

- Issues of comparable worth relative to gender are of concern in nursing, particularly in areas of salary and positions of prestige and responsibility.

- Nurses need to be alert to and employ strategies to combat sexual harassment.

- Gender-based differences in styles and patterns of communication can affect all areas of nursing practice, requiring attentiveness to effective communication with patients and colleagues in order to foster better patient outcomes.

- Sexism, occurring in both subtle and overt ways, continues to be an issue in nursing, and harassment and discrimination based on sexual orientation may be underrecognized.

DISCUSSION QUESTIONS AND ACTIVITIES

1. One frequently-cited political action strategy is to build coalitions with "powerful persons of like mind" (Hamilton, 1996). If nurses in your community are to become empowered, with whom would they build coalitions?

2. Considering Foolchand's (1995) strategies, in what ways does your school or curriculum address issues of improving racial equality in the nursing profession?

3. Patterson et al. (1995) discuss ways in which nursing students who are males learn to care. Read an article on how nursing students learn to care. Do men learn about, or express caring, differently than women? How does this relate to your experiences as a student nurse? How does this relate to Begany's (1994) images of nurturer or handmaiden?

4. What stereotypes of nurses are present in your community or national media? What types of *get well* cards are in your local card shop? What do you think it will take to change these and other stereotypes about nurses?

5. What is the gender makeup of your local nursing administration? How many women are in positions of authority or power within your health care setting?

What are their salary ranges? How do their salaries compare with men in positions of similar responsibility?

6. Observe gender based communication patterns between nurses and physicians. Consider your own style of communication with same gender and other gender friends and colleagues. What patterns do you identify? How might these patterns affect your professional interactions? Are there areas that need to be modified in order to promote more effective communication?

7. Explore various web sites to determine guidelines regarding sexual harassment that are offered by the American Nurse's Association, the Canadian Nurses Association, and other professional organizations. http://www.cna-nurses.ca and http://www.ana.org

REFERENCES

Achterberg, J. (1990). *Woman as healer*. Boston, MA: Shambhala.

American Assembly for Men in Nursing. (2001). *Membership* [Brochure]. Pensacola, FL: Author. (www.AAMN.org)

American Nurses Association. (2001). *Code of ethics for nurses*. Kansas City, MO: Author.

American Nurses Association. (1995). *Nursing's social policy statement* [Brochure]. Washington, DC: Author.

Amott, T., & Matthaei, J. (1996). *Race, gender, and work; A multicultural economic history of women in the United States* (2nd ed.). Boston: South End Press

Anderson, F., Maloney, J., Oliver, D., Brown, D., & Hardy, M. (1996). Nurse-physician communication: Perceptions of nurses at an army medical center. *Military Medicine, 161,* 411–415.

Baldwin, D. (1995). Territoriality and power in the health professions. In Final report of the Council on Graduate Medical Education, National Advisory Council on Nurse Education and Practice, *Report on primary care workforce projections* (pp. 1–36). Washington, DC: U.S. Department of Health and Human Services.

Begany, T. (1994). Your image is brighter than ever. *RN, 57,* 28–35.

Benokraitis, N. V., & Feagin, J. R. (1995). *Modern sexism: Blatant, subtle, and covert discrimination* (2nd ed.). Englewood Cliffs, NJ: Prentice-Hall.

Bernardi, A. (1996, Winter). Untitled. [Letter to the editor]. Interaction, *Newsletter of the American Assembly for Men in Nursing*, p. 3.

Bullough, V. (1990). Nightingale, nursing, and harassment. *Image, 22,* 4–7.

California bans prices based on gender. (1995, October 14). *The Dominion Post*, p. A2.

Campbell-Heider, N., & Hart, C. (1993). Updating the nurse's bedside manner. *Image, 25,* 133–139.

Chinn, P. L. (1991). *Anthology on caring*. New York: National League of Nursing Press.

Corser, W. D. (1998). A conceptual model of collaborative nurse-physician interactions: The management of traditional influences and personal tendencies. *Scholarly Inquiry for Nursing Practice, 12*(4), 343–346.

Ekstrom, D. N. (1999). Gender and perceived caring in nurse-patient dyads. *Journal of Advanced Nursing, 29*(6), 1393–1401.

Ellis, J., & Hartley, C. (2001). *Nursing in today's world* (7th ed.). Philadelphia, PA: Lippincott.

Feist-Price, S. (1994). Cross-gender mentoring relationships: Critical issues. *Journal of Rehabilitation, 60*, 13–17.

Fisher, M. (1999). Sex role characteristics of males in nursing. *Contemporary Nursing, 8*(3), 65–71.

Foolchand, M. (1995). Promoting racial equality in the nursing curriculum. *Nurse Education Today, 15*, 101–105.

Gilloran, A. (1995). Gender differences in care delivery and supervisory relationship: The case of psychogeriatric nursing. *Journal of Advanced Nursing, 21*, 652–658.

Grigsby, K., & Megel, M. (1995). Caring experiences of nurse educators. *Journal of Nursing Education, 34*, 411–418.

Hamilton, P. (1996). *Realities of contemporary nursing*. Menlo Park, CA: Addison-Wesley.

Henry, W. (1994, June 17). Pride and prejudice. *Time, 143*(26), 57–59.

JAMA (1996). The hospital hotel. *Journal of the American Medical Association, 275*, 324.

Kane, D & Thomas, B. (2000). Nursing and the "F" word. *Nursing Forum, 35*(2), 17–24.

Kavanagh, K. (1996). Social and cultural dimensions of health and health care. In J. Creasia & B. Parker, eds., *Conceptual foundations of nursing practice* (pp. 285–308). St. Louis, MO: Mosby.

Ketter, J. (1994, April). Sex discrimination targets men in some hospitals. *The American Nurse, 26*, 1, 24.

Laing, M. (1993). Gossip: Does it play a role in the socialization of nurses? *Image, 25*, 37–43.

Letizia, B. (1994, December). Ban on male nurses in labor and delivery is upheld. *RN, 57*, 16.

Lewenson. (1996). *Taking charge: Nursing suffrage & feminism in America, 1873–1920*. New York: National League of Nursing Press.

Madison, J & Minichiello, V. (2000). Recognizing and labeling sex-based and sexual harassment in the health care workplace. *Journal of Nursing Scholarship, 32*(4), 405–410.

National Council of State Boards of Nursing. (1992). *Profiles of member board: 1992*. Chicago: Author.

National League of Nursing (1995). 1995 *Nursing data review; NLN division of research*. New York: Author.

National Organization for Women. (1993). *Sexual harassment survival skills* [Brochure]. Morgantown, WV: Author.

Nightingale, F. (1859/1992). *Notes on nursing: What it is, and what it is not*. London: Harrison & Sons.

Paterson, B., Crawford, M., Saydak, M., Venkatesh, P., Tschikota, S., & Aronowitz, T. (1995). How male nursing students learn to care. *Journal of Advanced Nursing, 22*, 600–609.

Peter, E., & Gallop, R. (1994). The ethic of care: A comparison of nursing and medical students. *Image, 26*, 47–51.

Piercy, M. (1982). Councils. *Circles on the water*. New York: Knopf.

Propst, M. (1996). Registered nurses' practice and perspective toward sexuality in women's health. *Southern Nursing Research Society Abstracts*, 83.

Reskin, B., & Padavic, I. (1994). *Women and men at work*. Thousand Oaks, CA: Pine Forge Press.

Reverby, S. (1987). A caring dilemma: Womanhood and nursing in historical perspective. *Nursing Research, 36*, 5–10.

Shortell, S., Zimmerman, J., Rousseau, D., Gillies, R., Wagner, D., Draper, E., Knaus, W., & Duffy,

J. (1994). The performance of intensive care units: Does good management make a difference? *Medical Care, 32,* 508–525.

Spancraft, E. (1995, February). Banning male RNs from L & D is blatantly unfair [Letter to the editor]. *RN, 58,* 9.

Squires, T. (1995). Men in nursing. *RN, 58,* 26–28.

Stein, L. (1967). The nurse-doctor game. *Archives of General Psychiatry, 16,* 699–703.

Stein, L., Watts, D., & Howell, T. (1990). The doctor-nurse game revisited. *New England Journal of Medicine, 322,* 546–549.

Stevens, P. (1995). Structural and interpersonal impact of heterosexual assumptions on lesbian health care clients. *Nursing Research, 44,* 25–30.

Stromberg, A. (1988). Women in female-dominated professions. In A. Stromberg & S. Harkess, eds., *Women working: Theories, and facts in perspective* (pp. 206–224). Mountain View, CA: Mayfield.

Sullivan, E. J. (2000). Men in nursing: The importance of gender diversity. *Journal of Professional Nursing, 16*(5), 253–254.

Sweet, S., & Norman, I. (1995). The nurse-doctor relationship: A selective literature review. *Journal of Advanced Nursing, 22,* 165–170.

Tannen, D. (1990). *You just don't understand: Women and men in conversation.* New York: Ballantine.

Thompson, J. (1995, February). Banning male RNs from L & D is blatantly unfair [Letter to the editor]. *RN, 58,* 9.

Valentine, P. (1995). Management of conflict: Do nurses/women handle it differently? *Journal of Advanced Nursing, 22,* 142–149.

van Ooijen, E., & Charnock, A. (1995). How men and women view the world: A sexual perspective. *Nursing Times, 91,* 38–39.

Webster's college dictionary (1995). New York: Random House.

Williams, C. (1995). Hidden advantages for men in nursing. *Nursing Administration Quarterly, 19,* 63–70.

Zimmerman, J., Shortell, S., Rousseau, D., Duffy, J., Gillies, R., Knaus, W., Devers, K., Wagner, D., & Draper, E. (1993). Improving intensive care: Observations based on organizational case studies in nine intensive care units. *Critical Care Medicine, 21,* 1443–1451.

Zurlinden, J. (1997). *Lesbian and gay nurses.* Albany, NY: Delmar.

CHAPTER 18

Transcultural and Spiritual Issues

Written in collaboration with Mary Gail Nagai-Jacobson

> *God is a spirit, a mystery beyond human understanding, and therefore we can only approach that mystery through metaphor. Our metaphors come, of course, from human and cultural understandings of the good, the loving, the just. . . . More surely than anything else, we are defined by our stories—the cultural myths we hear from our earliest days.*
>
> **(Sewell, 1991, pp. 237, 261)**

OBJECTIVES

At the end of this chapter, the reader should be able to:

1. Describe factors associated with cultural sensitivity within nursing.

2. Discuss the influence of culture on health and health care decisions.

3. Identify approaches for dealing with transcultural issues in nursing.

4. Discuss issues related to the use of complementary therapies by patients.

5. Identify legal considerations related to transcultural issues.

6. Discuss the relationship between spirituality and health.

7. Describe issues associated with spirituality and religion.

8. Identify the nursing role in addressing patients' spiritual concerns.

9. Discuss considerations regarding nurturing one's spirit.

INTRODUCTION

The influence of culture, religion, and spirituality are major factors in the development of values. Because nurses deal with people from varied cultural and spiritual backgrounds, they must be alert for issues relating to these areas. This chapter presents general considerations regarding culture and spirituality and discusses related issues that may arise when caring for patients.

TRANSCULTURAL ISSUES

We live in a multicultural society, alive with diversity. Such diversity of people and backgrounds provides a richness to our lives, yet challenges our abilities to appreciate, rather than judge or fear, differences. **Diversity** is encountered wherever there are differences, whether these be gender, age, socioeconomic position, sexual orientation, health status, ethnicity, race, or culture (Kavanagh, 1993). Dealing with diversity is an essential component of nursing care. Nurses need competence in providing culturally appropriate care. **Cultural competence** (Waters, 1996; Engebretson & Headley, 2000) includes **cultural awareness**—knowledge about values, beliefs, behaviors, and the like of cultures other than one's own—and **cultural sensitivity**—the ability to incorporate the patient's cultural perspective into nursing assessments and to modify nursing care in order to be as congruent as possible with the patient's cultural perspective.

The same phenomenon may be viewed differently by people from different cultures, because culture teaches us to understand a perception of reality. For example, the *man in the moon* that most people in this country have been taught to "see" is identified in other cultures as a *frog in the moon, a woman in the moon,* or a *rabbit in the moon* (Tafoya, 1996). Another way of appreciating different perspectives is to consider what we see when we are in the valley, compared with what we see from halfway up the mountain or the view from the top of the mountain. Different perceptions of the same reality derive from the perspectives from which it is viewed. One view of reality is not more correct than the other; the different views merely come from different perspectives.

Ask Yourself

How Do You Deal with Diversity?

Consider a situation in which you were afraid of or judged someone you did not know because she or he was different from you.

- What about the person or situation triggered your judgment or fear?
- Why do you think you reacted to the person or situation the way you did?
- How and from whom did you learn to react in this way?
- What has helped you to understand diversity and overcome fear?
- How can nurses learn to appreciate rather than fear diversity among colleagues and patients?

Understanding Culture

Self-awareness is a key factor in dealing with transcultural issues. The best starting point for becoming sensitive to the culture of another is to understand our own culture and its influence on our perceptions and behaviors. **Culture** refers to the total lifeways of a group of interacting individuals, consisting of learned patterns of values, beliefs, behaviors, and customs shared by that group (Tripp-Reimer, 1987; Engebretson & Headley, 2000; Hopkins, 1997). These *learned patterns* are transmitted from one generation to the next in formal ways, such as through educational settings, and in informal ways, such as through role modeling. Unique cultural expressions can be observed within many groups of interacting individuals—for example, the culture of the deaf community, prison culture, or the culture of health care. We need to recognize that each of us is part of a culture and to identify values, beliefs, and behaviors that we hold dear, as these reflect our own cultural perspective. In this process we each must be alert to our own **ethnocentrism,** reflected in the tendency to judge behaviors of someone from another culture by the standards of our own culture.

In its *Position Statement on Cultural Diversity in Nursing Practice,* the American Nurses Association (ANA) (1991) stated that ethnocentric approaches to nursing practice were ineffective in meeting health and nursing needs of diverse cultural groups, and encouraged nurses in all settings to be knowledgeable about cultures and their impact on interactions with health care. Nurses must develop cultural sensitivity, which implies understanding behaviors and values of another culture within the context of that culture, without imposing our own cultural values on others. In this process we must avoid **stereotyping,** which is expecting all persons from a particular group to behave, think, or respond in a certain way based on preconceived ideas. Every culture contains variation, and some people within the group may not ascribe to all beliefs and values attributed to that culture.

Ask Yourself

How Might Ethnocentrism Affect Nursing Care?

Consider the varied meanings the following behaviors may have depending upon the cultural context in which they occur: direct eye contact may connote honesty or intrusion; a firm handshake may be viewed as confidence or hostility; and frequent bathing may be considered to be necessary or unhealthy.

- How might behaviors such as these be judged by people within the dominant culture in this country?

- How do practices and expectations within health care settings reflect ethnocentrism regarding behaviors such as these?

- How might ethnocentrism or stereotyping affect interaction with others, especially within a nursing setting?

Cultural Values and Beliefs

Because culture is one of the key organizing concepts of nursing, nurses need to be knowledgeable about:

> how cultural groups understand life processes; how cultural groups define health and illness; what cultural groups do to maintain wellness; what cultural groups believe to be the causes of illness; how healers cure and care for members of cultural groups; and how the cultural background of the nurse influences the way in which care is delivered. (ANA, 1991)

Cultural values and beliefs guide our thinking, being, and doing in patterned ways. Beliefs about health and practices related to health and healing are some of the patterns influenced by culture that are significant in providing health care. Such beliefs and practices manifest in both direct and subtle ways, and sensitivity to them can affect patient outcomes and satisfaction with care. It is helpful to recognize a distinction between **disease,** which is the biomedical explanation of sickness, and **illness,** which is a personal response to the disease flowing from how our culture teaches us to be sick (Burkhardt, 1985; Tafoya, 1996). Transcultural issues are often present in nursing situations, but may not be identified as such. Instead, patients may be labeled as stoic, uncooperative, noncompliant, strange, or "crazy" because of choices they make, and their health and care may be compromised. Leininger (1991) has delineated principles of transcultural care, human rights, and ethical considerations that offer guidance for nurses in dealing with transcultural issues, which are listed in Figure 18–1. Although she offers, these principles as a guide particularly for transcultural nurses, they apply as well to other nurses. In light of these principles, many nursing practices derived from the Western biomedical model may benefit from reevaluation.

Figure 18–1 **Transcultural Care Principles, Human Rights, and Ethical Considerations**

1. Human beings of any culture in the world have a right to have their cultural care values known, respected and appropriately used in nursing and other health care services.
2. Human cultures have diverse and universal modes of caring and healing practices that need to be recognized and used by professional nurses to function effectively and therapeutically with people of different cultures.
3. Care is the essence of nursing and a basic human need for growth, healing, well-being, recovery, and survival.
4. Cultural care is a critical component influencing human health, well-being, and recovery from illnesses or disabilities.
5. Every culture has at least two major types of health care systems namely, the *folk (generic, lay or indigenous) care system* and the *professional care system* which influences their health outcomes, and the transcultural nurse is

challenged to use this knowledge to guide nursing care decisions and actions.

6. All professional nurses are challenged to respect common human needs and humanistic aspects of people care worldwide, and also the divergent care expressions, meaning, and practices.

7. Transcultural nurses are expected to respect Western and non-Western cultures who often have different values, beliefs, and norms to assess and understand human beings.

8. Transcultural nursing principles and practices are the arching framework for all nursing care practices which differ from nursing practices that rely on traditional medical symptoms, diseases and treatment regimes.

9. Since transcultural nursing focuses upon *comparative cultural care* values, beliefs and practices of cultures, the nurse is expected to work with individuals, families, groups, cultures, subcultures and institutions that reflect cultural care variabilities.

10. Nurses with transcultural knowledge are expected to respond appropriately to *culture care differences* and *similarities* in order to ease or ameliorate a human condition or lifeway, and to help clients face death.

11. Ethical and moral differences and similarities exist among human cultures which necessitates that nurses recognize, respect and respond appropriately to such variabilities.

12. It is essential that transcultural nurses be open-minded and willing to learn from cultural informants about their human values, beliefs, needs and practices in order to make appropriate nursing care plans, judgments and actions.

13. The ability of the nurse to listen, use silence and envision the client's or family's human condition or cultural circumstance with its positive or less positive features is important in transcultural nursing.

14. Transcultural nursing often requires that nurses communicate with clients in their native language to know, learn and understand individuals, families and groups of different cultures.

15. Transcultural nurses are challenged to identify what constitutes ethical or moral principles and norms of cultures and not assume that all cultures are alike.

16. Transcultural nurses are expected to guide other nurses who have not been prepared in transcultural nursing in order to prevent marked ethnocentrism, cultural imposition practices, and inappropriate ethical and moral judgments about clients.

17. Transcultural nursing reflects that an individual or group of a designated culture are active participants and decision-makers in culture care practices in order to develop and maintain creative and effective professional care practices.

18. Clients of diverse or similar cultures have a right to have their caring life styles and expressions known and used in transcultural nursing in order to promote client health or well-being.

19. Transcultural nursing takes into account the world view, environmental context, ethnohistory, social structure features (including the religious, kinship, philosophic, economic, political, technological and cultural values), language, expressions, gender and age difference of people.

20. Transcultural nursing is concerned with the assessment of caregiver and carereceiver expressions, beliefs and lifeways that often go beyond nurse-client dyadic relationship to that of care relationships with families, groups, institutions and communities in order to facilitate congruent care practices and to avoid unfavorable culture care conflicts, stress and negligent care practices.

21. Since ethical, moral and legal systems of human values, and rights exist in all cultures, it is the task and responsibility of transcultural nurses to discover these dimensions with key and general informants and in diverse cultural contexts.

22. Human care rights tend to be covert and embedded in social structure, cultural values and world view of clients, and so the transcultural nurse is challenged to discover these dimensions mainly through qualitative research methods.

23. Transcultural nurses recognize that cultures are complex, dynamic and change over time and in varying ways.

24. Transcultural nurses recognize that many cultures and subcultures in the world have not been studied and yet nurses are expected to care for all peoples including minorities.

25. Transcultural nursing is a major breakthrough for new nursing knowledge and practices that do not follow the traditional nursing or medical disease, symptom and illness models.

Leininger, M. (1991). *Journal of Transcultural Nursing, 3,* 21–23. Reprinted with permission of the *Journal of Transcultural Nursing.*

Incorporating cultural assessment into care with patients is an important part of a comprehensive nursing assessment. This assessment facilitates better understanding of sometimes overlooked factors that influence health behaviors and decisions. Cultural assessment helps nurses to appropriately identify and understand the meaning of behaviors that might otherwise be judged negatively or be confusing to the nurse (Giger and Davidhizar, 1999; Engebretson & Headley, 2000; Breton, 2000). We must recognize that each person is culturally unique, and that not all persons in a particular cultural group believe or respond the same way. Cultural assessment includes exploration of six cultural phenomena that are evident in all cultural groups: communication, space, social organization, time, environmental control, and biological variation (Giger & Davidhizar, 1999; Engebretson & Headley, 2000). Such exploration enables nurses to identify areas where modifications in care can be incorporated so that care is more culturally congruent. Although the process may also reveal divergent beliefs that are difficult to accommodate within the current health care system, acknowledging differences may help the patient and family to feel more comfortable within the system. For example, when assessing eating patterns and food preferences, the nurse might discover that the patient commonly eats only two meals a day, consisting of burritos in the morning and rice and beans in the evening. Typical hospital food and a three-meals-a-day pattern might not be appetizing for this patient. The patient's nutrition may suffer, and she may perceive that she is not being fed. By arranging for the patient to have culturally similar foods at similar times, the nurse provides more culturally congruent care.

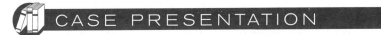

CASE PRESENTATION

Cultural Differences

Brenda White is a home health nurse caring for seventy-two-year old Mrs. Cortez, who is living with her daughter and family while recovering from a stroke. Part of the care involves working with the patient on coordination and strengthening exercises. Brenda has found Mrs. Cortez to be very cooperative and uncomplaining in doing the exercises under her direction, indicating that she would do what was needed to get well. One day Brenda's supervisor, Maria Lopez, tells her that the agency has received a complaint from Mrs. Cortez's family that Brenda is being too rough on the patient. Brenda responds that she does not understand this, because Mrs. Cortez has never complained. Brenda further explains that she was trying to have the patient work to her maximum capability and to give her instructions in a clear and direct manner. Ms. Lopez says that in her culture elders are considered very precious and are treated with gentleness and respect. Perhaps the family perceived that Brenda's direct ways indicated disrespect for their mother, even though the patient did not indicate this.

Think About It

How Can Nurses Develop Cultural Competence?

- How is cultural diversity evident in this situation?
- Where is there evidence of a lack of cultural competence?
- What might Brenda do to make her care more culturally sensitive?
- How do you think you would respond in a similar situation?
- How can nurses develop cultural competence?

Culture and the Health Care System

Concepts of health and healing, of right and wrong, of what is proper and what is not, are rooted in culture. Cultures have different explanatory models regarding health and illness that reflect their beliefs about the causes, symptoms, and treatments of illness, and response to dying and death. Our explanatory model helps us to recognize, respond to, interpret, cope with, and make sense of illness and other life experiences (Engebretson & Headley, 2000).

Transcultural issues arise when nurses, patients, and families hold differing views of what is important or necessary regarding health, recovery, illness, or the dying process. The contemporary health care system is not user-friendly when it comes to incorporating diversity. By virtue of its history, the system reflects predominantly middle-class, European American, Judeo-Christian, paternalistic values and perspectives (Kavanagh, 1993). This system includes the attitude that the health care provider knows what is "best for the patient," as viewed from the health provider's perspective.

The health provider's perspective generally derives from a combination of two cultural orientations. The primary cultural orientation is the biomedical model, and the secondary cultural orientation is the provider's personal cultural background. If the patient's perspective is different from this model and is not considered, dilemmas may emerge. Consider, for example, a situation in which the physician, who is schooled in the Western biomedical model, views death as "the enemy" to be overcome at all costs. The patient, who comes from a Native American culture, views death as a part of life that one prepares for by being in harmony with one's surroundings. Medical or surgical interventions that may prolong the patient's life a few weeks, which would be very important in the physician's world view, may be very low on the list of considerations for the patient. A patient who believes the suffering from his illness is a way of atoning for his sins may resist taking pain medication that health professionals deem important for his recovery.

We must be aware that the health care system is a different culture from that of most of the patients served by the system. The language, values, norms, behaviors, rituals, and environment are generally unfamiliar to those who seek its services. Even people who belong to the same dominant culture in society as their health care providers are often strangers when they enter the institutions of the system. For those who do not belong to the dominant culture, negotiating the system can be a formidable task. Lack of understanding of language, procedures, expectations, and other elements of the culture can lead to miscommunication, unclear decisions, and a sense of powerlessness or lack of control. Ethical or legal dilemmas may arise due to misunderstandings. Consider again the case of Mrs. Cortez. Misunderstanding of the nurse's intent might lead the family to decide to terminate nursing care or to bring legal action against the nurse because of their perception that their mother is being mistreated. Another example is a mentally alert ninety-year-old Appalachian woman who, after her doctor of thirty-five years retired, sought care from a new young physician. After a few visits she stopped going to see him, even though she was having serious health problems, because, in her perception, he did not do anything for her. Essentially, he did not talk with her nor spend the kind of time with her that her former physician had, and instead gave her medicines that she felt made her sick and that she did not need.

When we speak of values such as autonomy, beneficence, justice, or the right to self-determination, we must ask from whose perspective these values are understood—that of the nurse or that of the patient. This same question is appropriate regarding definitions of health. For example, many cultures place a higher emphasis on loyalty to the group than on the self-reliance and individualism valued within the broader culture in the United States (Andrews, 1999; Davis, 1999; Ludwick & Silva, 2000). Health care decisions in these cultures are often made by a group such as the family, community, or society, rather than by the individual. Cultural assessment provides insight into the congruence, or lack thereof, between patients' and nurses' values and understandings of health. Consider, for example, a situation in which the nurse believes that health includes being able to be a productive member of society and that health problems provide opportunities for one to grow and become more self-actualized. The patient, on the other hand, believes that his work-related injury is an act of *fate* and focuses on being free of pain and able to "get around." If the differing perceptions of health are not recognized and addressed, efforts to have the patient participate in rehabilitation and job retraining or to utilize nonpharmacological measures for pain control may meet with much resistance and patient dissatisfaction.

Complementary Therapies

Culture guides one's choice of when to go for health care, what kind of care to seek, to whom to go, and how long to participate in care. Many people who utilize conventional health care settings also utilize alternative or complementary therapies (Eisenberg, Kessler, Foster, Norlock, Calkins, & Delbanco, 1993; Eisenberg, Rogers, Ettner, Appel, Wilkey, Van Rompay, & Kessler, 1998). Such therapies may derive from traditions in the patient's own culture, or may be borrowed from traditions of another culture. Complementary therapies include a wide variety of modalities, such as relaxation techniques, healing touch and other energy-based healing techniques, spiritual healing, biofeedback, nutritional practices, herbal treatments, massage and other body work, meditation, prayer, homeopathy, acupuncture, and biofeedback.

These therapies are often used concurrently with conventional therapies, but they may be chosen in lieu of conventional therapies. In order to have a broad picture of the many factors affecting a patient's health and healing, we need to be aware of various therapies being utilized by the patient. We should incorporate discussion of complementary therapies into nursing assessment in an open way, since patients may be hesitant to bring up the subject. We do not need to ascribe to such therapies in order to become knowledgeable about them. Complementary therapies often derive from paradigms that differ from, and may not make sense in, the conventional medical model, yet may be very useful in the healing process. Hufford (1996) suggests that the patient has the major responsibility for seeking information regarding alternative therapies and making health choices in this regard, but that health care providers need to have some knowledge about risks and benefits involved. When patients are interested in complementary therapies, we must determine whether there are risks associated with their use. If there are significant risks involved, and the patient is committed to utilizing the therapy, we need to work with other health team members to minimize risks and maximize benefits. When there is not a strong commitment to the nonconventional modality, we should encourage ongoing discussion of known risks and benefits related to various options

(Hufford, 1996). When conventional health care providers can work with traditional systems and their healers, the overall care becomes more culturally congruent.

The principle of patient self-determination directs us to honor the right of persons to use both conventional and complementary therapies to address their health care needs (Burkhardt & Nagai-Jacobson, 1996). Respect for persons calls us to be open to views other than our own, and to appreciate that there are many paths to healing. Complementary modalities should never be discounted merely because they are not understood within the Western biomedical frame of reference. We need to respect convictions that derive from belief systems that are different from our own, and to be open to the contributions to health offered by other explanatory models. A nonjudgmental approach that respects differing values and beliefs and is sensitive to ethnocentric bias enhances the opportunity to explore jointly the efficacy of all options with the patient.

The area of informed consent presents some important questions relative to complementary therapies. Since noting alternative treatments is an important element of an informed consent, we must consider whether it is an ethical duty for practitioners of bioscientific medicine to include discussion of complementary therapies in discussion of therapeutic alternatives. Similarly, we must ask if practitioners of other healing modalities should be sure that their clients are aware of biomedical alternatives. Those who offer complementary therapies should explain the intervention and discuss risks, expected effects and benefits, and treatment options prior to initiating therapy. It is prudent to appraise other health team members of the use of complementary therapies, because they can affect conventional interventions in varying ways.

Practitioners of both conventional and complementary therapies need to be alert to potential threats to patient autonomy that flow from practitioner attitudes. When we assume that patient values and thought processes are the same as ours, we may believe that what we suggest is the only reasonable course of action. When patients choose another course of action, we may question their decision-making capacity or label them as unreasonable. In conventional practice, this may show up in referring to non-conventional therapies as quackery or non-scientific, trying to dissuade patients from using them, and even deriding the patient for making such choices. We must remember that a patient's choice of an option that may seem unreasonable from our perspective does not necessarily mean that they have not thought it through. Such differences often merely reflect a difference in values.

Think About It

How Should Nurses Deal with Complementary Therapies?

Conventional medicine and medical practitioners tend to be skeptical of healing modalities that have not been subjected to empirical scientific study; thus, discussion of nonconventional modalities is not included in lists of alternatives for patients, nor are these modalities available in most conventional health care settings.

- What do you think about this attitude toward complementary therapies?
- What experiences have you had with complementary therapies?
- How might attitudes toward complementary therapies affect the ability of nurses to provide culturally congruent care for their patients?
- What are the ethical implications related to limiting a patient's access to complementary therapies and practitioners within conventional health care institutions?
- What is your view of complementary therapies within nursing practice?

Factors important for the healing process are often culturally prescribed. For example, the involvement of family in the care of a sick member may be very important in some cultures. It can be quite distressing for nursing staff on a hospital unit when multiple family members "camp out" in a patient's room or the nearby hallway, or bring food from home that is not on a patient's diet. Providing culturally congruent care in such situations may include relaxing visiting regulations and collaborating with the family regarding appropriate foods from home. If the needs of one patient are different from those of the roommate, dilemmas may arise that require diplomatic interventions by the nurse.

Legal Considerations Related to Transcultural Issues

Cultural misunderstandings can provide fertile ground for litigation. Communication—verbal, nonverbal, and written—is always of utmost importance. When a patient's first language is different from that of the nurse, we must determine the extent of the patient's understanding of the nurse's language. When the patient uses another language (including sign language), having an interpreter fluent in the patient's language is essential. If the interpreter is a member of the patient's family, the translation may be filtered through the perspective of the family member. Consider, for example, an elderly Cambodian man who is in the hospital and not doing well. His grandson serves as interpreter. The grandson was born in this country and is embarrassed by his grandfather's "old" ways. When the man says that he needs a particular traditional herbal tea each afternoon in order to get well (which is available in a local ethnic store), the grandson translates this generically as "tea." Even though the nurse responds by making sure that the patient has tea each afternoon, the patient's needs are not met.

The language in which we explain procedures and of consent forms presents other issues. Be sure that the patient or family member is able to read the language in which the form is written, and that all terms used are understood. If the form needs to be interpreted for the patient, it is essential that the interpreter understands the procedure and that an appropriate person is available to clarify any areas of uncertainty. People may indicate that they understand when they do not, in order to avoid offending the nurse or being considered ignorant. One way of dealing with this is having patients describe in their own words what they have been told.

ISSUES RELATED TO SPIRITUALITY AND RELIGION

Spirituality is a universal human experience that transcends culture, although it may be colored and shaped by cultural experiences. Nurses at all levels of practice must be attentive to spirituality and recognize the individual as a body-mind-spirit being who experiences health concerns in all these dimensions. In the midst of advances in technology and scientific discoveries, which have increased our understanding of the nature of illness and disease, attunement to the role of spirituality in health and healing has diminished. Perhaps the limited scientific knowledge of former times made the role of the spirit and the intangible forces deriving from that spirit more apparent. Many persons were cared for in their homes, even in the case of serious illness. Touching, praying, and presence were a natural part of such environments. Historically, institutions such as hospitals were often staffed by religious orders concerned for both spiritual and physical needs.

Healing and health care has long been connected with the spirituality of a people. With indigenous peoples, healing rituals frequently are spiritual in nature. People seeking medical care continue to incorporate spiritual and religious rituals and practices into their care for self and others. It is noteworthy that the words health, holy, and whole all derive from the same old Saxon, *Hal*, and Greek, *Holos*, which mean whole. By their nature, then, health and healing are associated with that which is holy and whole. A question to ponder is whether contemporary health care culture, now vested in technology, managed care, mergers, and the like, can once again incorporate spirituality within its vision of healing.

Approaching Spirituality

By nature, humans are body-mind-spirit beings. The uniqueness of each person a nurse encounters encompasses the spiritual as well as physical, mental, and emotional manifestations of that person. **Spirituality** is the animating force, life principle, or essence of being that permeates life and is expressed and experienced in multifaceted connections with self, others, nature, and God or Life Force (Burkhardt, 1994; Burkhardt & Nagai-Jacobson, 1994; 2000; 2002). Meaning and purpose in life and life events flows from the spirit and is manifested in open or private ways. All persons are spiritual, whether they ascribe to a religious orientation or deny the existence of the Divine. Beliefs and values are molded and shaped by our spirituality as well as by societal and cultural conditioning.

Nursing espouses a holistic, body-mind-spirit view of persons. Understanding that persons are indeed body-mind-spirit beings, we recognize that spirituality is part of every encounter whether we are conscious of it or not. Holistic nursing care impels us to address spiritual as well as physical and mental concerns of patients. We must strive to become more aware of our own and others' spirituality in order to bring this essential aspect of care consciously into every nursing interaction.

Because spirituality is at once universal and often very personal and private, we may find this area difficult to approach. We must develop competence in addressing spiritual needs. Recognizing that spirituality is basic to health enables us to listen for language, observe behavior, and gather information related to spiritual concerns.

Spirituality assessment can provide us with information about how patients view life, death, health, and health concerns. Such assessment provides insight into important connections, beliefs, practices, or rituals that may influence a person's choices or affect healing. Processes that incorporate open-ended questions and allow patients to tell their stories are more effective than check-lists for spirituality assessment (Burkhardt & Nagai-Jacobson, 1994; 1997; 2000; 2002; Dossey, Keegan, & Guzzetta, 2000; Nagai-Jacobson & Burkhardt, 1996). Although expression of spiritual concerns may include talk of God or faith, patients communicate their spiritual needs and concerns in many other ways as well. They may express questions related to the meaning of present or past experiences, fears or worries about what is happening, or how they will find the strength they need. They may talk about important relationships, the need for reconciliation, experiences of peace or anxiety, or the desire to put their lives in order. Religious articles may be evident, or the nurse may observe the patient engaging in practices such as prayer or meditation. Effective spirituality assessment requires us to attend with our whole beings to indicators of spirituality occurring within routine interactions with patients. Opportunities to explore spirituality with patients present in many situations.

Think About It

Recognizing Spiritual Concerns

Spiritual issues reflect core experiences that often defy explanation. Such experiences may relate to suffering, forgiveness, hope, love, or mystery. In the midst of care with patients, nurses often hear comments or questions or observe behaviors reflective of spiritual concerns. Consider the following examples:

A patient or family member says:

"I don't know why God is doing this to me (or her)."

"I should have locked the gate."

"Will you pray for me?"

"I don't know why, but having surgery worries me."

"I wish I had been willing to go to the beach when he wanted to."

"I think I need to trust God and not take chemotherapy. God wants me to trust Him completely."

"Without my income I don't know how my family will make it."

"We told him not to buy that motorcycle."

"Do you believe in miracles?"

Patients or family members may be observed:

Reading a sacred text.

Wearing religious jewelry or articles of clothing.

Praying or meditating.

Staring out a window with a worried or pensive expression.

- How are spiritual concerns reflected in these comments or behaviors?

- What personal beliefs or experiences might affect your feelings and responses to comments or behaviors such as these?

- Describe aspects of each comment or behavior that might raise questions or concerns for you.

- How would you respond to each of these comments or behaviors? In which circumstances would you feel more comfortable or less comfortable?

Spirituality and Religion

Although spirituality may be expressed through religious beliefs and practices, it is not synonymous with these terms. **Religion** is the codification of beliefs and practices concerning the Divine and one's relationship with the Divine that are shared by a group of people. Religion may be quite intertwined within a dominant culture, as with Judaism in Israel or Hinduism in India, or it may be counterculture, as with the Amish in the United States. Some religions, such as many Christian sects, include people from different cultures. Religious teachings generally include rules regarding right and wrong and guidelines for dealing with issues related to these areas. Because religious beliefs and teachings flow from a particular world view, rules and values can be quite variable among different religions. A minor consideration within one religion or sect may constitute a serious dilemma in another. Norms for proper dress for women is one example. For instance, although most Christian denominations have few, if any, restrictions regarding womens' dress, some Christian sects teach that women should wear only skirts or dresses and not use makeup nor cut their hair. Orthodox Muslims have very strict rules regarding how women are to dress in public.

What is considered right or wrong within a particular religion is not always congruent with ethical perspectives of the greater society. Consider, for example, an infant girl brought to a hospital in the United States with severely infected wounds from trauma to her labial area following a clitorectomy procedure performed by her father.

Ask Yourself

How Does Spirituality Affect Your Nursing Practice?

- What religious or spiritual beliefs or practices are important to you?

- How has your spirituality or religious perspective been influential in your choice of nursing as a profession?

- How do you think your spirituality or religious perspective might affect or be incorporated into your nursing practice?

From the perspective of the nurse and the institution, this might be viewed as severe mutilation, constituting abuse, whereas the family would consider this an important religious practice. Another example is the Jehovah Witness belief that blood transfusions are wrong, and the ensuing dilemma when a transfusion is medically indicated as a life-saving measure.

Religiosity refers to beliefs and practices that are the expressive aspects of religion. These include, among others, prayer, ritual, dietary practices, modes of dress, and study of sacred texts. Awareness of religious practices and beliefs that are important to patients and families enables nurses to incorporate religious needs into care planning. Familiarity with beliefs and practices of different religions that may affect health care is important in order to be better able to incorporate particular needs into patient care (Andrews & Hanson, 1989). This information provides a basis from which nurses can explore with patients what is necessary to support or meet their spiritual needs, taking care not to presume a need until it is verified with the patient. For example, a Catholic patient may not wish to have a priest called, a Jewish patient may have no problem with eating ham, or a patient who lists no religious affiliation may practice daily meditation.

Although many people express their spirituality through religion, spiritual expression is not limited to this context. Many people will note that they believe in God but do not go to church. Instead, they pray on their own, or experience the Divine through nature, or relate to a Higher Power or Universal Being that is found in all of life. We must plan nursing care according to how each patient expresses and experiences spirituality.

Creating Sacred Space.   Addressing religious concerns within a health care setting does not require us to share the same religious perspective as our patients. What is necessary is that we create an environment that is open to a variety of religious and spiritual expression. Creating sacred space in the midst of science and technology can challenge our creativity. Nursing care may include providing the quiet a patient needs for meditation, arranging a private space for a particular ritual, contacting an appropriate spiritual support person, or ensuring that specific dietary requirements are met. Praying with or reading scripture to patients may be included in nursing care, providing it is done with the patient's permission and within the context of the patient's tradition. Prayer can be an important intervention, and research suggests that prayer reflecting an attitude of "Thy will be done" is particularly effective (Dossey, 1993; 1996). Dossey (1998) also reports evidence that prayer can be used with harmful intent or may reflect a goal different from that of the patient. He suggests that health care practitioners should consider obtaining permission from patients before praying for them. It is good for nurses who are so inclined to include prayer for patients in their personal prayer, with an openness to what is for the patient's highest good. Overall we need to be aware of acting out of our own spiritual or religious perspectives while taking care not to impose our views on another.

Dilemmas Related to Religious Beliefs.   When patients refuse conventional medical treatments based on religious beliefs or spiritual perspective, dilemmas can arise. Patients who decide to rely on prayer for healing, rather than chemotherapy for treatment of cancer, for example, may be considered irrational, and their competence to make decisions may be questioned. If an adult refuses a blood transfusion due to religious beliefs, after all risks have been explained, it is considered an informed decision. If a parent refuses a transfusion for a child based on the same belief, it may be taken to court as neglect or abuse. A woman who refuses to leave a dangerously abusive marriage because of religious convictions may find that frustrated health care providers are less responsive to her cries for help.

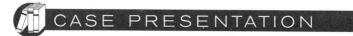

CASE PRESENTATION

When Religious Beliefs and Medical Care Conflict—Part 1

Suella is a thirty-three-year-old, unmarried woman who belongs to a Holiness church that includes the practice of snake handling. Three days ago she was bitten twice during a church service. Following the service she stayed with the preacher, who prayed with her for healing as is the custom in this church. The religion does not believe in taking antivenom. Suella's parents and siblings, who do not belong to the same church, brought her to the hospital in renal failure. Upon admission she was alert but lethargic, and repeatedly informed nurses that she did not want any blood, dialysis, feeding tube, or life support. She kept saying "My King will take care of me," insisting that her reliance was on God, and that she did not want antivenom. Upon her move to the intensive care unit, the attending physician documented the conversation with the patient, indicating that she did not want blood, dialysis, feeding tubes, CPR, or life support. The attending also consulted a renal physician, who ordered dialysis. A nurse who was getting ready to do the second dialysis treatment read the attending's note and recognized the ethical dilemma.

Think About It

Dealing with Conflicts between Religious Beliefs and Medical Care

- What should the nurse do in this situation?
- How do you think you would react to this patient's decisions?
- What principles would guide you in dealing with dilemmas arising from religious convictions?
- What personal religious or spiritual practices are important to your health?
- What personal convictions might affect your health care decisions?

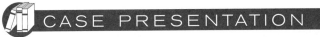

CASE PRESENTATION

When Religious Beliefs and Medical Care Conflict—Part 2

The nurse in this situation requested an ethics consult, and members of the hospital's ethics committee talked with the patient. Although the patient was lethargic, she could nod and reply yes and no when questioned. The patient reaffirmed her same wishes as noted on admission. When asked if she knew what would happen without treatment she stated "I'll die." The primary physician spoke to the patient again in the presence of an ethics member, at which time she once again reiterated her previous wishes. The physician discontinued all dialysis and set up a meeting with the family, after which the family spoke to the patient. Later that day the patient said she changed her mind and now wanted everything done. Ethics committee members were again called. When they asked the patient why she changed her mind, she responded "My family." Further exploration of what "everything" meant to the patient revealed that she was willing to have dialysis, blood, and tube feedings, but no CPR or intubation.

Think About It

When Family Members Have Different Religious Beliefs

- How would you, as the nurse, feel about following this patient's new directives?
- Do you see any new dilemmas resulting from the current situation?
- Is there any evidence of coercion in this situation? If so, how would you respond to that?
- How would your own spiritual perspective influence your care for this patient and family?

Nurturing Spirit

Caregiving is influenced by a nurse's spiritual, as well as physical and emotional, well-being. The ability to attend to spirituality with another requires that nurses first attend to their own spirits (Burkhardt & Nagai-Jacobson, 1997; 2000; 2002). Self-awareness, which includes appreciation of ourselves as a unique body-mind-spirit being, underlies our recognition of this same wholeness in others.

Just as sustenance and care are necessary for the health of body and mind, so too does the spirit require nurture. Caring for our spirit includes mindfulness and taking time to attend to our inner being. The spirit can be nurtured in many ways, and we must each discover what our own spirit needs in order to thrive. Prayer, meditation, music, religious worship, or shared ritual may be important. The spirit may be nurtured through special time with friends or family, or by giving ourself alone time at home, in nature, or in some other sacred space. Attending to our need for rest, play, or creative activity are other ways to care for spirit. The spirit can be nurtured in a very profound way through sharing our story. As we become more adept at nurturing our spirits, we are better able to recognize and support this process with patients and families.

SUMMARY

Attentiveness to spiritual and cultural aspects of care with patients is an important part of holistic nursing care. The diversity of cultures and spiritual expressions within our society requires that nurses be able to identify concerns and issues in these areas and address them competently and confidently. Familiarity with values, beliefs, and practices of various cultures and religions is a useful adjunct to careful cultural and spiritual assessments with patients. Self-awareness regarding our own cultural and spiritual values, beliefs, and expressions is necessary in order to address these areas with patients. Such awareness allows us to act from our own spiritual or cultural perspectives, while taking care not to impose these views on others. In this way care planning can more readily flow from assessments that identify issues and needs regarding the patient's cultural and spiritual expressions and experiences.

CHAPTER HIGHLIGHTS

- Since culture influences beliefs and behaviors regarding health and healing, cultural assessment is integral to a comprehensive nursing assessment.
- Providing effective nursing care within the diversity of our multicultural society requires cultural competence on the part of nurses. Cultural competence can help prevent dilemmas from arising when there are differences in cultural perspective between patient and nurse.
- The culture of health care institutions may vary greatly from that of the people served by these systems. Values such as autonomy, beneficence, or the right to self-determination need to be considered from the cultural perspectives of patient, family, and health care providers.
- Complementary therapies are used by many people encountered in conventional health care settings. Nursing care is enhanced when nurses are aware of various therapies being utilized by patients. Knowledge of and working with traditional healing systems and healers can help nurses promote more culturally congruent care.
- Communication is a key factor in providing culturally congruent and spiritually sensitive care and in averting associated legal and other dilemmas.
- Health and healing are associated with that which is holy and whole. Spirituality

has long been a component of healing and health care, since by nature, humans are body-mind-spirit beings.

- Grounded in a holistic view of persons, nursing care must include spirituality assessment and interventions addressing spiritual needs, recognizing that religious or spiritual perspective may influence health care choices.

- Expressions of spirituality are many and varied and may include, but are not limited to, the context of religion. Religious values are not always congruent with ethical perspectives of the greater society.

- Providing spiritual care requires that nurses be attentive to their own spirits and the spiritual concerns of patients and create an environment that is open to a variety of religious and spiritual expressions. Nurses need to be aware of acting from their own cultural, spiritual, or religious perspectives, while not imposing these views on others.

DISCUSSION QUESTIONS AND ACTIVITIES

1. Consider how your cultural, spiritual, or religious values affect personal choices regarding health and healing. Discuss this with other students, noting similarities and differences.

2. What aspects of the culture of the health care system are difficult for you as a nurse? Identify personal conflicts and the beliefs and values underlying them.

3. Recall a time when you or someone you know experienced a conflict with persons within the health care system. What values, beliefs, or understandings contributed to this conflict?

4. Discuss with other students nonconventional therapies, or folk remedies, that you or someone you know have used. Why was the therapy used? How did you know about the therapy? Was it used in place of or along with conventional therapies? What was the outcome? Research a complementary therapy through the National Center for Complementary and Alternative Medicine (www.nih. nccam.gov)

5. List ten things that nurture you spiritually. Consider how often you have done these in the past day, week, or month. Make a plan to include at least one each day for the next week.

6. Choose a religious tradition or a nonconventional therapy with which you are unfamiliar. Explore this tradition or therapy through readings and discussions with members, practitioners, or persons who have practiced the religion or utilized the therapy. Share your findings with classmates.

7. Discuss how nurses can create sacred space within health care settings.

8. Discuss patient health care choices or behaviors which are based on religious beliefs that might present a dilemma for you. Consider how you would approach the situation in a professional manner and describe the ethical stance that would guide your decisions.

REFERENCES

American Nurses Association. (1991). *Position paper on cultural diversity in nursing practice.* Kansas City, MO: Author.

Andrews, M. M. (1999). Cultural diversity in the health care workforce. In M. M. Andrews & J. S. Broyle, *Transcultural concepts in nursing care* (3rd ed., pp. 471–506).

Andrews, M. M., & Hanson, P. A. (1989). Religious beliefs: Implications for nursing practice. In J. S. Broyle & M. M. Andrews, eds., *Transcultural concepts in nursing care* (pp. 357–418). Glenview, IL: Scott, Foresman/Little, Brown College Division.

Breton, J. H. (2000). Treating beyond color: Health issues for minority women. *Advance for Nurse Practitioners,* (November), 65–68, 101.

Burkhardt, M. A. (1985). Nursing, health, and wholeness. *Journal of Holistic Nursing, 3,* 35–36.

Burkhardt, M. A. (1994). Becoming and connecting: Elements of spirituality for women. *Holistic Nursing Practice, 8,* 12–21.

Burkhardt, M. A., & Nagai-Jacobson, M. G. (1994). Reawakening spirit in clinical practice. *Journal of Holistic Nursing, 12,* 9–12.

Burkhardt, M. A., & Nagai-Jacobson, M. G. (1996). Patient self-determination and complementary therapies. *Bioethics Forum, 12*(4), 24–29.

Burkhardt, M. A., & Nagai-Jacobson, M. G. (1997). Spirituality and healing. In B. M. Dossey, ed., *AHNA core curriculum for holistic nursing* (pp. 42–51). Gaithersburg, MD: Aspen.

Burkhardt, M. A., & Nagai-Jacobson, M. G. (2000). Spirituality and health. In B. M. Dossey, L. Keegan, & C. E. Guzzetta, *Holistic nursing: A handbook for practice* (3rd ed., pp. 91–122). Gaithersburg, MD: Aspen.

Burkhardt, M. A., & Nagai-Jacobson, M. G. (2002). *Spirituality and healing: Living our connectedness.* Albany, NY: Delmar Publishers.

Davis, A. J. (1999). Global influence of American nursing: Some ethical issues. *Nursing Ethics: An International Journal for Health Care Professionals, 6*(2), 118–125.

Dossey, B. M., Keegan, L., & Guzzetta, C. E., (2000). *Holistic nursing: A handbook for practice.* Gaithersburg, MD: Aspen.

Dossey, L. (1993). *Healing words: The power of prayer and the practice of medicine.* San Francisco: HarperCollins.

Dossey, L. (1996). *Prayer is good medicine.* San Francisco: HarperCollins.

Dossey, L. (1998). *Be careful what you pray for: You just might get it.* San Francisco, CA: Harper San Francisco.

Engebretson, J. C. & Headley, J. A. (2000). Cultural diversity and care. In B. M. Dossey, L. Keegan, & C. E. Guzzetta, *Holistic nursing: A handbook for practice* (3rd ed., pp. 283–310). Gaithersburg, MD: Aspen.

Eisenberg, D. M., Kessler, R. C., Foster, C., Norlock, F. E., Calkins, D. R., & Delbanco, T. L. (1993). Unconventional medicine in the United States. *New England Journal of Medicine, 328,* 246–252.

Eisenberg, D. M., Rogers, B. D., Ettner, S., Appel, S., Wilkey, S., Van Rompay, M., & Kessler, R. C. (1998). Trends in alternative medicine use in the United States, 1990–1997. *Journal of the American Medical Association, 280*(18), 1569–1575.

Giger, J. N., & Davidhizar, R. E. (1995). *Transcultural nursing: Assessment and intervention* (2nd ed.). St. Louis, MO: Mosby.

Hopkins, W. E. (1997). *Ethical dimensions of diversity*. Thousand Oaks, CA: Sage.

Hufford, D. J. (1996, January 18–21). *Ethical dimensions of alternative medicine*. Presentation at the First Annual Alternative Therapies Symposium: Creating Integrated Healthcare, San Diego, CA.

Kavanagh, K. H. (1993). Transcultural nursing: Facing the challenges of advocacy and diversity/universality. *Journal of Transcultural Nursing, 5,* 4–13.

Leininger, M. (1991). Transcultural care principles, human rights, and ethical considerations. *Journal of Transcultural Nursing, 3,* 21–22.

Ludwick, R. & Silva, M. C. (August 14, 2000). Nursing around the world: Cultural values and ethical conflicts. *Online journal of issues in nursing*. Retrieved January 8, 2001 from the World Wide Web: http://www.nursingworld.org/ojin/ethicol/ethics_4.html

Nagai-Jacobson, M. G., & Burkhardt, M. A. (1996). Viewing persons as stories: A perspective for holistic care. *Alternative Therapies in Health and Medicine, 2,* 54–58.

Sewell, M., ed. (1991). *Cries of the spirit: A celebration of women's spirituality*. Boston: Beacon Press.

Tafoya, T. (1996, May). *Embracing the shadow: Mending the sacred hoop*. Paper presented at the South Texas AIDS Training (STAT) for Mental Health Providers: The Human, Transcultural, and Spiritual Dimensions of HIV/AIDS, San Antonio, TX.

Tripp-Reimer, T. (1987). Cultural assessment. In J. P. Bellak & P. A. Bamford, eds., *Nursing assessment: A multidimensional approach*. Boston: Jones & Bartlett.

Waters, C. (1996). Professional development in nursing—A culturally diverse postdoctoral experience. *Image, 28,* 47–50.

THE POWER TO MAKE
A DIFFERENCE

Part V discusses the importance of empowerment of nurses and patients. To deal with the complex issues facing nursing today, nurses are required to exercise integrity, accountability, and courage. Nurses have the responsibility, authority, and power to make principled choices. Additionally, empowerment of patients is an important element of nursing care that derives from an appreciation that patients have the ability to discern their needs and make decisions about their lives and health. Being an enabler of empowerment requires nurses to relinquish power and embrace the patient as an equal partner. Nurses can facilitate empowerment by working directly with patients and through addressing social, political, and environmental factors affecting empowerment of individuals and communities. In the midst of an ever changing and challenging health care environment in which issues of power and control continue to affect patient care, it is imperative that nurses be both empowered and competent enablers of patient empowerment.

CHAPTER 19

Empowerment
for Nurses

Written in collaboration with Barbara C. Banonis

> *Copper Woman warned Hai Nai Yu that the world*
> *would change and times might come when Knowing*
> *would not be the same as Doing. And she told her that*
> *Trying would always be very important.*
>
> **(Cameron, 1981, p. 53)**

OBJECTIVES

After completing this chapter, the reader should be able to:

1. Discuss the effect of mind sets on expectations regarding nursing practice and ethical stances.

2. Describe metaphors for nursing and discuss their impact on nursing ethics.

3. Explain the impact on nursing practice of perceptions about nursing from within and outside the profession.

4. Describe the concepts of power and empowerment.

5. Discuss personal empowerment and its importance within nursing.

6. Discuss the relationship among professional empowerment, principled behavior, and nursing practice.

7. Describe the role of diversity in empowerment.

8. Discuss the influence on professional practice of nursing's vision of nursing.

INTRODUCTION

Dealing in a principled way with issues facing nursing requires integrity, accountability, and courage. Discussion of issues in this book are grounded in the belief that: (1) nurses have the power to make choices and to act in responsible and principled ways, and (2) nurses have authority to make decisions and recommendations regarding activities that are within the scope of their practice. The parameters of nursing's power and authority, however, are not always clear. Many nurses feel constrained by the systems within which they work and by persisting paternalistic attitudes that promote disempowerment. This chapter discusses the concept of empowerment as a process through which nurses are enabled to clarify and claim their ability to make decisions regarding issues related to nursing practice. Elements of personal empowerment are addressed, and factors associated with professional empowerment are considered. The principles regarding empowerment for nurses that are discussed in this chapter apply as well to empowering patients, which is the focus of Chapter 20.

INFLUENCES ON NURSING'S PERCEPTIONS OF PRINCIPLED PRACTICE

Nurses, patients, and other health care providers may vary greatly in their perceptions of ideals for nursing and nursing practice. These perceptions influence expectations and decisions regarding care, authority, and accountability. Expectations regarding good nursing care or taking an ethical stance flow from such perceptions. We recognize that factors in our internal and external environments affect both personal and professional decision making. External environment factor include norms, ideals, and expectations of patients, families, other health care providers, and the professional and social systems within which we interact. The internal environment includes our *mind set* or inner world of personal beliefs and perceptions.

Influence of Mind Sets

Aroskar suggests that our mind sets, that is, our views and beliefs about the health care system, influence how we identify and respond to ethical issues and dilemmas in practice. For example, when nurses view health care in terms of medical cases focused on the cure of disease, the physician is seen as the dominant authority. Following the physician's orders (whether or not the nurse agrees with them) and loyalty to the physician and institution are considered the legitimate and ethical focus of nursing activities. Aroskar states that "this mind set may well impede efforts to achieve more ethical practice which requires critical, reflective thinking and challenges the decision-making structure of the present system" (1982, p. 26). If nurses view health care as a commodity in which nursing and medical care are sold to patients by institutions, the nurse's primary responsibility is to the employing institution. Within this view, needs of individual patients may be subordinated to the utilitarian goal focused on the good of the greatest number of people or the institutional goal of making a profit. Nurses who hold this view may not challenge the rightness or wrongness of nursing actions, provided they are congruent with goals and policies of the institution. This mind set finds fertile ground in managed care arenas. When nurses view health care as a basic human need and a right for each person, the nurse's primary responsibility is to the patient. The legitimate and ethical focus of nursing activities within this mind set must include attention to patient rights, safety, and overall well-being.

Metaphors of Nursing

Metaphors help us to understand a concept by comparing two things that are different, yet that share common characteristics. People often use *metaphors* to focus attention on particular aspects of reality in order to enhance understandings of roles, events, and experiences. Metaphors may also influence our perceptions of these events and experiences. For example, likening nurses to *angels in white* calls attention to nursing roles of caring, protecting, and serving; yet viewing nurses as angels may set up the expectation that they be somewhat distant and above human frailties. Metaphors that have been associated with nursing reflect different ideas about nursing roles and responsibilities in health care. These metaphors also suggest different approaches to determining an appropriate ethical stance for nursing care delivery.

Winslow discusses the impact on nursing ethics of a shift from a military metaphor for nursing, which stresses loyalty, to a legal metaphor for nursing as advocate for patient rights. The military metaphor is associated with obedience to higher authority, a view of disease as the enemy, discipline, respect for those of higher rank, uniform dress, and, above all, loyalty. Winslow notes that "loyalty meant refusal to criticize the nurse's hospital or training school, fellow nurses, and most importantly, the physician under whom the nurse worked . . . being loyal to the physician by preserving the patient's confidence was the same as being loyal to the patient" (1984, p. 33). Ethical imperatives that flow from this metaphor include following physician orders, even if the nurse questions their appropriateness, upholding the patient's faith in the physician, even if the nurse questions the doctor's competence, and being loyal to health care colleagues, even at the expense of the patient.

In the early history of nursing, following the physician's order without question would have absolved the nurse from guilt, even in the event of a harmful outcome for the patient. Today, however, this is not the case. Nursing's move from vocation to profession requires that nurses be more personally accountable for their actions. Court rulings have held nurses legally responsible for their decisions and actions. Legal decisions, changes in the health care delivery system, and feminist awarenesses within the nursing profession have encouraged the transition from the metaphor of loyal soldier to that of patient advocate. Winslow (1984) notes that a significant revision in nursing's self-image began in the 1960s and 1970s. Greater emphasis on consumerism and patient rights, coupled with growing dissatisfaction with increased costs and depersonalization of health care, helped to open the door for nurses to expand their roles as patient advocates. As advocates for patient rights, nurses are responsible to those who require nursing care. This obliges nurses to be alert to situations in which patients may be endangered by incompetent, unethical, or illegal practice by any member of the health care team or the health care system and to take appropriate actions to safe-guard the patient (American Nurses Association, 1985; 2001). Current nursing codes and standards that stress responsibility to patients through collegial membership in the health team reflect ethical imperatives flowing from the metaphor of advocacy.

Loyalty remains a valued virtue for nurses within the advocacy metaphor. Although ideally the nurse's first loyalty is to the patient, circumstances of conflicting loyalty may occur. Loyalty to colleagues and to employers is also important, and nurses may at times be faced with making difficult decisions between advocacy for patients or loyalty to colleagues. Such situations require personal integrity, knowledge, and courage on the part of the nurse.

How nurses picture nursing and the vision they hold of their role in health care influences their ability to practice in a holistic, patient-focused way. Nursing's self-image is evident in metaphors nurses use to describe their roles and their practice. In studying metaphors nurses use to capture their experience of nursing, Hartrick and Schreiber (1998) discovered a wide variety of images reflecting the tasks and responsibilities of nursing; the pivotal role nurses play in the system; the experience of empowerment and powerlessness; personal development and discovery; and the relational and caring nature of nursing. They note that the images of nursing reflected in these metaphors illuminate the complexities and ambiguities of nursing practice. These images highlight as well the influence of social, organizational, and cultural constraints on nurses. These constraints often prompt nurses to feel unable to practice nursing in a way that is consistent with their values.

Think About It

How Do Mind Sets Affect Perceptions?

You are the vice president for nursing at a large medical center. Recently one of the physicians, who holds a lot of power in the system and is generally very open and easy to work with, expressed considerable displeasure about the refusal of a particular nurse to carry out a medical order and referring concerns about certain physician practice decisions to the ethics committee. The physician says that you should fire the nurse for insubordination. You are aware that the nurse's decisions were reasonable, in the patient's interest, and based on sound principles and standards of nursing practice.

- How would you respond to the physician?

- Where do you see potential for conflicting loyalties in this situation?

- Discuss how differing perceptions of nursing might affect this situation.

- Describe what you see as the most realistic outcome in this situation. What about the ideal outcome?

How Nursing Is Perceived by Others

Factors such as mind sets and metaphors influence our perceptions of and choices regarding principled behavior. Perceptions of others also affect our considerations regarding appropriate or ethical nursing actions. Although nursing as a profession has claimed the metaphor of advocate in lieu of that of loyal soldier, many nurses within the profession have not fully embrace the change. Operationalizing the advocacy role may put nurses at risk in some institutions and situations, as demonstrated in cases such as that of Jolene Tuma discussed in Chapter 11. Although nursing has made a paradigm shift regarding its role and responsibilities, awareness of nursing's current professional imperatives is often lacking among patients, families, physicians, and health care administrators. The role of nursing as perceived by many outside of the profession remains embedded in the loyal soldier metaphor, and health care as medical cases or commodity mind sets. As a result, many physicians still expect nurses to follow their bidding and take offense when nurses challenge their decisions or actions. The hierarchical, patriarchal system remains the norm in many health care institutions. Since physicians are perceived to be of higher rank, their influence often holds more sway than that of nurses who may challenge them. Although patients and families often have more continual and direct contact with nurses, they may not fully understand that the nurse is their advocate. Instead, they often function from the mind set that the physician is the captain of a ship in which the nurse is a member of the crew. Images in the media that depict nurses in ancillary, subordinate roles also affect perceptions of patients and others regarding expectations of nurses.

UNDERSTANDING POWER AND EMPOWERMENT

Nurses have the power to make a difference by acting in principled ways in all areas of their lives and practice. However, as has been evident throughout the discussions in this book, many factors mitigate against nurses claiming this power. Nurses need to develop skills in dealing with these factors in order to function fully in their legitimate roles within health care. Nurses must be aware of values, beliefs, and other factors affecting personal decision making, and expand their knowledge of ethical principles, legal considerations, and issues facing nursing. Understanding **power** and **empowerment** can help in developing strategies for action in this regard.

Although the word *power* is often understood in terms of strength, force, or control, a primary dictionary definition of the term, derived from its Latin root potere, is "the ability to do or act, capability of doing or accomplishing something" (*The Random House Dictionary of the English Language*, 1987). To have power, then, implies having the ability to do or act; and to *empower* would be to facilitate the ability of another person to do or to act.

Rodwell suggests that empowerment is a "helping process whereby groups of individuals are enabled to change a situation, given skills, resources, opportunities and authority to do so. It is a partnership which respects and values self and others—aiming to develop positive beliefs in self and the future" (1996, p. 309). Similarly, Ellis-Stoll and Popkess-Vawter (1998) describe empowerment as a participative process, or partnership between a nurse and patient, which is designed to assist in changing unhealthy behaviors. This partnership is viewed by some as a social process of recognizing, promoting, and enhancing patient's abilities to meet their own needs, solve their own problems, and mobilize the necessary resources in order to feel in control of their own lives (Connelly, Keele, Kleinbeck, Schneider, & Cobb, 1993; Fulton, 1997). Bolton & Brookings (1998) describe empowerment as the capacity of disenfranchised people to understand and become active participants in the matters that affect their lives, suggesting that a personal attitude that change is possible is important for empowerment to occur. Gurka (1995) reflects that empowerment is a philosophy or world view flowing from belief in each person's inherent worth and process of self-discovery which involves creating a vision, taking risks, making choices, and behaving in authentic ways. Empowerment requires respect for an individual's personal beliefs and goals and trust in the person's ability to make decisions, take action, and be accountable for the actions. Although sharing of knowledge through education is important for empowerment, the literature clearly indicates that emotional and social support is essential as well.

In-depth analyses of the concept suggests that empowerment is both process and outcome, taking different forms within different people and contexts (Gibson, 1991; Hawks, 1992; Rodwell, 1996; Ellis-Stoll & Popkess-Vawter, 1998; Ryles, 1999). Because of this, empowerment needs to be defined by the people concerned. Empowerment is a transactional process involving relationship with others. This relationship includes mutually beneficial interactions aimed at strengthening rather than weakening; power sharing through mutual sharing of knowledge, resources, and opportunities; and respect for self and others. Empowerment is nurtured by collaborative efforts that focus on solutions rather than problems, and on strengths, rights, and abilities rather than deficits. Empowerment derives from a feminine perspective of *power with or power to*, which implies sharing responsibility, knowledge, and resources; collaboration for goal achievement; incorporating diversity; valuing the contributions of each person; and valuing the process. In contrast is the masculine view of *power over* that incorporates a sense of paternalistic control, struggle for and protection of limited resources, separation of leaders and followers, expediency and results even at the expense of persons (Chinn, 1995).

Empowerment can seem like a rather abstract term, and you may be wondering what being empowered looks and feels like. Certainly, two people in the same circumstances can have different experiences of empowerment. Nurse scholars use a variety of descriptive terms when discussing people who are empowered. These include: positive self-concept, personal satisfaction, self-efficacy, sense of mastery regarding self and the environment, sense of control, sense of connectedness, self-development, feeling of hope, the ability to make changes, self-determination, action orientation, authority, autonomy, capability of social intercourse, caring, choosing, self-confidence, courage, decision-making ability, emancipatory power, endurance, expertise, freedom, influence, instrumental exercise of power, participation, resilience, rights, self-control, solidarity, strength, sturdiness, taking a position, assertiveness, coercion, enabling, and freedom to make choices (Bolton & Brookings, 1998; Byrne, 1998; Chavasse, 1992; Connelly, Keele, Kleinbeck, Schneider, & Cobb, 1993; Ellis-Stoll

& Popkess-Vawter, 1998; Fulton, 1997; Hartrick & Schreiber, 1998; Hawks, 1992; Jones, O'Toole, Hoa, Chau, & Muc, 2000; Klakovich, 1995; Kuokkanen & Leino-Kilpi, 2000; Laschinger, Wong, McMabon, & Kaufmann, 1999; Rodwell, 1996; Ryles, 1999; Wallerstein & Bernstein, 1988). Although not all of these attributes are necessarily part of every experience of empowerment, they provide markers that help us identify the process and presence of empowerment.

Empowerment implies choice on the part of those being empowered. We cannot empower another, because to presume to do so removes the element of choice. Individuals and groups must ultimately motivate and empower themselves. This process requires self-awareness, positive self-esteem, commitment to self and others, and the desire and ability to make decisions. Responsibility and accountability for our actions and having the authority to act are implicit in the ability to choose.

Through the empowerment process, we can enable others to develop awareness of areas that need change, foster a desire to take action, and share resources, skills, and opportunities that support the change. Rodwell (1996) notes that it is self-awareness and resources, rather than the services provided to persons, that self-empower. Enhanced self-esteem, personal satisfaction, sense of connectedness, the ability to set and reach goals, a sense of control over life and change processes, and a sense of hope and direction are outcomes of empowerment.

Ask Yourself

What Makes You Feel Empowered?

- Consider a situation in which you felt empowered. Describe factors contributing to your sense of empowerment.
- Recall a time when you felt disempowered. What contributed to this sense? How might you have felt more empowered in the situation?

PERSONAL EMPOWERMENT

Nursing's power to make a difference in care with patients derives from many factors. In order to serve as credible models of empowerment for others, we must demonstrate congruence between values and behaviors in our own lives. Personal integrity implies an ability to be honest with and care for ourselves, as well as respond to the needs of others. Often nurses, and especially women, have learned to value care for others before or instead of care for self. A true value for human life must include value for our own life as well. The biblical adage is: "Love thy neighbor *as* thyself," not instead of thyself or before thyself (Leviticus 19:18). We must attend to ourselves and treat ourselves with the same respect and dignity as we treat others. Personal empowerment begins with actions that support the meeting of our own needs and self-actualization. It is from our personal stores of creativity, empowerment, and health that we are able to inspire, teach, and assist others in achieving their potential.

In principle many nurses would agree with the concept of care for self; however, actions often conflict with this acknowledged belief. Nurses often agree to work additional hours even when they are exhausted; consume large amounts of caffeine and sugar to boost waning energy; go home to care for children, spouse, and friends; and collapse into bed only to get up and do it all again the next day because they feel limited power to do otherwise. What causes a person to behave in a way that conflicts with their stated values? Often the person has learned conflicting messages. A belief in caring for ourselves may conflict with a learned belief that caring for others is more admirable or important than caring for ourselves.

Some people feel very little control over any area of their lives. Others may feel empowered to make decisions in some situations but not in others—for example, a person may actively make decisions in the home environment while feeling like a pawn of the system at work. The sense of power that nurses have in their personal lives may affect their perception of empowerment in the professional arena. Burnout, job dissatisfaction, and limited professional commitment affect the quality of patient care, and are often associated with feelings of powerlessness (Moss, 1995). Attributes of empowerment noted in the previous section reflect important considerations for self-empowerment on both personal and professional levels.

The ability to facilitate empowerment in others requires us to attend to personal empowerment. This means valuing ourselves and "listening inwardly to your own senses as well as listening intently and actively to others, consciously taking in and forming strength" (Chinn, 1995, p. 3). Self-awareness is necessary, since self-perception has a direct link to quality of patient care (Moss, 1995). Such awareness requires attentiveness to factors that influence our thoughts, feelings, actions, and reactions in the present circumstance and reflective considerations of such influences on past experiences. Empowerment involves taking ownership of our inner life and recognizing that we have full control over our thoughts, feelings, and actions.

Owning our thoughts involves recognizing old or repetitive thought patterns and changing those that are no longer supporting a creative, actualizing life. Self-critical, judgmental, and negative thinking are particularly confining. Old thinking can be updated with new knowledge. Questioning the origin of particular thoughts can reveal ideas that were true at one time but are no longer true. For example, a child who was always told that she did not know enough to make a decision, and that mother knew best, may become an adult who still consults her mother before making decisions. Seeking alternative views of situations, and learning logical or critical thinking skills, are other ways to restructure thought patterns.

Feelings are transient signals that alert us to what is supportive or offensive in a situation. Owning feelings means acknowledging and investigating the internal source of the message, rather than blaming other persons or situations for our feelings. People may experience different feelings in similar situations. For example, a death can elicit feelings of sadness, despair, hope, relief, joy, and others, depending upon the unique inner response of each person. Feelings and the reactions they elicit are in the person, not in the event.

We need to name and take ownership of personal values and to claim our ability to make choices. When experiencing a lack of control in life, we should identify both internal and external barriers to having control, consider whether we want control, and explore what we need to do and are willing to risk in order to take control. Consciously acting based upon clear evaluation of the current situation, rather than acting automatically, is one way to own our behavior. Taking ownership of behavior requires being able to see options. Believing there are no options can result in feeling powerless, trapped, or victimized. Even when we do not believe we can change a current unacceptable situation immediately, we can make a plan for change and set that plan into motion one step at a time. A *victim* waits and hopes something or someone else will change; makes excuses for not taking action (time, cost, fatigue, and the like); blames people, places, or things for their situation; is trapped and unaware of options. An *empowered person* decides to be accountable for personal responses, makes plans, considers options, develops strategies for change, and acts on plans by doing what is necessary to succeed.

Personal empowerment "is growth of personal strength, power, and ability to enact one's own will and love for self in the context of love and respect for others . . . [and] is only possible when individuals express respect and reverence for all other forms of life and ground the energy of the Self as one with the earth" (Chinn, 1995, p. 3). A commitment to personal growth and self-care, developing a positive sense of self, awareness of strengths and abilities as well as limitations, and drawing on our supports and sources of connectedness foster this process. It is essential that we trust ourselves and our knowledge and abilities and are courageous in taking risks. Empathy with others, appreciation of diversity, tolerance, flexibility, and willingness to compromise empower a person. Empowerment requires being true to ourselves and our values in the midst of a loving response to the choices of others. Congruence among our being, knowing, and doing reflects personal integrity. This means that our actions flow from our essence, and our choices derive from what we know to be good and true.

PROFESSIONAL EMPOWERMENT

Professional empowerment is built upon the foundational elements of personal accountability and support of nursing colleagues. In order to deal in a principled way with issues and dilemmas arising within health care settings, nurses must feel personally and professionally empowered to act on sometimes difficult choices. Many factors affect nursing actions in the professional arena, including personal attitudes and self-concept; the structural and functional interrelatedness of health care systems; political, economic, and social forces; and interactions with patients and colleagues. Barriers to empowerment exist within the community of nursing and are also imposed from external sources. Curtin reminds us that "many nurses are unwilling to assume responsibility for decision making and that nursing has failed to develop an adequate support system for nurses" (1982, p. 10).

Empowerment requires nurses to become knowledgeable about and address system issues as well as interpersonal issues. Such issues include recognizing the need for changing the power base within the current health care system, moving from a paternalistic, hierarchical model of control toward one that values collaboration, and the power of the collective. Nurses must become involved in shared decision making and in forming institutional policies as part of this process (Chandler, 1991; Gaul, 1995; Moss, 1995).

The effect of nurses' empowerment in the health care environment can have personal, institutional, and patient care implications. In terms of nursing management and health systems, some authors view empowerment as a method for delegating authority and sharing power and a strategy for improving productivity of nurses. Laschinger and colleagues (1999) report that empowered nurses are more likely to initiate and sustain independent behaviors to accomplish task objectives in the face of difficulty, thereby increasing work effectiveness. One study suggests a link between staff nurses' perceptions of their work effectiveness and workplace empowerment (Laschinger and Wong, 1999). The authors identify three factors that have a positive impact on empowerment: access to the structures of information, support, and resource. Moss (1995) relates empowerment to increased efficiency, job satisfaction, and better patient care. In contrast, Moss notes that feelings of powerlessness are associated with job dissatisfaction and low levels of professional commitment, which are barriers to quality patient care. This author links nurses' perceptions of themselves to quality of patient care, reflecting that nurses who are burned out and dissatisfied are more inclined to give only the most routine care. Klakovich (1995) proposes that only an empowered work force can be effective in today's recent innovations of patient-focused care, case management, and shared governance. Inherent in this perspective is a sense that each person is free to make choices, and that those who are empowered, both internally and by the system, feel more in control of their lives, are able to act in appropriate, meaningful ways and to do what they truly want to do.

When nurses feel disempowered in their work settings, they can choose the *victim* stance, which relinquishes power to the system, or they can challenge the system. Dealing with the system requires skills in conflict management, negotiation, and effective communication. Challenging the system can take many forms. Being a change agent begins with the nurse's personal presence and attitude. For example, one nurse described how her commitment to caring for the whole person was challenged when she began working in a level III trauma center. Feeling constantly criticized by co-workers as she incorporated emotional and spiritual support into her care, she made the choice to act out of her values as a holistic nurse and return a loving spirit to the injustice of their criticism. She noted that this choice came as a great challenge, and that it was often difficult to go to work under the scrutiny focused in her direction. However, she used each opportunity of conversation to suggest that they work together to unite the staff with an attitude of mutual caring, support, and nurturance. Her presence was reflected in her choice to stand in her power and speak her truth. Although this was not easy, living her values contributed to a change in attitude within the whole staff, particularly regarding how they supported and cared for each other.

Nurses can address social and economic constraints on nursing and health care through their involvement in professional organizations and through becoming politically active. Participation on institution boards or committees that focus on patient care and professional practice concerns is another way to challenge the system, as is speaking out about unsafe or questionable practices. Speaking out is sometimes referred to as **whistle blowing.**

Unity in Diversity

Empowerment incorporates divergent and conflicting solutions to problems based on value in support of others rather than in divisiveness (Chinn, 1995; Gibson, 1991). It implies embracing diversity and moving from fear of that which is different to appreciation of the strength derived from and unity contained in diversity. Nurses need to recognize that systems exert control, in part, by fostering divisiveness among workers in order to deter unity of opposition to system policies. When nurses unite with and support colleagues who challenge harmful or potentially harmful practices, they are personally and professionally empowered.

Challenging unjust, unprofessional, or unethical practices is not an easy decision, and may entail risk for nurses. Feeling empowered to take a stand requires personal integrity and support from others. Support that enables nurses to be true advocates for patients may come from colleagues, from professional organizations, and from the legal protection of *whistleblower laws*. Tressman notes that nearly three-quarters of the states have enacted or introduced **whistleblower** legislation or regulations in recent years. For nurses who are considering taking action or speaking out, she offers these suggestions:

- Determine if you are ready, both personally and professionally, to take action through personal reflection and consultation with others
- Consult a lawyer
- Contact your state nurses' association for information about the status of whistleblower legislation in your state, and for guidance in the whistleblower process
- Use a journal to document instances that give you concern and that compromise care, creating a paper trail that includes dates, times, and outcomes of unsafe or inappropriate care. Make a copy of all documentation
- Fill out "assignment despite objection" forms when you are working in situations that are unsafe
- Speak only the truth, state only the facts, and follow the institution's chain of command to the letter before contacting an outside agency
- If you decide to contact an outside agency, send all documents via certified mail with a return receipt
- Be professional when dealing with the administration and refrain from making it personal. Presuming that administrators with integrity will act on your concerns quickly, do not wait too long for results
- Build leadership skills and unity among your colleagues
- Work with your state nurses' and national nurses' associations to help pass or strengthen whistleblower laws in your state and nationally (2000, p. 22).

Nurses need to be willing to struggle with difficult questions and arrive at decisions that flow from their internal values and perspective, rather than looking for the *right* answer from an external source. Empowerment implies accountability for our own choices and actions. Jameton (1984) reflects that people pretend they are forced to do things when they are not. He gives the example of a nurse who instructs a patient to take a medication because the physician ordered it, noting that both patient and nurse pretend that they must act because of the physician's order, although each could make another choice. Reflecting that nurses who choose to work in systems such as hospitals are accountable for their actions despite the existence of systemic problems affecting health care, Jameton writes,

> If one fails to resist exploitation, incompetence, and corrupt practices, one becomes responsible for them. If one resists them, one enters into conflict with conventional conceptions of behavior for employees and thereby risks reprisals. One has to choose between complicity and self-sacrifice, or enter the uncomfortable middle ground of irony. Ethics does not give a clear answer as to which one must choose. Instead, one is free to move in the direction of the kind of world one personally desires to create. (1984, p. 289)

We must decide whether we prefer a world in which we are empowered in the professional arena, or one in which we are controlled by others. The choices we make influence the outcome.

RE-VISIONING NURSING

Empowerment within the profession requires a renewed vision of nursing. As nurses we need to redefine nursing according to our own vision, rather than accepting the definition imposed by the dominant groups in health care, that is, physicians and institutions. When nurses draw pictures of their vision of nursing, what emerges are images of caring, light, comfort, and love. These images reflect the heart of the vision of nursing within nurses. Making choices based on the vision and values of the profession fosters congruence between nursing's knowing and doing, which strengthens personal and professional effectiveness. In contrast, nurses who work in situations in which they feel a lack of synchronicity with their values often experience burnout, become nasty, take on attributes and values of the dominant group, and look for someone to blame (behaviors reflective of oppressed groups). Remaining in a victim role involves a choice to give away our power and allow someone else to define our reality. Redefining nursing according to nursing's own vision is an act of empowerment.

Empowerment involves risk and commitment and requires both courage and compassion. Curtin (1996) illustrates this through a parable about a baby eagle who, after falling from his nest and breaking his wing, was found by a mountain climber who took him home, nursed the broken wing, and put him in with the chickens. Not knowing what or how to eat, the eagle learned from the chickens how to peck at the feed on the ground. Even as he grew larger and stronger he continued to peck away like the chickens and forgot that he was an eagle. When a friend of the climber noted that the eagle should be flying up in the mountains with other eagles, the climber responded that the eagle knew he had good situation with free food and a warm coop, and would not fly away even if he could. The friend offered to teach the eagle to fly and took him to the top of the barn, telling him that he was an eagle and could fly and be free. The eagle heard this but remembered what happened the last time he tried to fly, and, seeing the chickens below, remembered the food and shelter, and would not fly. The friend tried another approach of taking the eagle to the mountains, teaching him how to spread and flap his wings, and encouraging his efforts, telling him repeatedly that he was an eagle and could fly. Finally the eagle took the risk and flew, delighting in the experience; but as he flew over the chicken yard, he remembered that he was hungry and returned to peck for food with the chickens. This distressed the friend who disparaged the eagle for continuing to act like a chicken when he could be free. Eventually a new plan was devised in which the friend carefully crept up to the eagle and, putting a hood over his head, carried him to an area where there were other eagles. The eagle saw their nests and watched them hunt, eat, feed their young, and fly. The friend showed him the beauty of his homeland, encouraged him to hunt and fly, and reminded him that he was an EAGLE. After several days the eagle got the idea, and when the friend took him to the top of the highest mountain, he took off and soared high, never looking back, and never eating chicken feed again, because he was an EAGLE, and he knew it. (Summarized from Curtin, 1996.)

Curtin relates the insights of this parable to empowerment for nurses. The story demonstrates that empowerment is not easy for either the one trying to empower or the one being empowered, but that it is important not to give up. We must also realize that empowerment costs money, time, and effort.

> It (empowerment) isn't easy. Telling the eagle to fly wasn't enough. It isn't easy. Changing the eagle's environment and even teaching him to fly wasn't enough. It isn't easy. You have to start at the beginning and recreate an attitude in a new environment. It's tough on the eagle too. The eagle was frightened: he had been hurt. The eagle knew the old, safe ways of pecking and free grain and warm nest. And he could have that with no effort! It was hard for the eagle to believe that the easy way sooner or later would destroy him. And it was really tough on the eagle when [the friend] blamed him for being what he'd been taught to be all his life. (Curtin, 1996, p. 210)

Curtin notes that neither freedom nor risk are easy, and that they are not for everyone. It is important, however, not to "blame the chickens for what they are. It's unfair—and it's a waste of time. But never give up on the eagles. They can fly—and they will" (p. 210). Empowerment for nurses means recognizing *who* we are, knowing that, like the eagle, we have both the ability and the freedom to fly!

SUMMARY

Empowerment is a multifaceted concept. Awareness of attitudes about nursing's role in health care and factors that shape these attitudes enables nurses to identify more effectively that which supports or diminishes both personal and professional empowerment. Attentiveness to personal empowerment, which includes integrity, accountability, and courage, is foundational for addressing empowerment issues within the profession. No one can empower another. However, we can facilitate the inner process of empowerment when knowledge and resources are offered within an environment of mutual respect and support. Empowerment for nurses requires remembering *who* we are, recognizing that *knowing* must be the same as *doing*, and following our own vision of nursing.

CHAPTER HIGHLIGHTS

- Mind sets regarding health care influence how nurses identify and respond to ethical issues and dilemmas in practice settings.
- Nursing's contemporary self-perception reflects the legal metaphor of patient advocate rather than the military metaphor of loyal soldier. Each of these metaphors implies different ethical imperatives for nursing.
- Current nursing codes and standards of practice reflect ethical imperatives that flow from the advocacy metaphor.
- Empowerment, which is both process and outcome, derives from a feminine perspective of *power to or power with*, reflecting a supportive partnership based on mutual love and respect that enables people to change situations given necessary resources, knowledge, skills, and opportunities. Empowerment comes from within a person and involves choice; we cannot empower another.
- The ability to deal with health care issues and dilemmas in a principled way derives from personal and professional empowerment and requires attentiveness to intrapersonal, interpersonal, and systems issues.
- Personal empowerment requires self-awareness and is characterized by maintaining personal integrity in the midst of a loving response to the choices of others. Self-concept and sense of power in a nurse's personal life affects nursing care and a nurse's ability to enable empowerment in others.
- Recognizing unity in diversity and incorporating divergent views and solutions empowers nurses and others.
- Defining nursing according to nursing's own vision is an act of empowerment that implies accountability for our own choices and actions, with awareness that each choice helps create the kind of world and environment within which nurses must practice.

DISCUSSION QUESTIONS AND ACTIVITIES

1. Talk with both retired and practicing nurses about ethical imperatives that guide (or guided) their nursing practice. Identify mind sets and metaphors reflective of these imperatives.

2. Where in your life do you feel most personally empowered? Discuss the circumstances surrounding your feelings of empowerment with other students.

3. Review Chapters 5 and 6 and reflect on how your values and current phase of development affect your sense of personal empowerment.

4. Describe a situation in which you took ownership for your own thoughts, feelings, or actions. Describe a time when you found yourself blaming others or assuming a victim stance. Discuss with classmates factors prompting each stance and how you felt in each situation.

5. Discuss differences in others that might engender fear or caution in you and limit your ability to embrace the diversity.

6. What aspects of empowerment do you think are most important in nursing practice settings? Support your perspective.

7. Interview practicing nurses regarding personal and professional power, including situations where they feel empowered to make decisions, where they derive authority to make decisions, and situations in which they have experienced dilemmas around the issue of power. Ask them to describe their ideal image of nursing and compare that to their current reality.

8. Illustrate your vision of nursing and develop strategies for making nursing's self-vision better known to others. Implement one strategy.

REFERENCES

American Nurses Association. (1985). *Code for nurses with interpretive statements*. Washington, DC: Author.

American Nurses' Association. (2001). *Code of Ethics for Nurses*. Kansas City, MO: Author.

Aroskar, M. A. (1982). Are nurses' mind sets compatible with ethical practice? *Topics in Clinical Nursing, 4,* 22–32.

Bolton, B., & Brookings, J. (1998). Development of a measure of intrapersonal empowerment. *Rehabilitation Psychology, 43*(2), 131–142.

Byrne, C. (1999). Facilitating empowerment groups: Dismantling professional boundaries. *Issues in Mental Health Nursing, 19,* 55–71.

Cameron, A. (1981). *Daughters of copper woman*. Vancouver, BC: Press Gang.

Chandler, G. E. (1991). Creating an environment to empower nurses. *Nursing Management, 22,* 20–23.

Chavasse, J. M. (1992). New dimensions of empowerment in nursing—and challenges. *Journal of Advanced nursing, 17,* 1–2.

Chinn, P. (1995). *Peace and power: Building communities for the future*. New York: National League of Nursing Press.

Connelly, L. M., Keele, B. S., Kleinbeck, V. M., Schneider, J. K., & Cobb, A. K. (1993). A place to be yourself: Empowerment from the client's perspective. *IMAGE: Journal of Nursing Scholarship, 25*(4), 297–303.

Curtin, L. (1982). Autonomy, accountability and nursing practice. *Topics in Clinical Nursing, 4,* 7–14.

Curtin, L. (1996). *Nursing into the 21st century*. Springhouse, PA: Springhouse.

Ellis-Stoll, C. C., & Popkess-Vawter, S. (1998). A concept analysis on the process of empowerment. *Advances in Nursing Science, 21*(2), 62–68.

Fulton, Y. (1997). Nurses' views on empowerment: A critical social theory perspective. *Journal of Advanced Nursing, 26*, 529–536.

Gaul, A. L. (1995). Casuistry, care, compassion, and ethics data analysis. *Advances in Nursing Science, 17*, 47–57.

Gibson, C. H. (1991). A concept analysis of empowerment. *Journal of Advanced Nursing, 16*, 354–361.

Gurka, A. M. (1995). Transformational leadership: Qualities and strategies for the CNS. *Clinical Nurse Specialist, 9*, 169–174.

Hartrick, G., & Schreiber, R. (1998). Imaging ourselves: Nurses' metaphors of practice. *Journal of Holistic Nursing, 16*(4), 420–434.

Hawks, J. H. (1992). Empowerment in nursing education: Concept analysis and application to philosophy, learning and instruction. *Journal of Advanced Nursing, 17*, 609–618.

Jameton, A. (1984). *Nursing practice: The ethical issues.* Englewood Cliffs, NJ: Prentice-Hall.

Jones, P. S., O'Toole, M. T., Hoa, N., Chau, T. T., & Muc, P. D. (2000). Empowerment of nursing as a socially significant profession in Vietnam. *Journal of Nursing Scholarship, 32*(3), 317–321.

Klakovich, M. (1995). Development and psychometric evaluation of the reciprocal empowerment scale. *Journal of Nursing Management, 3*(2), 127–143.

Kuokkanen, L., & Leino-Kilpi, H. (2000). Power and empowerment in nursing: Three theoretical approaches. *Journal of Advanced Nursing, 31*(1), 235–241.

Laschinger, H. K., & Wong, C. (1999). Staff nurse empowerment and collective accountability: Effect on perceived productivity and self-rated work effectiveness. *Nursing Economics, 17*(6), 308–316.

Laschinger, H. K., Wong, C., McMahon, L., & Kaufmann, C. (1999). Leader behavior impact on staff nurse empowerment, job tension, and work effectiveness. *JONA, 29*(5), 28–39.

Moss, M. T. (1995). Foundations of nursing empowerment. *Nursing Economics, 13*, 112–114.

Rodwell, C. M. (1996). An analysis of the concept of empowerment. *Journal of Advanced Nursing, 23*, 305–313.

Ryles, S. M. (1999). A concept analysis of empowerment: Its relationship to mental health nursing. *Journal of Advanced Nursing, 29*(3), 600–607.

The Random House dictionary of the English language, second edition unabridged. (1987). New York: Random House.

Tressman, S. (2000). Speaking out: Two nurses tell their stories. *The American Nurse, 32*(4), 1–2, 22.

Wallerstein, N., & Bernstein, E. (1988). Empowerment education: Freire's ideas adapted to health education. *Health Education Quarterly, 15*(4), 379–394.

Winslow, G. R. (1984). From loyalty to advocacy: A new metaphor for nursing. *The Hastings Center Report, 14*, 32–40.

CHAPTER **20**

Enabling Patient Empowerment

Power is the energy from which action arises.
(Chinn, 1995, p. 8)

OBJECTIVES

After completing this chapter, the reader should be able to:

1. Discuss the meaning of patient empowerment.

2. Discuss the nursing role in empowerment of patients.

3. Describe attitudes of nurses that enable empowerment.

4. Identify nursing knowledge and skills basic to empowerment.

5. Describe factors that enhance or block patient empowerment.

6. Discuss approaches to fostering empowerment with patients.

INTRODUCTION

The concept of empowerment relates to the principle of autonomy and to the nursing role of patient advocate. Fostering empowerment in others requires nurses to be attentive to both personal and professional empowerment. This chapter focuses on nursing's role in facilitating empowerment of patients. Understanding of power and empowerment, discussed in Chapter 19, apply to patients as well as nurses. The discussion of empowerment in this chapter flows from these same understandings.

PATIENTS AND EMPOWERMENT

The concept of empowering patients has emerged as nursing has directed its ethical focus to advocacy for patients. Adherence to principles discussed throughout this book, particularly respect for persons, autonomy, justice, and beneficence, makes it incumbent upon nurses to involve patients in making decisions about their health and care. Some patients have both desire and skills to take charge of their lives, some have desire but need to improve their skills, while others have limitations in ability and desire. Negotiating within a system that has traditionally placed decision making authority and power primarily within the hands of physicians requires skill, support, and a strong sense of personal empowerment. Factors discussed in Chapter 19 regarding personal empowerment for nurses apply as well to patients. Patient empowerment is both a process and outcome in which nurses have an active role.

NURSES AND PATIENT EMPOWERMENT

We cannot empower another, as that would strip them of their ability to choose. Although empowerment is something that comes from within a person, nurses can serve as enablers of the process. Enabling the empowerment process requires a paradigm shift away from the paternalistic attitude of knowing what is best for the patient. Instead we recognize and accept that patients are essentially responsible for their own health and have the ability to discern what they need, make decisions, and direct their own destinies. In order to make appropriate decisions, however, people may need information and support.

Gibson describes empowerment in the health care arena as "a social process of recognizing, promoting and enhancing people's abilities to meet their own needs, solve their own problems and mobilize the necessary resources in order to feel in control of their own lives . . . a process of helping people to assert control over the factors which affect their health" (1991, p. 339). In light of this description and nursing's focus on patient advocacy, nurses are called to be enablers of the empowerment process with patients, families, and communities. Certain attitudes, knowledge, and skills are basic to fulfilling this role.

Attitudes of Nurses That Enable Empowerment

A view of the nurse as a partner, facilitator, and resource rather than merely one who provides services for patients is basic to enabling empowerment with patients

(Gibson, 1991; Ellis-Stoll & Popkess-Vawter, 1998; Fulton, 1997). Nurses must learn to surrender their need for control, developing instead attitudes of collaboration and mutual participation in decision making. This requires self-reflection on the part of the nurse, through which the nurse confronts personal values and subtle, and not so subtle, benefits gained from being in a position of power. It is essential that nurses make a commitment to being with patients as they struggle with their questions and issues and seek meaning in the process. Relinquishing control also means that nurses need to accept decisions made by patients and families, even when they are different from what the nurse might do or suggest. Respect for persons, which includes valuing others and mutual trust, is key (Gibson, 1991; Rodwell, 1996; Ellis-Stoll & Popkess-Vawter, 1998; Ryles, 1999).

Nursing Knowledge and Skills Necessary for Enabling Empowerment

Information presented throughout this book provides a foundation for facilitating the empowerment process. Attention to ethical principles and processes of decision making fosters empowerment. Awareness of the development of values and their impact on choices allows nurses to be more clear about their own perspectives, so as to foster integrity and avoid imposing personal values on others. Knowledge of social, cultural, political, economic, and other forces affecting a person's options and health choices is essential.

Empowerment is an interactive process. As in many other areas of nursing, effective communication is necessary for facilitating empowerment. The ability to listen with our whole being and to trust intuitive as well as intellectual understanding is important. Reflective listening allows us to help people to recognize their own strengths, abilities, and personal power. Active listening also helps people develop awareness of root causes of problems and to determine their readiness to take action for change. If it is determined that the patient does not want to be empowered, nursing interventions need to be provided in a style of empowerment rather than control (Gibson, 1991). This means approaching patients with an attitude of trust in their abilities to know, at some place within themselves, what they need, and to incorporate behaviors such as offering choices about aspects of care over which they can have control.

Having opportunities and resources necessary for understanding and changing our world is part of the empowerment process. Nurses must have knowledge of factors affecting a patient's health and health care decisions in order to help provide or share the necessary resources. Such knowledge includes awareness of patient and family values and decision-making style; cultural context; social, political, and economic influences on our options; and health care system constraints. We also recognize that individual responsibility for health is necessarily tempered by social and environmental factors. Gibson (1991) suggests that nurses need to focus health promotion efforts on the macro social level, attending to conditions that control, influence, and produce health or illness in people. Efforts as individuals, within professional organizations, and within communities, aimed at providing access to health care for all, provide a broad base of support for empowerment.

Nurses must approach patients as equal partners. Skillful collaboration and negotiation, which incorporate power sharing and mutually beneficial interactions, enable empowerment. Relinquishing professional power returns power to the patient.

ENHANCING PATIENT CAPACITY FOR DECISION MAKING

The ability to make decisions regarding our life and destiny requires a basic level of cognitive functioning and sense of control over life and change processes. Empowerment originates in self-esteem; is developed through love, a sense of connectedness, responsibility, and opportunities for choice; and is supported through perceived meaning and hope in life (Rodwell, 1996).

Helping patients to know who they are facilitates empowerment. The process of self-discovery enables patients to decide what they want to do based on appreciation of who they are. Thus "the patient's empowerment to make decisions comes from the deepest understanding of the self" (Purtilo & Meier, 1993). This may require facilitating a patient's self-awareness on many levels, such as identifying personal values, sources of these values, where and with whom they feel connected, and where and how they experience control in life. Utilizing the decision making process discussed in Chapter 6 can facilitate empowerment with patients.

Determining whether a person functions primarily from a sense of internal or external locus of control can be useful. **Locus of control** refers to beliefs about the ability to control events in our life. People who believe that they are able to influence or control things that happen to them are considered to have an **internal locus of control.** On the other hand, people who feel that forces outside of themselves direct or rule their lives, whether these be generalized forces such as fate or other persons who are perceived as more powerful, are considered to have an **external locus of control.** Persons who are internally motivated are more likely to perceive themselves as having power to make choices and control their lives, and to be motivated to make necessary changes. Those who are externally motivated tend to be more fatalistic, expecting their lives to be controlled by powerful others, and less likely to enact personal power (Dawson, 1994; Miller, 1993).

Ask Yourself

How Does Locus of Control Affect Empowerment?

- Reflect on how you have thought through significant decisions in your life. Do you consider that you are more internally or externally motivated? Give specific examples to support your self-assessment.

- In working with patients what would you consider indications of internal and external locus of control?

- How would your approach to facilitating empowerment be different with persons who exhibit internal locus of control compared to those with external locus of control?

Barriers to Empowerment

Empowerment involves a willingness to take risks, to move beyond that which is known and perhaps comfortable, to the unknown. It often requires a change in self-perception, developing a different vision of who we are. This can stimulate anxiety and fear. Nurses need to recognize such barriers and appreciate that not everyone wants to take the risks and assume the responsibility that empowerment demands. Paternalistic attitudes within the health care system have fostered reliance on health care providers to determine what patients need for health. Other barriers include patient lack of knowledge of resources or strategies that promote empowerment, dependency, apathy, mistrust, and being labeled by staff (Connelly, Keele, Kleinbeck, Schneider, & Cobb, 1993). Social, cultural, economic, or political factors can present barriers such as limitation of resources, control of knowledge about options, locking people into traditional roles and expectations, social labeling that stereotypes and devalues certain people or behaviors, and restriction of access to resources. Lack of empowerment of professionals and their inability to relinquish power to patients affect patient empowerment as well. Honoring patient decisions may be very threatening to nurses who do not appreciate that patients know what they need.

FOSTERING PATIENT EMPOWERMENT

We can facilitate empowerment in others by being role models of self-empowerment. As noted previously, belief that patients have the right and ability to make choices regarding their health, and other areas of their lives, is basic to empowerment. Patients need to be given opportunities for choice regarding small as well as major decisions. This means that there needs to be participatory decision making, involving collaboration and negotiation, in all areas of health care. For example, involving patients in making decisions about when they will bathe, what foods to include in their diet, or when to take their medications is as important to empowerment as their participation in decision making regarding life support measures. Because of social, environmental, and other factors, some people have had limited opportunities for making choices and may need education, practice, and nurture in this area. Offering options and developing strategies to enhance the patient's ability to set and reach goals are important parts of the nursing role. Connelly et al. (1993) suggest that choosing implies having both the freedom and the courage to choose from different options. Support is an important part of the encouraging process.

Support can take many forms. We provide support by determining what patients identify as empowering to them and encouraging these choices, behaviors, or attitudes. Caring relationships, in which experiences are shared and patients are accepted for who they are, offer support. Having at least one other person who supports a choice made or a stance that a person takes enhances the likelihood that the person will follow through on the decision.

Considering options and making choices implies having both knowledge and availability of needed resources. Enabling empowerment may require us to provide or help patients discover how to access resources. In some instances this may mean becoming politically and socially active regarding health care issues affecting vulnerable populations. We need to develop strategies that enhance a patient's ability to acquire necessary knowledge. This may mean working with patients or communities to identify both health concerns and socioculturally relevant approaches to dealing with these concerns. We foster empowerment by promoting processes that encourage mutually respectful exchange of ideas and analysis of concerns and potential solutions. Success in achieving goals must be defined from the perspective of the patient or community.

❓ Think About It

Outcomes of Patient Empowerment

Upholding the view that patients know what they need opens nurses to the probability that some patients will make decisions that are not consistent with what the nurse or other health team members think is best. Such decisions may have a relatively minor impact on a patient's or family's health and well-being or may be judged to have potentially serious outcomes for the patient or family.

- What factors need to be considered when dealing with decisions involving differing values between patients and nurses?
- Give examples of situations in which patient empowerment might potentiate an ethical dilemma for you.
- If you feel a patient is making an unwise decision, how would you respond?
- Discuss your view regarding any limits or constraints on patient empowerment.

SUMMARY

Patient empowerment is an important element of nursing care that derives from an appreciation that patients have the ability to discern their needs and make decisions about their lives and health. Being an enabler of empowerment requires that nurses learn to relinquish power and embrace the patient as an equal partner. Self-awareness, respect for others, and effective communication skills serve as foundations for the process. Knowledge about and availability of resources, support, and opportunities for choice are necessary for empowerment. Nurses can facilitate empowerment by working directly with patients and through addressing social, political, and environmental factors affecting empowerment of individuals and communities. In the midst of an ever changing and challenging health care environment in which issues of power and control continue to affect patient care, nurses must be competent enablers of patient empowerment.

CHAPTER HIGHLIGHTS

- Patient empowerment, which is both a process and an outcome, relates to ethical principles and flows from nursing's focus on patient advocacy.

- Although nurses cannot empower patients, they can be enablers of empowerment, a process that requires recognition and acceptance that patients have the ability to discern what they need, to make decisions, and to direct their own destinies.
- Empowerment is interactive and requires knowledge of personal values and needs for control, mutual trust and respect, effective communication and reflective listening skills, and a willingness to accept patient decisions regardless of whether the nurse thinks they are best.
- Fostering patient empowerment requires knowledge of social, political, cultural, economic, and environmental factors affecting a person's options and health choices and may involve addressing health promotion efforts on the macro social level.
- Empowerment is fostered through self-discovery, enhanced self-esteem, a sense of connectedness, support, opportunities for choice, and having needed resources, knowledge, and skills.
- Empowerment strategies that mesh with a person's or community's sociocultural context are more effective.

DISCUSSION QUESTIONS AND ACTIVITIES

1. Describe a personal experience as a patient within the health care system in which you felt that you were empowered. What contributed to the empowerment process for you?

2. Describe a patient or family with whom you have worked who exhibited empowerment. Give specific examples of evidences of empowerment from your perspective.

3. Observe practicing nurses in a clinical setting and describe attitudes and behaviors that foster or block empowerment with patients.

4. Discuss factors within the health care system that inhibit patient empowerment.

5. Describe the relationship between patient empowerment and principled behavior in nursing.

6. Describe a situation in which you believe you fostered empowerment with a patient or family. How did you enable the process? Describe the outcome.

7. What would indicate to you that a patient might not want to be empowered? How would you approach and work with this patient?

REFERENCES

Chinn, P. L. (1995). *Peace & power: Building communities for the future* (4th ed.). New York: National League of Nursing Press.

Connelly, L. M., Keele, B. S., Kleinbeck, S. V. M., Schneider, J. K., & Cobb, A. K. (1993). A place to be yourself: Empowerment from the client's perspective. *Image, 25,* 297–303.

Dawson, M. S. (1994). Using locus of control to empower student nurses to be professional. *Nursing Forum, 29,* 10–15.

Ellis-Stoll, C. C., & Popkess-Vawter, S. (1998). A concept analysis on the process of empowerment. *Advances in Nursing Science, 21*(2), 62–68.

Fulton, Y. (1997). Nurses' views on empowerment: A critical social theory perspective. *Journal of Advanced Nursing, 26,* 529–536.

Gibson, C. H. (1991). A concept analysis of empowerment. *Journal of Advanced Nursing, 16,* 354–361.

Miller, C. M. (1993). Trajectory and empowerment theory applied to care of patients with multiple sclerosis. *Journal of Neuroscience Nursing, 25,* 343–348.

Purtilo, R. B., & Meier, R. H. (1993). Team challenges: Regulatory constraints and patient empowerment. *American Journal of Physical Medicine & Rehabilitation, 72,* 327–330.

Rodwell, C. M. (1996). An analysis of the concept of empowerment. *Journal of Advanced Nursing, 23,* 305–313.

Ryles, S. M. (1999). A concept analysis of empowerment: Its relationship to mental health nursing. *Journal of Advanced Nursing, 29*(3), 600–607.

APPENDIX **A**

Code of Ethics for Nurses (2001)

Reprinted with permission of the American Nurses Association, 2001

PREFACE

Ethics is an integral part of the foundation of nursing. Nursing has a distinguished history of concern for the welfare of the sick, injured and vulnerable and for social justice. This concern is embodied in the provision of nursing care to individuals with the community. Nursing encompasses the prevention of illness, the alleviation of suffering, and the protection, promotion and restoration of health in the care of individuals, families, groups and communities. Nurses act to change those aspects of social structures that detract from health and well-being. Individuals who become nurses are expected not only to adhere to the ideals and moral norms of the profession but also to embrace them as a part of what it means to be a nurse. The ethical tradition of nursing is self-reflective, enduring, and distinctive. A code of ethics makes explicit the primary goals, values, and obligations of the profession.

The Code of Ethics for Nurses serves the following purposes:

- It is a succinct statement of the ethical obligations and duties of every individual who enters the nursing profession.
- It is the profession's nonnegotiable ethical standard.
- It is an expression of nursing's own understanding of its commitment to society.

There are numerous approaches for addressing ethics; these include adopting or ascribing to ethical theories, including humanist, feminist, and social ethics, adhering to ethical principles, and cultivating virtues. The Code of Ethics for Nurses reflects all of these approaches. The words "ethical" and "moral" are used throughout the Code of Ethics. "Ethical" is used to refer to reasons for decisions about how one ought to act, using the above mentioned approaches. In general, the word "moral" overlaps with "ethical" but is more aligned with personal belief and cultural values. Statements that describe activities and attributes of nurses in this Code of Ethics are to be understood as normative or prescriptive statements expressing expectations of ethical behavior.

The Code of Ethics uses the term *patient* to refer to recipients of nursing care. The derivation of this word refers to "one who suffers," reflecting a universal aspect of human existence. Nevertheless, it is recognized that nurses also provide services to those seeking health as well as those responding to illness, to students and to staff, in health care facilities as well as in communities. Similarly, the term *practice* refers to the actions of the nurse in whatever role the nurse fulfills, including direct patient care provider, educator, administrator, researcher, policy developer, or other. Thus, the values and obligations expressed in this Code of Ethics applies to nurses in all roles and settings.

The Code of Ethics for Nurses is a dynamic document. As nursing and its social context change, changes to the Code of Ethics are also necessary. The Code of Ethics consists of two components: the provisions and the accompanying interpretive statements. There are nine provisions. The first three describe the most fundamental values and commitments of the nurse; the next three address boundaries of duty and loyalty, and the last three address aspects of duties beyond individual patient encounters. For each provision, there are interpretive statements that provide greater specificity for practice and are responsive to the contemporary context of nursing. Consequently, the interpetive statements are subject to more frequent revision than are the provisions. Additional ethical guidance and detail can be found in ANA or constituent member association position statements that address clinical, research, administrative, educational or public policy issues.

The Code of Ethics for Nurses with Interpretive Statements provides a framework for nurses to use in ethical analysis and decision-making. The Code of Ethics establishes the ethical standard for the profession. It is not negotiable in any setting nor is it subject to revision or amendment except by formal process of the House of Delegates of the ANA. The Code of Ethics for Nurses is a reflection of the proud ethical heritage of nursing, a guide for nurses now and in the future.

1 The nurse, in all professional relationships, practices with compassion and respect for the inherent dignity, worth and uniqueness of every individual, unrestricted by considerations of social or economic status, personal attributes, or the nature of health problems.

1.1 Respect for human dignity

A fundamental principle that underlies all nursing practice is respect for the inherent worth, dignity, and human rights of every individual. Nurses take into account the needs and values of all persons in all professional relationships.

1.2 Relationships to patients

The need for health care is universal, transcending all individual differences. The nurse establishes relationships and delivers nursing services with respect for patient needs and values, and without prejudice. An individual's lifestyle, value system and religious beliefs should be considered in planning health care with and for each patient. Such consideration does not suggest that the nurse necessarily agrees with or condones certain individual choices, but that the nurse respects the patient as a person.

1.3 The nature of health problems

The nurse respects the worth, dignity and rights of all human beings irrespective of the nature of the health problems. The worth of the person is not affected by disease, disability, functional status, or proximity to death. This respect extends to all who require the services of the nurse for the promotion of health, the prevention of illness, the restoration of health, the alleviation of suffering, and the provision of supportive care to those who are dying.

The measures nurses take to care for the patient enable the patient to live with as much physical, emotional, social and spiritual well-being as possible. Nursing care aims to maximize the values that the patient has treasured in life and extends supportive care to the family and significant others. Nursing care is directed toward meeting the comprehensive needs of patients and their families across the continuum of care. This is particularly vital in the care of patients and their families at the end of life to prevent and relieve the cascade of symptoms and suffering that are commonly associated with dying.

Nurses are leaders and vigilant advocates for the delivery of dignified and humane care. Nurses actively participate in assessing and assuring the responsible and appropriate use of interventions in order to minimize unwarranted or unwanted treatment and patient suffering. The acceptability and importance of carefully considered decisions regarding resuscitation status, withholding and withdrawing life-sustaining therapies, forgoing medically provided nutrition and hydration, aggressive pain and symptom management and advance directives are increasingly evident. The nurse should provide interventions to relieve pain and other symptoms in the dying patient even when those interventions entail risks of hastening death. However, nurses may not act with the sole intent of ending a patient's life even though such action may be motivated by compassion, respect for autonomy and quality of life considerations. Nurses have invaluable experience, knowledge and insight into care at the end of life and should be actively involved in related research, education, practice and policy development.

1.4 The right to self-determination

Respect for human dignity requires the recognition of specific patient rights, particularly self-determination. Self-determination, also known as autonomy, is the philosophical basis for informed consent in health care. Patients have the moral and legal right to determine what will be done with their own person; to be given accurate, complete, and understandable information in a manner that facilitates an informed judgment; to be assisted with weighing the benefits, burdens and available options in their treatment, including the choice of no treatment; to accept, refuse or terminate treatment without deceit, undue influence, duress, coercion or penalty; and to be given necessary support throughout the decision-making and treatment process. Such support would include the opportunity to make decisions with family and significant others and the provision of advice and support from knowledgeable nurses and other health professionals. Patients should be involved in planning their own health care to the extent they are able and choose to participate.

Each nurse has an obligation to be knowledgeable about the moral and legal rights of all patients to self-determination. The nurse preserves, protects and supports those interests by assessing the patient's comprehension of both the information presented and the implications of decisions. In sitautions in which the patient lacks the capacity to make a decision, a designated surrogate decision-maker should be consulted. The role of the surrogate is to make decisions as the patient would based upon the patient's previously expressed wishes and known values. In the absence of a designated surrogate decision-maker, decisions should be made in the best interests of the patient, considering the patient's personal values to the extent they are known. The nurse supports patient self-determination by participating in discussions with surrogates, providing guidance and referral to other resources as necessary, and identifying and addressing problems in the decision-making process. Support of autonomy in the broadest sense also includes recognition that people of some cultures place less weight on individualism and choose to defer to family or community values in decision making. Respect not just for the specific decision but also for the patient's method of decision making is consistent with the principle of autonomy.

Individuals are interdependent members of the community. The nurse recognizes that there are situations in which the right to individual self-determination may be outweighed or limited by the rights, health and welfare of others, particularly in relation to public health considerations. Nonetheless, limitation of individual rights must always be considered a serious deviation from the standard of care, justified only when there are no less restrictive means available to preserve the rights of others and the demands of justice.

1.5 Relationships with colleagues and others

The principle of respect for persons extends to all individuals with whom the nurse interacts. The nurse maintains compassionate and caring relationships with colleagues and others with a commitment to the fair treatment of individuals, to integrity-preserving compromise, and to resolving conflict. Nurses function in many roles, including direct care provider, administrator, educator, researcher and consultant. In each of these roles, the nurse treats colleagues, employees, assistans, and students with respect and compassion. This standard of conduct precludes any and all prejudicial actions, any form of harassment or threatening behavior, or disregard for the effect of one's actions on others. The nurse values the distinctive contribution of individuals or groups, and collaborates to meet the shared goal of providing quality health services.

2 The nurse's primary commitment is to the patient, whether an individual, family, group or community.

2.1 Primacy of the patient's interests

The nurse's primary commitment is to the recipient of nursing and health care services—the patient—whether the recipient is an individual, a family, a group, or a community. Nursing holds a fundamental commitment to the uniqueness of the individual patient; therefore, any plan of care must reflect that uniqueness. The nurse strives to provide patients with opportunities to participate in planning care, assures that patients find the plans acceptable and supports the implementation of the plan. Addressing patient interests requires recognition of the patient's place in the family or other networks of relationship. When the patient's wishes are in conflict with others, the nurse seeks to help resolve the conflict. Where conflict persists, the nurse's commitment remains to the identified patient.

2.2 Conflict of interest for nurses

Nurses are frequently put in situations of conflict arising from competing loyalties in the workplace, including situations of conflicting expectations from patients, families, physicians, colleagues, and in many cases, health care organizations and health plans. Nurses must examine the conflicts arising between their own personal and professional values, the values and interests of others who are also responsible for patient care and health care decisions, as well as those of patients. Nurses strive to resolve such conflicts in ways that ensure patient safety, guard the patient's best intersts and preserve the professional integrity of the nurse.

Situations created by changes in health care financing and delivery systems, such as incentive systems to decrease spending, pose new possibilities of conflict between economic self-interest and professional integrity. Bonuses, sanctions, and incentives tied to financial targets are examples of features of health care systems that may present such conflict. Conflicts of interest may arise in any domain of nursing activity including clinical practice, administration, education or research. Advance practice nurses who bill directly for services and nursing executives with budgetary responsibilities must be especially cognizant of the potential for conflicts of interest. Nurses should disclose to all relevant parties (e.g., patients, employers, colleagues) any perceived or actual conflict of interest and in some situations should withdraw from further participation. Nurses in all roles must seek to ensure that employment arrangements are just and fair and do not create an unreasonable conflict between patient care and direct personal gain.

2.3 Collaboration

Collaboration is not just cooperation, but it is the concerted effort of individuals and groups to attain a shared goal. In health care, that goal is to address the health needs of the patient and the public. The complexity of health care delivery systems require a multi-disciplinary approach to the delivery of services that has the strong support and active participation of all the health professions. Within this context, nursing's unique contribution, scope of practice, and relationship with other health professions needs to be clearly articulated, represented and preserved. By its very nature, collaboration requires mutual trust, recognition, and respect among the health care team, shared decision making about patient care, and open dialogue among all parties who have an interest in and a concern for health outcomes. Nurses should work to assure that the relevant parties are involved and have a voice in decision-making about patient care issues. Nurses should see that the questions that need to be addressed are asked and the information needed for informed decision-making is available and provided. Nurses should actively promote the collaborative multi-disciplinary planning required to ensure the availability and accessibility of quality health services to all persons who have needs for health care.

Intra-professional collaboration within nursing is fundamental to effectively address the health needs of patients and the public. Nurses engaged in non-clinical roles such as administration or research, while not providing direct care, nonetheless are collaborating in the provision of care through their influence and direction of those who do. Effective nursing care is accomplished through the interdependence of nurses in differing roles—those who teach the needed skills, set standards, manage the environment of care, or expand the boundaries of knowledge used by the profession. In this sense, nurses in all roles share a responsibility for the outcomes of nursing care.

2.4 Professional boundaries

When acting within the role of a professional, the nurse recognizes and maintains boundaries that establish appropriate limits to relationships. While the nature of nursing work has an inherently personal component, nurse-patient relationships and nurse-colleague relationships have, as their foundation, the purpose of preventing illness, alleviating suffering, and protecting, promoting, and restoring the health of patients. In this way, nurse-patient and nurse-colleague relationships differ from those that are purely personal and unstructured, such as friendship. The intimate nature of nursing care, the involvement of nurses in important and sometimes highly stressful life events, and the mutual dependence of colleagues working in close concert all present the potential for blurring of limits to professional relationships. Maintaining authenticity and expressing oneself as an individual while remaining within the bounds established by the purpose of the relationship can be especially difficult in prolonged or long-term relationships. In all encounters, nurses are responsible for retaining their professional boundaries. When these boundaries are jeopardized, the nurse should seek assistance from peers or supervisors or take appropriate steps to remove herself or himself from the situation.

3 The nurse promotes, advocates for and strives to protect the health, safety and rights of the patient.

3.1 Privacy

The nurse safeguards the patient's right to privacy. The need for health care does not justify unwanted intrusion into the patient's life. The nurse advocates for an environment that provides for sufficient physical privacy, including auditory privacy for discussions of a personal nature and policies and practices that protect the confidentiality of information.

3.2 Confidentiality

Associated with the right to privacy, the nurse has a duty to maintain donfidentiality of all patient information. The patient's well-being could be jeopardized and the fundamental trust between patient and nurse destroyed by unnecessary access to data or by the inappropriate disclosure of patient identifiable information. The rights, well-being, and safety of the individual patient should be the primary factors in arriving at any professional judgment concerning the disposition of confidential information received from or about the patient, whether oral, written or electronic. The standard of nursing practice and the nurse's responsibility to provide quality care require that relevant data be shared with those members of the health care team who have a need to know. Only information pertinent to a patient's treatment and welfare is disclosed and only to those directly involved with the patient's care. Duties of confidentiality, however, are not absolute and may need to be modified in order to protect the patient, other innocent parties and in circumstances of mandatory disclosure for public health reasons.

Information used for purposes of peer review, third-party payments, and other quality improvement or risk management mechanisms may be disclosed only under defined policies, mandates, or protocols. These written guidelines must assure that the rights, well-being, and safety of the patient are protected. In general, only that information directly relevant to the task or specific responsibility should be disclosed. When using electronic communications, special effort should be made to maintain data security.

3.3 Protection of participants in research

Stemming from the right to self-determination, each individual has the right to choose whether or not to participate in research. It is imperative that the patient or legally authorized surrogate receive sufficient information that is material to an informed decision, to comprehend that information, and to know how to discontinue participation in research without penalty. Necessary information to achieve an adequately informed consent includes the nature of participation, potential harms and benefits, and available alternatives to taking part in the research. Additionally, the patient should be informed of how the data will be protected. The patient has the right to refuse to participate in research or to withdraw at any time without fear of adverse consequences or reprisal.

Research should be conducted and directed only by qualified persons. Prior to implementation, all research should be approved by a qualified review board to ensure patient protection and the ethical integrity of the research. Nurses should be cognizant of the special concerns raised by research involving vulnerable groups, including children, prisoners, students, the elderly, and the poor. The nurse who participates in research in any capacity should be fully informed about both the subject's and the nurse's rights and obligations in the particular research study and in research in general. Nurses have the duty to question and, if necessary, to report and to refuse to participate in research they deem morally objectionable.

3.4 Standards and review mechanisms

Nursing is responsible and accountable for assuring that only those individuals who have demonstrated the knowledge, skill, practice experiences, commitment and integrity essential to professional practice are allowed to enter into and continue to practice within the profession. Nurse educators have a responsibility to ensure that basic competencies are achieved and to promote a commitment to professional practice prior to entry of an individual into practice. Nurse administrators are responsible for assuring that the knowledge and skills of each nurse in the workplace are assessed prior to the assignment of responsibilities requiring preparation beyond basic academic programs.

The nurse has a responsibility to implement and maintain standards of professional nursing practice. The nurse should participate in planning, establishing, implementing, and evaluating review mechanisms designed to safeguard patients and nurses, such as peer review processes or committees, credentialing processes, quality improvement initiatives, and ethics committees. Nurse administrators must ensure that nurses have access to and inclusion on institutional ethics committees. Nurses must bring forward difficult issues related to patient care and/or institutional constraints upon ethical practice for discussion and review. The nurse acts to promote inclusion of appropriate others in all deliberations related to patient care.

Nurses should also be active participants in the development of policies and review mechanisms designed to promote patient safety, reduce the likelihood of errors, and address both environmental system factors and human factors that present increased risk to patients. In addition, when errors do occur, nurses are expected to follow institutional guidelines in reporting errors committed or observed to the appropriate supervisory personnel and for assuring responsible disclosure of errors to patients. Under no circumstances shoud the nurse participate in, or condone through silence, either an attempt to hide an error or a punitive response that serves only to fix blame rather than correct the conditions that led to the error.

3.5 Acting on questionable practice

The nurse's primary commitment is to the health, well-being, and safety of the patient across the life span and in all settings in which health care needs are addressed. As an advocate for the patient, the nurse must be alert to and take appropriate action regarding any instances of incompetent, unethical, illegal or impaired practice by any member of the health care team or the health care system or any action on the part of others that places the rights or best interests of the patient in jeopardy. To function effectively in this role, nurses must be knowledgeable about the Code of Ethics, standards of practice of the profession, relevant federal, state and local laws and regulations, and the employing organization's policies and procedures.

When the nurse is aware of inappropriate or questionable practice in the provision or denial of health care, concern should be expressed to the person carrying out the questionable practice. Attention should be called to the possible detrimental effect upon the patient's well-being or best interests as well as the integrity of nursing practice. When factors in the health care delivery system or health care organization threaten the welfare of the patient, similar action should be directed to the responsible administrator. If indicated, the problem should be reported to an appropriate higher authority within the institution or agency, or to an appropriate external authority.

There should be established processes for reporting and handling incompetent, unethical, illegal or impaired practice within the employment settings so that such reporting can go through official channels, thereby reducing the risk of reprisal against the reporting nurse. All nurses have a responsibility to assist those who identify potentially questionable practice. State nurses associations should be prepared to provide assistance and support in the development and and evaluation of such processes and reporing procedures. When incompetent, unethical, illegal or impaired practice is not corrected within the employment setting and continues to jeopardize patient well-being and safety, the problem should be reported to other appropriate authorities such as practice committees of the pertinent professional organizations, the legally constituted bodies concerned with licensing of specific categories of health workers and professional practitioners, or the regulatory agencies concerned with evaluating standards of practice. Some situations may warrant the concern and involvement of all such groups. Accurate reporting and factual documentation, and not merely opinion, undergird all such responsible actions. When a nurse chooses to engage in the act of responsible reporting about situations that are perceived as unethical, incompetent, illegal or impaired, the professional organization has a responsibility to provide the nurse with support and assistance and to protect the practice of those nurses who choose to voice their concerns. Reporting unethical, illegal, incompetent or impaired practices, even when done appropriately, may present substantial risks to the nurse; nevertheless, such risks do not eliminate the obligation to address serious threats to patient safety.

3.6 Addressing impaired practice

Nurses must be vigilant to protect the patient, the public and the profession from potential harm when a colleague's practice, in any setting, appears to be impaired. The nurse extends compassion and caring to colleagues who are in recovery from illness or when illness interferes with job performance. In a situation where a nurse suspects another's practice may be impaired, the nurse's duty is to take action designed both to protect patients and to assure that the impaired individual receives assistance in regaining optimal function. Such action should usually begin with consulting supervisory personnel and may also include confronting the individual in a supportive manner and with the assistance of others or helping the individual to access appropriate resources. Nurses are encouraged to follow guidelines outlined by the profession and policies of the employing organization to assist colleagues whose job performance may be adversely affected by mental or physical illness or by personal circumstances. Nurses in all roles should advocate for colleagues whose job performance may be impaired to ensure that they receive appropriate assistance, treatment and access to fair institutional and legal processes. This includes supporting the return to practice of the individual who has sought assistance and is ready to resume professional duties.

If impaired practice poses a threat or danger to self or others, regardless of whether the individual has sought help, the nurse must take action to report the individual to persons authorized to address the problem. Nurses who advocate for others whose job performance creates a risk for harm should be protected from negative consequences. Advocacy may be a difficult process and the nurse is advised to follow workplace policies. If workplace policies do not exist or are inappropriate—that is, they deny the nurse in question access to due legal process or demand resignation—the reporting nurse may obtain guidance from the professional association, state peer assistance programs, employee assistance program or a similar resource.

4 The nurse is responsible and accountable for individual nursing practice, and determines the appropriate delegation of tasks consistent with the nurse's obligation to provide optimum patient care.

4.1 Acceptance of accountability and responsibility

Individual registered nurses bear primary responsibility for the nursing care that their patients receive and are individually accountable for their own practice. Nursing practice includes direct care activities, acts of delegation, and other responsibilities such as teaching, research, and administration. In each instance the nurse retains accountability and responsibility for the quality of practice and for conforming with standards of care.

Nurses are faced with decisions in the context of the increased complexity and changing patterns in the delivery of health care. As the scope of nursing practice changes, the nurse must exercise judgment in accepting responsibilities, seeking consultation, and assigning activities to others who carry out nursing care. For example, some advanced practice nurses have the authority to issue prescription and treatment orders to be carried out by other nurses. These acts are not acts of delegation. Both the advanced practice nurse issuing the order and the nurse accepting the order are responsible for the judgments made and accountable for the actions taken.

4.2 Accountability for nursing judgment and action

Accountability means to be answerable to one's self and others for one's own actions. In order to be accountable, nurses act under a code of ethical conduct that is grounded in the moral principles of fidelity and respect for the dignity, worth, and self-determination of patients. Nurses are accountable for judgments made and actions taken in the course of nursing practice, irrespective of health care organizations' policies or providers' directives.

4.3 Responsibility for nursing judgment and action

Responsibility refers to the specific accountability or liability associated with the performance of duties of a particular role. Nurses accept or reject specific role demands based upon their education, knowledge, competence, and extent of experience. Nurses in administration, education and research also have obligations to the recipients of nursing care. Although nurses in administration, education and research have relationships with patients that are less direct, in assuming the responsibilities of a particular role, they share responsibility for the care provided by those whom they supervise and instruct. The nurse must not engage in practices prohibited by law or delegate activities to others that are prohibited by practice acts of other health care providers.

The individual nurse is responsible for assessing his or her own competence. When the needs of the patient are beyond the qualifications and competencies of the nurse, consultation and collaboration must be sought from qualified nurses, other health professionals, or other appropriate sources. Educational resources should be sought by nurses and provided by institutions to maintain and advance the competence of nurses. Nurse educators act in collaboration with their students to assess the learning needs of the student, the effectiveness of the teaching program, the identification and utilization of appropriate resources, and the support needed for the learning process.

4.4. Delegation of nursing activities

Since the nurse is accountable for the quality of nursing care given to patients, nurses are accountable for the assignment of nursing responsibilities to other nurses and the delegation of nursing care activities to other health care workers. While delegation and assignment are used here in a generic moral sense, it is understood that individual states may have a particular legal definition of these terms.

The nurse must make reasonable efforts to assess individual competency when assigning selected components of nursing care to other healthcare workers. This assessment involves evaluating the knowledge, skills and experience of the individual to whom the care is assigned, the complexity of the assigned tasks, and the health status of the patient. The nurse is also responsible for monitoring the activities of these individuals and evaluating the quality of the care provided. Nurses may not delegate responsibilities such as assessment and evaluation; they may delegate tasks. The nurse must not knowingly assign or delegate to any member of the nursing team a task for which that person is not prepared or qualified. Employer policies or directives do not relieve the nurse of responsibiilty for making judgments about the delegation and assignment of nursing care tasks.

Nurses functioning in management or administrative roles have a particular responsibility to provide an environment that supports and facilitates appropriate assignment and delegation. This includes providing appropriate orientation to staff, assisting less experienced nurses in developing necessary skills and competencies, and establishing policies and procedures that protect both the patient and nurse from the inappropriate assignment or delegation of nursing responsibilities activities or tasks.

Nurses functioning in educator or preceptor roles may have a less direct relationship with patients. However, through assignment of nursing care activiteis to learners they share responsibility and accountability for the care provided. It is imperative that the knowledge and skills of the learner be sufficient to provide the assigned nursing care and that appropriate supervision be provided to protect both the patient and the learner.

5 The nurse owes the same duties to self as to others, including the responsibility to preserve integrity and safety, to maintain competence, and to continue personal and professional growth.

5.1 Moral self-respect

Moral respect accords moral worth and dignity to all human beings irrespective of their personal attributes or life situation. Such respect extends to oneself as well; the same duties that we owe to others we owe to ourselves. Self-regarding duties refer to a realm of duties that primarily concern oneself and include professional growth and maintenance of competence, preservation of wholeness of character, and personal integrity.

5.2 Professional growth and maintenance of competence

Though it has consequences for others, maintenance of competence and ongoing professional growth involves the control of one's own conduct in a way that is primarily self-regarding. Competence affects one's self-respect, self-esteem, professional status, and the meaningfulness of work. In all nursing roles, evaluation of one's own performance, coupled with peer review, is a means by which nursing practice can be held to the highest standard.s Each nurse is responsible for participating in the development of criteria for evaluation of practice and for using those criteria in peer and self-assessment.

Continual professional growth, particularly in knowledge and skill, requires a commitment to lifelong learning. Such learning includes, but is not limited to, continuing education, networking with professional colleagues, self-study, professional reading, certification and seeking advanced degrees. Nurses are required to have knowledge relevant to the current scope and standards of nursing practice, changing issues, concerns, controversies, and ethics. Where the care required is outside the competencies of the individual nurse, consultation should be sought or the patient should be referred to others for appropriate care.

5.3 Wholeness of character

Nurses have both personal and professional identities that are neither entirely separate, nor entirely merged, but are integrated. In the process of becoming a professional, the nurse embraces the values of the profession, integrating them with personal values. Duties to self involve an authentic expression of one's own moral point-of-view in practice. Sound ethical decision making requires the respectful and open exchange of views between and among all indivdiuals with relevant interests. In a community of moral discourse, no one person's view should automatically take precedence over that of another. Thus the nurse has a responsibility to express moral perspectives, even when they differ from those of others, and even when they might not prevail.

This wholeness of character encompasses relationships with patients. In situations where the patient requests a personal opinion from the nurse, the nurse is generally free to express an informed personal opinion as long as this preserves the voluntariness of the patient and maintains appropriate professional and moral boundaries. It is essential to be aware of the potential for undue influence attached to the nurse's professional role. Assisting patients to clarify their own values in reaching informed decisions may be helpful in avoiding unintended persuasion. In situations where nurses' responsibilities include care for those whose personal attributes, condition, lifestyle or situation is stigmatized by the community and are personally unacceptable, the nurse still renders respectful and skilled care.

5.4 Preservation of integrity

Integrity is an aspect of wholeness of character and is primarily a self-concern of the individual nurse. An economically constrained health care environment presents the nurse with particularly troubling threats to integrity. Threats to integrity may include a request to deceive a patient, to withhold information, or to falsify records, as well as verbal abuse from patients or coworkers. Threats to integrity may also include an expectation that the nurse will act in a way that is inconsistent with the values or ethics of the profession, or more specifically a request that is in direct violation of the Code of Ethics. Nurses have a duty to remain consistent with both their personal and professional values and to accept compromise only to the degree that it remains an integrity-preserving compromise. An integrity-preserving compromise does not jeopardize the dignity or well-being of the nurse or others. Integrity-preserving compromise can be difficult to achieve, but is more likely to be accomplished in situations where there is an open forum for moral discourse and an atmosphere of mutal respect and regard.

Where nurses are placed in situations of compromise that exceed acceptable moral limits or involve violations of the moral standards of the profession, whether in direct patient care or in any other forms of nursing practice, they may express their conscientious objection to participation. Where a particular treatment, intervention, activity, or practice is morally objectionable to the nurse, whether intrinsically so or because it is inappropriate for the specific patient, or where it may jeopardize both patients and nursing practice, the nurse is justified in refusing to participate on moral grounds. Such grounds exclude personal preference, prejudice, convience or arbitrariness. Conscientious objection may not insulate the nurse against formal or informal penalty. The nurse who decides not to take part because of conscientious objection must communicate this decision in appropriate ways. Whenever possible, such a refusal should be made known in advance and in time for alternate arrangements to be made for patient care. The nurse is obliged to provide for the patient's safety, to avoid abandonment, and to withdraw only when assured that alternative sources of nursing care are available to the patient.

Where patterns of institutional behavior or professional practice compromise the integrity of all its nurses, nurses should express their concern or conscientious objection collectively to the appropriate body or committee. In addition, they should express their cocnern, resist, and seek to bring about a change in those persistent activities or expectations in the practice setting that are morally objectionable to nurses and jeopardize either patient or nurse well being.

6 The nurse participates in establishing, maintaining and improving healthcare environments and conditions of employment conducive to the provision of quality health care and consistent with the values of the profession through individual and collective action.

6.1 Influence of the environment on moral virtues and values

Virtues are habits of character that predispose persons to meet their moral obligations; that is, to do what is right. Excellences are habits of character that predispose a person to do a particular job or task well. Virtues such as wisdom, honesty and courage are habits or attributes of the morally good person. Excellences such as compassion, patience and skill are habits of character of the morally good nurse. For the nurse, virtues and excellences are those habits that affirm and promote the values of human dignity, well-being, respect, health, independence and other values central to nursing. Both virtues and excellences, as aspects of moral character, can be either nurtured by the environment in which the nurse practices or they can be diminished or thwarted. All have a responsibility to create, maintain, and contribute to environments that support the growth of virtues and excellences and enable nurses to fulfill their ethical obligations.

6.2 Influence of the environment on ethical obligations

All nurses, regardless of role, have a responsibility to create, maintain, and contribute to environments of practice that support nurses in fulfilling their ethical obligations. Environments of practice include observable features, such as working conditions, and written policies and procedures setting out expectations for nurses, as well as less tangible characteristics such as informal peer norms. Organizational structures, role descriptions, health and safety initiatives, grievance mechanisms, ethics committees, compensation systems, and disciplinary procedures all contribute to environments that can either present barriers or foster ethical practice and professional fulfillment. Environments in which employees are provided fair hearing of grievances, are supported in practicing according to standards of care, and are justly treated allow the realization of the values of the profession and are consistent with sound nursing practice.

6.3 Responsibility for the health care environment

The nurse is responsible for contributing to a moral environment that encourages respectful interactions with colleagues, support of peers, and identification of issues that need to be addressed. Nurse administrators have a particular responsibility to assure that employees are treated fairly and that nurses are involved in decisions related to their practice and working conditions. Acquiescing and accepting unsafe or inappropriate practices, even if the individual does not participate in the specific practice, is equivalent to condoning unsafe practice. Nurses should not remain employed in facilities that routinely violate patient rights or require nurses to severely and repeatedly compromise standards of practice or personal morality.

As with concerns about patient care, nurses should address concerns about the health care environment through appropriate channels. Organizational changes are difficult to accomplish and may require persistent efforts over time. Toward this end, nurses may participate in collective action such as collective bargaining or workplace advocacy, preferably through a professional association such as the state nurses association, in order to address the terms and conditions of employment. Agreements reached through such action must be consistent with the profession's standards of practice, the state law, regulating practice and the Code of Ethics for Nursing. Conditions of employment must contribute to the moral environment, the provision for quality patient care and professional satisfaction for nurses.

The professional association also serves as an advocate for the nurse by seeking to secure just compensation and humane working conditions for nurses. To accomplish this, the professional associaiton may engage in collective bargaining on behalf of nurses. While seeking to assure just economic and general welfare for nurses, collective bargaining, nonetheless, seeks to keep the interests of both nurses and patients in balance.

7 The nurse participates in the advancement of the profession through contributions to practice, education, administration, and knowledge development.

7.1 Advancing the profession through active involvement in nursing and in health care policy

Nurses should advance their profession by contributing in some way to the leadership, activities, and the viabiilty of their professional organizations. Nurses can also advance the profession by serving in leadership or mentorship roles or on committees within their places of employment. Nurses who are self-employed can advance the profession by serving as role models for professional integrity. Nurses can also advance the profession through participation in civic activities related to health care or through local, state, national, or international initiatives. Nurse educators have a specific responsibility to enhance students' commitment to professional and civic values. Nurse administrators have a responsibility to foster an emplooyment environment that facilitates nurses' ethical integrity and professionalism, and nurse researchers are responsible for active contribution to the body of knowledge supporting and advancing nursing practice.

7.2 Advancing the profession by developing, maintaining, and implementing professional standards in clinical, administrative, and educational practice

Standards and guidelines reflect the practice of nursing grounded in ethical commitments and a body of knowledge. Professional standards and guidelines for nurses must be developed by nurses and reflect nursing's responsibility to society. It is the responsibility of nurses to identify their own scope of practice as permitted by professional practice standards and guidelines, by state and federal laws, by relevant societal values, and by the Code of Ethics.

The nurse as administrator or manager must establish, maintain, and promote conditions of employment that enable nurses within that organization or community setting to practice in accord with accepted standards of nursing practice and provide a nursing and health care work environment that meets the standards and guidelines of nursing practice. Professional autonomy and self-regulation in the control of conditions of practice are necessary for implementing nursing standards and guidelines and assuring quality care for those whom nursing serves.

The nurse educator is responsible for promoting and maintaining optimum standards of both nursing education and of nursing practice in any settings where planned learning activities occur. Nurse educators must also ensure that only those students who possess knowledge, skills and the competencies that are essential to nursing graduate from their nursing programs.

7.3 Advancing the profession through knowledge development, dissemination, and application to practice

The nursing profession should engage in scholarly inquiry to identify, evaluate, refine and expand the body of knowledge that forms the foundation of its discipline and practice. In addition, nuring knowledge is derived from the sciences and from the humanities. Ongoing scholarly activities are essential to fulfilling a profession's obligations to society. All nurses working alone or in collaboration with others can participate in the advancement of the profession through the development, evaluation, dissemination, and application of knowledge in practice. However, an organizational climate and infrastructure conducive to scholarly inquiry must be valued and implemented for this to occur.

8 **The nurse collaborates with other health professionals and the public in promoting community, national, and international efforts to meet health needs.**

8.1 Health needs and concerns

The nursing profession is committed to promoting the health, welfare, and safety of all people. The nurse has a responsibility to be aware not only of specific health needs of individual patients, but also of broader health concerns such as world hunger, environmental pollution, lack of access to health care, violation of human rights, and inequitable distribution of nursing and health care resources. The availability and accessibility of high-quality health services to all people requires both inter-disciplinary planning and collaborative partnerships among health professionals and others at the community, national, and international levels.

8.2 Responsibilities to the public

Nurses, individually and collectively, have a responsibility to be knowledgeable about the health status of the community and existing threats to health and safety. Through support of and participation in community organizations and groups, the nurse assists in efforts to educate the public, facilitates informed choice, identifies conditions and circumstances that contribute to illness, injury, and diseae, fosters healthy life styles, and participates in institutional and legislative efforts to promote health and meet national health objectives. In addition, the nurse suports initiatives to address barriers to health, such as poverty, homelessness, unsafe living conditions, abuse and violence and lack of access to health services.

The nurse also recognizes that health care is provided to culturally diverse populations in this country and in all parts of the world. In providing care, the nurse should avoid imposition of the nurse's cultural values upon others. The nurse should affirm human dignity and show respect for the values and practices associated with different cultures and use approaches to care that reflect awareness and sensitivity.

9 **The profession of nursing, as represented by associations and their members, is responsible for articulating nursing values, for maintaining the integrity of the profession and its practice, and for shaping social policy.**

9.1 Assertion of values

It is the responsibility of a professional association to communicate and affirm the values of the profession to its members. It is essential that the professional organization encourages discourse that supports critical self-reflection and evaluation within the profession. The organization also communicates to the public the values that nursing considers central to social change that will enhance health.

9.2 The profession carries out its collective responsibility through professional associations

The nursing profession continues to develop ways to clarify nursing's accountability to society. The contract between the profession and society is made explicit through such mechanisms as (a) The Code of Ethics for Nurses, (b) the standards of nursing practice, (c) the ongoing development of nursing knowledge derived from nursing theory, scholoarship, and research in order to guide nursing actions, (d) educational requirements for practice, (e) certification, and (f) mechanisms for evaluating the effectiveness of professional nursing actions.

9.3 Intraprofessional integrity

A professional association is responsible for expressing the values and ethics of the profession and also for encouraging the professional organization and its members to function in accord with those values and ethics. Thus, one of its fundamental responsibilities is to promote awareness of and adherence to the Code of Ethics and to critique the activities and ends of the professional association itself. Values and ethics influence the power structures of the association in guiding, correcting, and directing its activities. Legitimate concerns for the self-interest of the association and the profession are balanced by a commitment to the social goods that are sought. Through critical self-reflection and self-evaluation, associations must foster change within themselves, seeking to move the professional community towards its stated ideals.

9.4 Social reform

Nurses can work individually as citizens or collectively through political action to bring about social change. It is the responsibility of a professional nursing association to speak for nurses collectively in shaping and reshaping health care within our nation, specifically in areas of health care policy and legislation that affect accessibility, quality, and the cost of health care. Here, the professional association maintains vigilance and takes action to influence legislators, reimbursement agencies, nursing organizations, and other health professions. In these activities, health is understood as being broader than delivery and reimbursement systems, but extending to health-related sociocultural issues such as violation of human rights homelessness, hunger, violence and the stigma of illness.

APPENDIX B

A Patient's Bill of Rights
American Hospital Association

Reprinted with permission of the American Hospital Association,
copyright © 1992

INTRODUCTION

Effective health care requires collaboration between patients and physicians and other health care professionals. Open and honest communication, respect for personal and professional values, and sensitivity to differences are integral to optimal patient care. As the setting for the provision of health services, hospitals must provide a foundation for understanding and respecting the rights and responsibilities of patients, their families, physicians, and other caregivers. Hospitals must ensure a health care ethic that respects the role of patients in decision making about treatment choices and other aspects of their care. Hospitals must be sensitive to cultural, racial, linguistic, religious, age, gender, and other differences as well as the needs of persons with disabilities.

The American Hospital Association presents *A Patient's Bill of Rights* with the expectation that it will contribute to more effective patient care and be supported by the hospital on behalf of the institution, its medical staff, employees, and patients. The American Hospital Association encourages health care institutions to tailor this bill of rights to their patient community by translating and/or simplifying the language of this bill of rights as may be necessary to ensure that patients and their families understand their rights and responsibilities.

PATIENT BILL OF RIGHTS*

1. The patient has the right to considerate and respectful care.

2. The patient has the right to and is encouraged to obtain from physicians and other direct caregivers relevant, current, and understandable information concerning diagnosis, treatment, and prognosis.

Except in emergencies when the patient lacks decision-making capacity and the need for treatment is urgent, the patient is entitled to the opportunity to discuss and request information related to the specific procedures and/or treatments, the risks involved, the possible length of recuperation, and the medically reasonable alternatives and their accompanying risks and benefits.

Patients have the right to know the identity of physicians, nurses, and others involved in their care, as well as when those involved are students, residents, or other trainees. The patient also has the right to know the immediate and long-term financial implications of treatment choices, insofar as they are known.

3. The patient has the right to make decisions about the plan of care prior to and during the course of treatment and to refuse a recommended treatment or plan of care to the extent permitted by law and hospital policy and to be informed of the medical consequences of this action. In case of such refusal, the patient is entitled to other appropriate care and services that the hospital provides or transfer to another hospital. The hospital should notify patients of any policy that might affect patient choices within the institution.

4. The patient has the right to have an advance directive (such as a living will, health care proxy, or durable power of attorney for health care) concerning treatment or designating a surrogate decision maker with the expectation that the hospital will honor the intent of that directive to the extent permitted by law and hospital policy.

Health care institutions must advise patients of their rights under state law and hospital policy to make informed medical choices, ask if the patient has an advance directive, and include that information in patient records. The patient has the right to timely information about hospital policy that may limit its ability to implement fully a legally valid advance directive.

5. The patient has the right to every consideration of privacy. Case discussion, consultation, examination, and treatment should be conducted so as to protect each patient's privacy.

6. The patient has the right to expect that all communications and records pertaining to his/her care will be treated as confidential by the hospital, except in cases such as suspected abuse and public health hazards when reporting is permitted or required by law. The patient has the right to expect that the hospital will emphasize the confidentiality of this information when it releases it to any other parties entitled to review information in these records.

---

* These rights can be exercised on the patient's behalf by a designates surrogate or proxy decision maker if the patient lacks decision-making capacity, is legally incompetent or is a minor.

7. The patient has the right to review the records pertaining to his/her medical care and to have the information explained or interpreted as necessary, except when restricted by law.

8. The patient has the right to expect that, within its capacity and policies, a hospital will make reasonable response to the request of a patient for appropriate and medically indicated care and services. The hospital must provide evaluation, service, and/or referral as indicated by the urgency of the case. When medically appropriate and legally permissible, or when a patient has so requested, a patient may be transferred to another facility. The institution to which the patient is to be transferred must first have accepted the patient for transfer. The patient must also have the benefit of complete information and explanation concerning the need for, risks, benefits, and alternatives to such a transfer.

9. The patient has the right to ask and be informed of the existence of business relationships among the hospital, educational institutions, other health care providers, or payers that may influence the patient's treatment and care.

10. The patient has the right to consent to or decline to participate in proposed research studies or human experimentation affecting care and treatment or requiring direct patient involvement, and to have those studies fully explained prior to consent. A patient who declines to participate in research or experimentation is entitled to the most effective care that the hospital can otherwise provide.

11. The patient has the right to expect reasonable continuity of care when appropriate and to be informed by physicians and other caregivers of available and realistic patient care options when hospital care is no longer appropriate.

12. The patient has the right to be informed of hospital policies and practices that relate to patient care, treatment, and responsibilities. The patient has the right to be informed of available resources for resolving disputes, grievances, and conflicts, such as ethics committees, patient representatives, or other mechanisms available in the institution. The patient has the right to be informed of the hospital's charges for services and available payment methods.

The collaborative nature of health care requires that patients, or their families/surrogates, participate in their care. The effectiveness of care and patient satisfaction with the course of treatment depend, in part, on the patient fulfilling certain responsibilities. Patients are responsible for providing information about past illnesses, hospitalizations, medications, and other matters related to health status. To participate effectively in decision making, patients must be encouraged to take responsibility for requesting additional information or clarification about their health status or treatment when they do not fully understand information and instructions. Patients are also responsible for ensuring that the health care institution has a copy of their written advance directive if they have one. Patients are responsible for informing their physicians and other caregivers if they anticipate problems in following prescribed treatment.

Patients should also be aware of the hospital's obligation to be reasonably efficient and equitable in providing care to other patients and the community. The hospital's rules and regulations are designed to help the hospital meet this obligation. Patients and their families are responsible for making reasonable accommodations to the needs of the hospital, other patients, medical staff, and hospital employees. Patients are responsible for providing necessary information for insurance claims and for working with the hospital to make payment arrangements, when necessary.

A person's health depends on much more than health care services. Patients are responsible for recognizing the impact of their life-style on their personal health.

CONCLUSION

Hospitals have many functions to perform, including the enhancement of health status, health promotion, and the prevention and treatment of injury and disease; the immediate and ongoing care and rehabilitation of patients; the education of health professionals, patients, and the community; and research. All these activities must be conducted with an overriding concern for the values and dignity of patients.

APPENDIX C

Code of Ethics
for Registered Nurses
Canadian Nurses Association

Reprinted with permission of the Canadian Nurses Association, copyright © 1997

PREAMBLE

The *Code of Ethics for Registered Nurses* gives guidance for decision-making concerning ethical matters, serves as a means for self-evaluation and reflection regarding ethical nursing practice, and provides a basis for peer review initiatives. The code not only educates nurses about their ethical responsibilities, but also informs other health care professionals and members of the public about the moral commitments expected of nurses.

The Canadian Nurses Association (CNA) periodically revises its code to address changing societal needs, values, and conditions that challenge the ability of nurses to practice ethically. Examples of such factors are: the consequences of economic constraints; increasing use of technology in health care; and, changing ways of delivering nursing services, such as the move to care outside the institutional setting. This revised *Code of Ethics for Registered Nurses* provides nurses with direction for ethical decision-making and practice in everyday situations as they are influenced by current trends and conditions. It applies to nurses in all practice settings, whatever their position and area of responsibility.

Ethical problems and concerns, as well as ethical distress at the individual level, can be the result of decisions made at the institutional, regional, provincial and federal levels. Differing responsibilities, capabilities and ways of working toward change also exist at the client, institutional and societal levels. For all contexts the code offers guidance on providing care that conforms with ethical practice, and on actively influencing and participating in policy development, review and revision.

The complex issues in nursing practice have both legal and ethical dimensions. The laws and ethics of health care overlap, as both are concerned that the conduct of health professionals show respect for the well-being, dignity and liberty of clients. An ideal system of law would be compatible with ethics, in that adherence to the law ought never require the violation of ethics. Still, the domains of law and ethics remain distinct, and the code addresses ethical responsibilities only.

ELEMENTS OF THE CODE

A value is something that is prized or held dear; something that is deeply cared about. This code is organized around seven primary values that are central to ethical nursing practice:

- **Health and well-being**
- **Choice**
- **Dignity**
- **Confidentiality**
- **Fairness**
- **Accountability**
- **Practice environments that are conducive to safe, competent and ethical care.**

Each value is articulated by responsibility statements that clarify its application and provide more direct guidance. Where it is clear that an action or inaction would involve an **ethical violation** (i.e., the neglect of a moral obligation), the level of guidance is prescriptive. The statement is intended to tell the nurse and others what is ethically acceptable and what is not. Where the situation involves an **ethical problem** or dilemma, guidance is advisory. No ready-made answers can be offered and thoughtful consideration is required to increase the quality of decision-making. Where the situation provokes feelings of guilt, concern, or distaste, it is a situation of ethical distress. In instances of **ethical distress** the level of guidance is more limited but there remains a responsibility for the nurse to examine the situation in light of the provisions of the code. Decisions will be influenced by the particular circumstances of the situation. Ethical reflection and judgement are required to determine how a particular value or responsibility applies in a particular nursing context.

There is room within the profession for disagreement among nurses about the relative weight of different ethical values and principles. More than one proposed intervention may be ethical and reflective of good practice. Discussion is extremely helpful in the resolution of ethical issues. As appropriate, clients, colleagues in nursing and other disciplines, professional nurses' associations and other experts are included in discussions about ethical problems. In addition to this code, legislation, and the standards of practice, policies, and guidelines of professional nurses associations may also assist in problem-solving.

The values articulated in this code are grounded in the professional nursing relationship with clients and indicate what nurses care about in that relationship. For example, to identify health and well-being as a value is to say that nurses care for and about the health and well-being of their clients. The nurse-client relationship presupposes a certain measure of trust on the part of the client. Care and trust complement one another in professional nursing relationships. Both hinge on the values identified in the code. By upholding these values in practice, nurses earn and maintain the trust of those in their care. For each of the values, the scope of responsibilities identified extends beyond individuals to include families, communities and society.

HEALTH AND WELL-BEING

Nurses value health and well-being and assist persons to achieve their optimum level of health in situations of normal health, illness, injury, or in the process of dying.

1. Nurses provide care directed first and foremost toward the health and well-being of the client.

2. Nurses recognize that health is more than the absence of disease or infirmity and assist clients to achieve the maximum level of health and well-being possible.

3. Nurses recognize that health status is influenced by a variety of factors. In ways that are consistent with their professional role and responsibilities, nurses are accountable for addressing institutional, social, and political factors influencing health and health care.

4. Nurses support and advocate a full continuum of health services including health promotion and disease prevention initiatives, as well as diagnostic, restorative, rehabilitative and palliative care services.

5. Nurses respect and value the knowledge and skills other health care providers bring to the health care team and actively seek to support and collaborate with others so that maximum benefits to clients can be realized.

6. Nurses foster well-being when life can no longer be sustained, by alleviating suffering and supporting a dignified and peaceful death.

7. Nurses provide the best care circumstances permit even when the need arises in an emergency outside an employment situation.

8. Nurses participate, to the best of their abilities, in research and other activities that contribute to the ongoing development of nursing knowledge. Nurses participating in research observe the nursing profession's guidelines, as well as other guidelines, for ethical research.

CHOICE

Nurses respect and promote the autonomy of clients and help them to express their health needs and values, and to obtain appropriate information and services.

1. Nurses seek to involve clients in health planning and health care decision-making.

2. Nurses provide the information and support required so that clients, to the best of their ability, are able to act on their own behalf in meeting their health and health care needs. Information given is complete, accurate, truthful, and understandable. When they are unable to provide the required information, nurses assist clients in obtaining it from other appropriate sources.

3. Nurses demonstrate sensitivity to the willingness/readiness of clients to receive information about their health condition and care options. Nurses respect the wishes of those who refuse, or are not ready, to receive information about their health condition.

4. Nurses practice within relevant legislation governing consent or choice. Nurses seek to ensure that nursing care is authorized by informed choice, and are guided by this ideal when participating in the consent process in cooperation with other members of the health team.

5. Nurses respect the informed decisions of competent persons to refuse treatment and to choose to live at risk. However, nurses are not obliged to comply with clients' wishes when doing so would require action contrary to the law. If the care requested is contrary to the nurse's moral beliefs, appropriate care is provided until alternative care arrangements are in place to meet the client's needs.

6. Nurses are sensitive to their position of relative power in professional relationships with clients and take care to foster self-determination on the part of their clients. Nurses are sufficiently clear about personal values to recognize and deal appropriately with potential value conflicts.

7. Nurses respect decisions and lawful directives, written or verbal, about present and future health care choices affirmed by a client prior to becoming incompetent.

8. Nurses seek to involve clients of diminished competence in decision-making to the extent that those clients are capable. Nurses continue to value autonomy when illness or other factors reduce the capacity for self-determination, such as by providing opportunities for clients to make choices about aspects of their lives for which they maintain the capacity to make decisions.

9. Nurses seek to obtain consent for nursing care from a substitute decision-maker when clients lack the capacity to make decisions about their care, did not make their wishes known prior to becoming incompetent, or for any reason it is unclear what the client would have wanted in a particular circumstance. When prior wishes of an incompetent client are not known or are unclear, care decisions must be in the best interest of the client and are based on what the client would want, as far as it is known.

DIGNITY

Nurses value and advocate the dignity and self-respect of human beings.

1. Nurses relate to all persons receiving care as persons worthy of respect and endeavor in all their actions to preserve and demonstrate respect for each individual.

2. Nurses exhibit sensitivity to the client's individual needs, values, and choices. Nursing care is designed to accommodate the biological, psychological, social, cultural, and spiritual needs of clients. Nurses do not exploit clients' vulnerabilities for their own interests or gain, whether this be sexual, emotional, social, political, or financial.

3. Nurses respect the privacy of clients when care is given.

4. Nurses treat human life as precious and worthy of respect. Respect includes seeking out and honoring clients' wishes regarding quality of life. Decision-making about life-sustaining treatment carefully balances these considerations.

5. Nurses intervene if others fail to respect the dignity of clients.

6. Nurses advocate the dignity of clients in the use of technology in the health care setting.

7. Nurses advocate health and social conditions that allow persons to live with dignity throughout their lives and in the process of dying. They do so in ways that are consistent with their professional role and responsibilities.

CONFIDENTIALITY

Nurses safeguard the trust of clients that information learned in the context of a professional relationship is shared outside the health care team only with the client's permission or as legally required.

1. Nurses observe practices that protect the confidentiality of each client's health and health care information.

2. Nurses intervene if other participants in the health care delivery system fail to respect client confidentiality.

3. Nurses disclose confidential information only as authorized by the client, unless there is substantial risk of serious harm to the client or other persons, or a legal obligation to disclose. Where disclosure is warranted, both the amount of information disclosed and the number of people informed is restricted to the minimum necessary.

4. Nurses, whenever possible, inform their clients about the boundaries of professional confidentiality at the onset of care, including the circumstances under which confidential information might be disclosed without consent. If feasible,

when disclosure becomes necessary, nurses inform clients what information will be disclosed, to whom, and for what reasons.

5. Nurses advocate policies and safeguards to protect and preserve client confidentiality and intervene if the security of confidential information is jeopardized because of a weakness in the provisions of the system, e.g., inadequate safeguarding guidelines and procedures for the use of computer databases.

FAIRNESS

Nurses apply and promote principles of equity and fairness to assist clients in receiving unbiased treatment and a share of health services and resources proportionate to their needs.

1. Nurses provide care in response to need regardless of such factors as race, ethnicity, culture, spiritual beliefs, social or marital status, gender, sexual orientation, age, health status, lifestyle or the physical attributes of the client.

2. Nurses are justified in using reasonable means to protect against violence when they anticipate acts of violence toward themselves, others or property with good reason.

3. Nurses strive to be fair in making decisions about the allocation of services and goods that they provide, when the distribution of these is within their control.

4. Nurses put forward, and advocate, the interests of all persons in their care. This includes helping individuals and groups gain access to appropriate health care that is of their choosing.

5. Nurses promote appropriate and ethical care at the institutional/agency and community levels by participating, to the extent possible, in the development, implementation, and ongoing review of policies and procedures designed to make the best use of available resources and of current knowledge and research.

6. Nurses advocate, in ways that are consistent with their role and responsibilities, health policies and decision-making procedures that are fair and comprehensive, and that promote fairness and inclusiveness in health resource allocation.

ACCOUNTABILITY

Nurses act in a manner consistent with their professional responsibilities and standards of practice.

1. Nurses comply with the values and responsibilities in this *Code of Ethics for Registered Nurses* as well as with the professional standards and laws pertaining to their practice.

2. Nurses conduct themselves with honesty and integrity.

3. Nurses, whether they are engaged in clinical, administrative, research or educational endeavors, have professional responsibilities and accountabilities toward

safeguarding the quality of nursing care clients receive. These responsibilities vary but are all oriented to the expected outcome of safe, competent and ethical nursing practice.

4. Nurses, individually or in partnership with others, take preventive as well as corrective action to protect clients from unsafe, incompetent or unethical care.

5. Nurses base their practice on relevant knowledge, and acquire new skills and knowledge in their area of practice on a continuing basis, as necessary for the provision of safe, competent and ethical nursing care.

6. Nurses, whether engaged in clinical practice, administration, research or education, provide timely and accurate feedback to other nurses about their practice, so as to support safe and competent care and contribute to ongoing learning. By so doing, they also acknowledge excellence in practice.

7. Nurses practice within their own level of competence. They seek additional information or knowledge; seek the help, and/or supervision and help, of a competent practitioner; and/or request a different work assignment, when aspects of the care required are beyond their level of competence. In the meantime, nurses provide care within the level of their skill and experience.

8. Nurses give primary considerations to the welfare of clients and any possibility of harm in future care situations when they suspect unethical conduct or incompetent or unsafe care. When nurses have reasonable grounds for concern about the behavior of colleagues in this regard, or about the safety of conditions in the care setting, they carefully review the situation and take steps, individually or in partnership with others, to resolve the problem.

9. Nurses support other nurses who act in good faith to protect clients from incompetent, unethical or unsafe care, and advocate work environments in which nurses are treated with respect when they intervene.

10. Nurses speaking on nursing and health-related matters in a public forum or a court provide accurate and relevant information.

PRACTICE ENVIRONMENTS CONDUCIVE TO SAFE, COMPETENT AND ETHICAL CARE

Nurses advocate practice environments that have the organizational and human support systems, and the resource allocations necessary for safe, competent and ethical nursing care.

1. Nurses collaborate with nursing colleagues and other members of the health team to advocate health care environments that are conducive to ethical practice and to the health and well-being of clients and others in the setting. They do this in ways that are consistent with their professional role and responsibilities.

2. Nurses share their nursing knowledge with other members of the health team for the benefit of clients. To the best of their abilities, nurses provide mentorship

and guidance for the professional development of students of nursing and other nurses.

3. Nurses seeking professional employment accurately state their area(s) of competence and seek reasonable assurance that employment conditions will permit care consistent with the values and responsibilities of the code, as well as with their personal ethical beliefs.

4. Nurses practice ethically by striving for the best care achievable in the circumstances. They also make the effort, individually or in partnership with others, to improve practice environments by advocating on behalf of their clients as possible.

5. Nurses planning to participate in job action, or who practice in environments where job action occurs, take steps to safeguard the health and safety of clients during the course of the action.

APPENDIX D

ICN Code of Ethics for Nurses

International Council of Nurses

Reproduced with permission from the International Council of Nurses, 2000.

Nurses have fundamental responsibilities to promote health, to prevent illness, to restore health and to alleviate suffering.

The need for nursing is universal. Inherent in nursing is respect for human rights, incliding the right to life, to dignity and to be treated with respect. Nursing care is unrestricted by considerations of nationality, race, creed, colour, age, sex, politics or social status.

Nurses render health services to the individual, the family and the community and coordinate their services with those of related groups.

NURSES AND PEOPLE

The nurse's primary responsibility is to those people requiring nursing care.

In providing care, the nurse promotes an environment in which human rights values, customs and spiritual beliefs of the individual family and community are respected.

The nurse ensures that the individual receives sufficient information on which to base consnt for care and related treatment.

The nurse holds in confidence personal information and uses judgment in sharing this information.

The nurse shares with society the responsibility for initiating and supporting action to meet the health and social needs of the public, in particular those of vulnerable populations.

The nurse also shares responsibility to sustain and protect the natural environment from depletion, pollution, degradation and destruction.

NURSES AND PRACTICE

The nurse carries personal responsibility and accountability for nursing practice, and for maintaining competence by continual learning.

The nurse maintains a standard of personal health such that the ability to provide care is not compromised.

The nurse uses judgment regarding individual competence when accepting and delegating responsibilities.

The nurse at all times maintains standards of personal conduct which reflect well on the profession and enhance public confidence.

The nurse, in providing care, ensures that use of technology and scientific advances are compatible with the safety, dignity and rights of people.

NURSES AND CO-WORKERS

The nurse sustains a cooperative relationship with co-workers in nursing and other fields.

The nurse takes appropriate action to safeguard the individual when his care is endangered by a co-worker or any other person.

NURSES AND THE PROFESSION

The nurse plays the major role in determining and implementing desirable standards of nursing practice management, research and education.

The nurse is active in developing a core of research-based professional knowledge.

The nurse, acting through the professional organization, participates in creating and maintaining equitable social and economic working conditions in nursing.

Glossary

Accountability The state of being answerable to someone for something one has done.

Active voluntary euthanasia An act in which the physician both provides the means of death for a patient, such as a lethal dose of medication, and administers it.

Activism A passionate approach to everyday activities that is committed to seeking a more just social order through critical analysis, provocation, transformation, and rebalancing of power.

Act-utilitarianism A basic type of utilitarianism that suggests people choose actions that will, in any given circumstance, increase the overall good.

Administrative law The branch of law that consists mainly of the legal powers granted to administrative agencies by the legislature, and the rules that the agencies make to carry out their powers.

Advance directives Instructions that indicate which health care interventions to initiate or withhold, or which designate someone who will act as a surrogate in making such decisions, in the event that a person loses decision making capacity.

Allocative policies Policies designed to provide net benefits to some distinct group or class of individuals or organizations, at the expense of others, in order to ensure that public objectives are met.

Anonymity A situation in which even the researcher cannot link information with a particular participant in a study.

Appeals to conscience Personal and subjective beliefs, founded on a prior judgment of rightness or wrongness, that are motivated by personal sanction, rather than external authority.

Assault The unjustifiable attempt or threat to touch a person without consent that results in fear of immediately harmful or threatening contact.

Assisted suicide A situation in which patients receive the means of death from someone, such as a physician, but activate the process themselves.

Authority The state of having legitimate power and sovereignty.

Autonomy An ethical principle that literally means self-governing. It denotes having the freedom to make independent choices.

Axiology The branch of philosophy that studies the nature and types of values.

Battery The unlawful touching of another or the carrying out of threatened physical harm including every willful, angry, and violent or negligent touching of another's person, clothes, or anything attached to his or her person or held by him or her.

Belmont Report   Policies developed by the United States National Commission for the Protection of Human Subjects of Biomedical and Behavioral Research (1978) regarding ethical principles for research with human subjects.

Beneficence   The ethical principle that requires one to act in ways that benefit another. In research, this implies the protection from harm and discomfort, including a balance between the benefits and risks of a study.

Cartesian philosophy   A widespread belief during the Renaissance related to Descartes's proposal that the universe is a physical thing, and all therein is analogous to machines that can be analyzed and understood, and that the mind and body are separate entities.

Categorical imperative   The Kantian maxim stating that no action can be judged as right which cannot reasonably become a law by which every person should always abide.

Character ethics   Theories of ethics, sometimes called virtue ethics, that are related to the concept of innate moral virtue.

Cheating   Dishonesty and deception regarding examinations, projects, or papers.

Civil law   (Also called private law) The law that determines a person's legal rights and obligations in many kinds of activities involving other people.

Code of nursing ethics   Explicit declaration of the primary goals and values of the profession that indicate the profession's acceptance of the responsibility and trust with which it has been invested by society.

Coercion   Actual or implied threat of harm or penalty for not participating in a research project, or offering excessive rewards for participation in the project.

Common law   A system of law, also known as case law, based largely on previous court decisions. In this system, decisions are based upon earlier court rulings in similar cases, or precedents. Over time, these precedents take on the force of law.

Communitarian theories   Theories of justice that place the community, rather than the individual, the state, the nation, or any other entity, at the center of the value system; that emphasize the value of public goods; and that conceive of values as rooted in communal practices.

Compassion   A focal virtue combining an attitude of active regard for another's welfare with an imaginative awareness and emotional response of deep sympathy, tenderness, and discomfort at the other person's misfortune or suffering.

Competence   A person's ability to make meaningful life decisions. A declaration of incompetence involves legal action with a ruling by a judge that the person is unable to make such life decisions.

Complementary therapies   Therapeutic interventions that derive from traditions other than conventional Western medicine which are used by patients with or without the knowledge of conventional medical practitioners.

Confidentiality   The ethical principle that requires nondisclosure of private or secret information with which one is entrusted. In research, confidentiality refers to the researcher's assurance to participants that information provided will not be made public or available to anyone other than those involved in the research process without the participant's consent.

Consequentialism   A theory of ethics, sometimes called utilitarianism.

Constitutional law   A formal set of rules and principles that describe the powers of a government and the rights of the people.

Contract   An agreement between two or more people that can be enforced by law.

Contract law   A type of law that deals with the rights and obligations of people who make contracts.

Cosmology   A branch of philosophy that describes the structure, origin, and processes of the universe.

Covert values   Expectations that are not in writing that are often identified only through participation in, or controversies within, an organization or institution.

Criminal law   A type of law that deals with crimes, or actions considered harmful to society.

Cultural awareness   Knowledge about values, beliefs, behaviors, and the like of cultures other than one's own.

Cultural competence   Skill in dealing with transcultural issues, which is demonstrated through cultural awareness and cultural sensitivity.

Cultural sensitivity   The ability to incorporate a patient's cultural perspective into nursing assessments, and to modify nursing care in order to be as congruent as possible with the patient's cultural perspective.

Culture   The total lifeways of a group of interacting individuals, consisting of learned patterns of values, beliefs, behaviors, and customs shared by that group.

Decision making capacity   The ability of a person to understand all information about a health condition, to communicate understanding and choices, and to reason and deliberate; and, the possession of personal values and goals that guide the decision.

Declaration of Helsinki   Principles issued by the World Medical Assembly to guide clinical research in 1964; revised in 1975.

Defamation   Harm that occurs to a person's reputation and good name, diminishes others' value or esteem, or arouses negative feelings toward the person by the communication of false, malicious, unprivileged, or harmful words.

Deontology   Related to the term duty, deontology is a group of ethical theories based upon the rationalist view that the rightness or wrongness of an act depends upon the nature of the act, rather than the consequences that occur as a result of it.

Discernment   A focal virtue of sensitive insight, acute judgment, and understanding that eventuates in decisive action.

Disease   The biomedical explanation of sickness.

Distributive justice   Application of the ethical principle of justice that relates to fair, equitable, and appropriate distribution in society, determined by justified norms that structure the terms of social cooperation. Its scope includes policies that allot diverse benefits and burdens such as property, resources, taxation, privileges, and opportunities.

Diversity The experience within nursing of differences among colleagues and patients in areas such as gender, age, socioeconomic position, sexual orientation, health status, ethnicity, race, or culture.

Do not resuscitate (DNR) orders Written directives placed in a patient's medical chart indicating that cardiopulmonary resuscitation is to be avoided.

Durable power of attorney Allows a competent person to designate another as a surrogate or proxy to act on her or his behalf in making health care decisions in the event of the loss of decision making capacity.

Egalitarian theories Theories of justice that promote ideals of equal distribution of social benefits and burdens, and recognize the social obligation to eliminate or reduce barriers that prevent fair equality of opportunity.

Empirical Knowledge gained through the processes of observation and experience.

Empowerment A helping process and partnership, enacted in the context of love and respect for self and others, through which individuals and groups are enabled to change situations, and are given skills, resources, opportunities, and authority to do so. It involves creating a vision, taking risks, making choices, and behaving in authentic ways.

Ethical dilemma Occurs when there are conflicting moral claims.

Ethical principles Basic and obvious moral truths that guide deliberation and action. Major ethical principles include autonomy, beneficence, nonmaleficence, veracity, confidentiality, justice, fidelity, and others.

Ethical treatment of data Implies integrity of research protocols and honesty in reporting findings.

Ethic of caring An approach to ethical decision making grounded in relationship and mutual responsibility, in which choices are contextually bound and strategies are focused on maintaining connections and not hurting anyone.

Ethic of justice An approach to ethical decision making, based on objective rules and principles in which choices are made from a stance of separateness.

Ethics A formal process for making logical and consistent decisions based upon moral beliefs.

Ethnocentrism Judging behaviors of someone from another culture by the standards of one's own culture.

Eugenics Meaning "good birth," eugenics is based in the belief that some human traits are more desirable for society than others, and that society should weed out what proponents consider to be undesirable traits. Proponents of eugenics advocate policies that encourage so called "genetically superior" people to have children, while discouraging so called "genetically inferior" people from having children, through practices such as forced sterilization.

Euthanasia Causing the painless death of a person in order to end or prevent suffering.

Expertise   The characteristic of having a high level of specialized skill and knowledge.

External locus of control   The belief that forces outside of oneself direct or rule one's life, whether these be generalized forces such as fate or other persons who are perceived as more powerful.

External standards of nursing practice   Guides for nursing care that are developed by non-nurses, legislation, or institutions.

Faith   A generic feature of the human struggle to find and maintain meaning flowing from an integration of ways of knowing and valuing.

False imprisonment   The unlawful, unjustifiable detention of a person within fixed boundaries, or an act intended to result in such confinement.

Felonies Serious crimes that carry significant fines and jail sentences. Examples of felonies include first- and second-degree murder, arson, burglary, extortion, kidnaping, rape, and robbery.

Fidelity   An ethical principle related to the concept of faithfulness and the practice of promise-keeping.

Forgery   Includes fraud or intentional misrepresentation.

Formalism   A term often used to refer to deontology.

Fraud   A deliberate deception for the purpose of securing an unfair or unlawful gain.

Full disclosure   Indicates that a research participant must be fully informed of the nature of a study, anticipated risks and benefits, time commitment, expectations of the participant and the researcher, and the right to refuse to participate.

Genetic diagnosis   A process of biopsy of embryos to determine the presence of genetic flaws and gender prior to implantation.

Genetic engineering   The ability to genetically alter organisms for a variety of purposes, particularly to promote their health and strength.

Genetic screening   A process for determining whether persons are predisposed to certain diseases, and whether couples have the possibility of giving birth to a genetically-impaired infant.

Grassroots lobbying   Lobbying efforts that involve mobilizing a committed constituency to influence the opinions of policy makers.

Guardian *ad litem*   A court appointed guardian for a particular action or proceeding; such a guardian may not oversee all of the person's affairs.

Health policies   Authoritative decisions focusing on health that are made in the legislative, executive, or judicial branches of government and are intended to direct or influence the actions, behaviors, or decisions of others; their lifestyles and personal behaviors; and improvements in the availability, accessibility, and quality of their health care services.

Illness   A personal response to disease flowing from how one's culture teaches one to be sick.

Informed consent A process by which patients are informed of the possible outcomes, alternatives, and risks of treatments and required to give their consent freely. This implies legal protection of a patient's right to personal autonomy by providing the opportunity to choose a course of action regarding plans for health care, including the right to refuse medical recommendations and to choose from available therapeutic alternatives. *In research*, this refers to consent to participate in a research study after the research purpose, expected commitment, risks and benefits, any invasion of privacy, and ways that anonymity and confidentiality will be addressed have been explained.

Integrity Refers to adherence to moral norms that is sustained over time. Implicit in integrity is trustworthiness and a consistency of convictions, actions, and emotions.

Intentional torts Willful or intentional acts that violate another person's rights or property.

Internal locus of control The belief that one is able to influence or control things that happen in one's life.

Internal standards of nursing practice Standards of nursing practice that are developed within the profession of nursing.

Invasion of privacy Includes intrusion on the patient's physical and mental solitude or seclusion, public disclosure of private facts, publicity that places the patient in a false light in the public eye, or appropriation for the defendant's benefit or advantage of the patient's name or likeness.

Journals Personal written records kept on a periodic or regular basis containing factual material and subjective interpretations of events, thoughts, feelings, and plans.

Judicial decisions Authoritative court decisions that direct or influence the actions, behaviors, or decisions of others.

Justice An ethical principle that relates to fair, equitable, and appropriate treatment in light of what is due or owed to persons, recognizing that giving to some will deny receipt to others who might otherwise have received these things. *In research*, justice implies the rights of fair treatment and privacy, including anonymity and confidentiality.

Kantianism A deontological theory of ethics based upon the writings of the philosopher Immanuel Kant.

Law The system of enforceable principles and processes that governs the behavior of people in respect to relationships with others and with the government.

Libel Printed defamation by written words and images that injure a person's reputation or cause others to avoid, ridicule, or view the person with contempt.

Libertarian theories Theories of distributive justice that propose that the just society protects the rights of property and liberty of each person, allowing citizens to improve their circumstances by their own effort.

Living wills Legal documents developed voluntarily by persons, giving directions to health care providers related to withholding or withdrawing life support if certain conditions exist.

Lobbying The art of persuasion—attempting to convince a legislator, a government official, the head of an agency, or a state official to comply with a request—whether it is convincing them to support a position on an issue or to follow a particular course of action.

Locus of control   Beliefs about the ability to control events in one's life.

Loyalty   Showing sympathy, care, and reciprocity to those with whom we appropriately identify; working closely with others toward shared goals; keeping promises; making mutual concerns a priority; sacrificing personal interests to the relationship; and giving attention to these over a substantial period of time.

Malpractice   The form of negligence in which any professional misconduct, unreasonable lack of professional skill, or nonadherence to the accepted standard of care causes injury to a patient or client.

Managed care   An integrated form of health care delivery and financing that represents attempts to control costs by modifying the behavior of providers and patients.

Material rules   Rules by which distributive justice decisions regarding entitlement are made.

Medical futility   Situations in which medical interventions are judged to have no medical benefit, or in which the chance for success is low.

Misdemeanor   A criminal offense of a less serious nature than a felony, usually punishable by a fine or short jail sentence, or both.

Moral development   A product of the sociocultural environment in which one lives and develops that reflects the intellectual and emotional process through which one learns and incorporates values regarding right and wrong.

Moral distress   The reaction to a situation in which there are moral problems that seem to have clear solutions, yet one is unable to follow one's moral beliefs because of external restraints. This may be evidenced in anger, frustration, dissatisfaction, and poor performance in the work setting.

Moral integrity   A focal virtue that relates to soundness, reliability, wholeness, an integration of character, and fidelity in adherence to moral norms sustained over time.

Moral outrage   A state which occurs when someone else in the health care setting performs an act the nurse believes to be immoral. In cases of moral outrage, the nurse does not participate in the act and therefore does not feel responsible for wrong, but feels powerlessness to prevent it.

Moral philosophy   The philosophical discussion of what is considered to be good or bad, right or wrong.

Moral thought   Individuals' cognitive examination of right and wrong, good and bad.

Moral uncertainty   A state which occurs when one senses that there is a moral problem, but is not sure of the morally correct action; when one is unsure what the moral principles or values apply; or when one is unable to define the moral problem.

Moral values   Preferences or dispositions reflective of right or wrong, should or should not, in human behavior.

Naturalism   A view of moral judgment that regards ethics as dependent upon human nature and psychology.

Negligence   The omission to do something that a reasonable person, guided by those ordinary considerations that ordinarily regulate human affairs, would do, or doing something that a reasonable and prudent person would not do.

Noncompliance   Denoting an unwillingness on the part of the patient to participate in health care activities that have been recommended by health care providers.

Nonmaleficence   An ethical principle related to beneficence that requires one to act in such a manner as to avoid causing harm to another, including deliberate harm, risk of harm, and harm that occurs during the performance of beneficial acts.

Nuremberg Code   A set of principles for the ethical conduct of research against which the experiments in the Nazi concentration camps could be judged.

Nurse practice acts   Legislative statutes within each state that define nursing, describe boundaries of practice, establish standards for nurses, and protect the domain of nursing.

Nursing process   A model commonly used for decision making in nursing.

Nursism   A form of sexism that maligns the caring role in society and leads to discrimination in nursing by virtue of the role undertaken, regardless of gender.

Obligation   Being required to do something by virtue of a moral rule, a duty, or some other binding demand, such as a particular role or relationship.

Overt values   Values of individuals, groups, institutions, and organized systems that are explicitly communicated through philosophy and policy statements.

Palliative care   A comprehensive, interdisciplinary, and total care approach, focusing primarily on comfort and support of patients and families who face illness that is chronic or not responsive to curative treatment.

Parentalism   A nongender term that parallels the meaning of paternalism, while avoiding gender bias.

Partisan   Adherence to the ideology of a particular political party.

Paternalism   A gender-biased term that literally means acting in a "fatherly" manner, the traditional view of which implies well-intended actions of benevolent decision making, leadership, protection, and discipline, which, in the health care arena, manifest in the making of decisions on behalf of patients without their full consent or knowledge.

Patient Self-Determination Act   A federal law requiring institutions such as hospitals, nursing homes, health maintenance organizations, and home care agencies receiving Medicare or Medicaid funds to provide written information to adult patients regarding their rights to make health care decisions.

Philosophy   The intense and critical examination of beliefs and assumptions.

Plagiarism   Taking another's ideas or work and presenting them as one's own.

Plaintiff   The term used for the complaining or injured party in a lawsuit.

Policy formulation   A phase of the policy-making process that includes such actions as agenda setting and the subsequent development of legislation.

Policy implementation   A phase of the policy-making process that follows enactment of legislation and includes taking actions and making additional decisions necessary to implement legislation such as rule making and policy operation.

Policy modification   A phase of the policy-making process that exists to improve or perfect legislation previously enacted.

Political   Relates to the complex process of policy making within the government.

Political issues   Those issues that are regulated or influenced by decisions within either the executive, judicial, or legislative branches of government.

Political parties   Organized groups with distinct ideology that seek to control government.

Power   The ability to do or act; the capability of doing or accomplishing something.

Practical dilemma   A situation in which moral claims compete with nonmoral claims.

Practical imperative   The Kantian maxim requiring that one treat others always as ends and never as a means.

Precedents   Court rulings upon which subsequent rulings in similar cases are based. Over time these precedents take on the force of law.

Principles   Basic and obvious truths that guide deliberation and action.

Private law (Also called civil law)   The law that determines a person's legal rights and obligations in many kinds of activities involving other people.

Profession   A complex, organized occupation preceded by a long training program geared toward the acquisition of exclusive knowledge necessary to provide a service that is essential or desired by society, leading to a monopoly that provides autonomy, public recognition, prestige, power, and authority for the practitioner.

Public law   Law that defines a person's rights and obligations in relation to government, and describes the various divisions of government and their powers.

Quality of life   A subjective appraisal of factors that make life worth living and contribute to a positive experience of living.

Racism   The assumption that members of one race are superior to those of another.

Rationalism   A view of moral judgment that regards truth as necessary, universal, and superior to the information received from the senses, having an origin in the nature of the universe or in the nature of a higher being.

Regulatory policies   Policies that are designed to influence the actions, behaviors, and decisions of others through directive techniques.

Religion   The codification of beliefs and practices concerning the Divine and one's relationship with the Divine that are shared by a group of people.

Religiosity   Beliefs and practices that are the expressive aspects of religion.

Respect for human dignity   Implies the rights of patients to full disclosure and self-determination regarding participation in research and in making health care choices.

Respect for persons   An attitude by which one considers others to be worthy of high regard.

Right to fair treatment   Assures equitable treatment of participants in the research selection process, during the study, and after the completion of the study.

Right to privacy   The right to be left alone or to be free from unwanted publicity. *In research*, this is the right of research participants to determine when, where, and what kind of information is shared, with an assurance that information and observations are treated with respect and kept in strict confidence.

Rules or **regulations**   Policies that are established to guide the implementation of laws and programs.

Rule-utilitarianism   A type of utilitarianism that suggests people choose rules that, when followed consistently, will maximize the overall good.

Self-awareness   Conscious awareness of one's thoughts, feelings, physical, and emotional responses, and insights in various situations.

Sexism   The assumption that members of one sex are superior to those of the other.

Sexual harassment   All unwelcome sexual advances, request for sexual favors, and other conduct of a sexual nature.

Slander   Defamation that occurs when one speaks unprivileged or false words about another.

Spectrum of urgency   A spectrum depicting the degree of urgency in health care decision making, ranging from minor and nonurgent to severe and very urgent.

Spirituality   The animating force, life principle, or essence of being that permeates life and is expressed and experienced in multifaceted connections with self, others, nature, and God or Life Force.

Standards of nursing practice   Written documents outlining minimum expectations for nursing care.

Statutes or **laws**   Legislation that has been enacted by legislative bodies and approved by the executive branch of government.

Statutory (legislative) law   Formal laws written and enacted by federal, state, or local legislatures.

Stereotyping   Expecting all persons from a particular group to behave, think, or respond in a certain way based on preconceived ideas.

Sympathy   Sharing, in imagination, of others' feelings.

Theory   A proposed explanation for a class of phenomena.

Tort   A wrong or injury that a person suffers because of someone else's action, either intentional or unintentional. The action may cause bodily harm; damage a person's property, business, or reputation; or make unauthorized use of a person's property.

Trustworthiness   A focal virtue that results in recognition by others of one's consistency and predictability in following moral norms.

Unintentional torts   Torts that occur when an act or omission causes unintended injury or harm to another person.

Utilitarianism   A moral theory which holds that an action is judged as good or bad in relation to the consequence, outcome, or end result derived from it.

Utilitarian theories   Theories of distributive justice that distribute resources based on the premise of the greatest good for the greatest numbner of people. These theories place social good before individual rights.

Utility   The property of usefulness in any object, whereby it tends to produce benefit, advantage, pleasure, good, or happiness or prevent mischief, pain, evil, or unhappiness.

Values   Ideals, beliefs, customs, modes of conduct, qualities, or goals that are highly prized or preferred by individuals, groups, or society.

Values clarification   Refers to the process of becoming more conscious of and naming what one values or considers worthy.

Values conflict   Internal or interpersonal conflict that occurs in circumstances in which personal values are at odds with those of patients, colleagues, or the institution.

Veracity   Truth-telling.

Victim blaming   Holding the people burdened by social conditions accountable for their own situations and responsible for needed solutions.

Virtue ethics   Theories of ethics, usually attributed to Aristotle, which represent the idea that an individual's actions are based upon innate moral virtue.

Whistle blowing   Speaking out about unsafe or questionable practices affecting patient care or working conditions. This should be resorted to only after a person has unsuccessfully used all appropriate organizational channels to right a wrong, and has a sound moral justification for taking this action.

Whistleblowers   Persons who alert the public about serious wrongdoing created or concealed within an organization, such as unsafe conditions, incompetence, or professional misconduct.

Index